D1605033

handbook of Canine Electrocardiography

GARY R. BOLTON, D.V.M.

Associate Professor of Small Animal Medicine and Cardiology,
New York State Veterinary College, Cornell University

1975   W. B. SAUNDERS COMPANY • Philadelphia • London • Toronto

W. B. Saunders Company: West Washington Square
Philadelphia, Pa. 19105

12 Dyott Street
London, WC1A 1DB

833 Oxford Street
Toronto, Ontario M8Z 5T9, Canada

Library of Congress Cataloging in Publication Data

Bolton, Gary R

Handbook of canine electrocardiography.

Includes index.

1. Dogs — Diseases.   2. Dogs — Physiology.   3. Veterinary
electrocardiography.   I. Title.

SF991.B67   636.7'08'96120754   75–17749

ISBN 0–7216–1838–3

Handbook of Canine Electrocardiography   ISBN 0-7216-1838-3

© 1975 by W. B. Saunders Company. Copyright under the International Copyright
Union.   All rights reserved.   This book is protected by copyright.   No part of it may be
reproduced, stored in a retrieval system, or transmitted in any form or by any means,
electronic, mechanical, photocopying, recording, or otherwise, without written permission
from the publisher. Made in the United States of America. Press of W. B. Saunders
Company. Library of Congress catalog card number 74-17749.

Last digit is the print number: 9   8   7   6   5   4   3   2   1

To my parents, Mr. and Mrs. Robert Bolton

PREFACE

Electrocardiography is a diagnostic clinical tool that has received inadequate recognition in the field of veterinary medicine until recently. In spite of the fact that necessary equipment is minimal, the "mystique" of this science has dissuaded many clinicians from utilizing it as a diagnostic aid.

This text attempts to dispel that "mystique," explain principles, and present case examples in a clear and concise way so that practitioners can use electrocardiography in their daily work.

Common and general abnormalities are presented here. Unusual problems are referenced for more detailed study in other texts.

The author welcomes comments and constructive criticisms to make this text more useful to veterinary clinicians.

GARY R. BOLTON

ACKNOWLEDGMENTS

I would like to thank Dr. Stephen Ettinger for the excellent training that I received from him when we were at the Animal Medical Center. I would also like to thank Dr. Ettinger and Dr. Peter Suter for generously allowing me to use several illustrations from their text, *Canine Cardiology*.

Special thanks is given to Dr. Joel Edwards and Dr. James Dorney for reviewing the entire manuscript, and to Dr. David Taylor for reviewing portions of it.

Many of the exceptional electrocardiograms in this text were supplied by my generous colleagues Dr. William Thomas, Dr. Robert Lynk, Dr. Edward Grano, Dr. Michael Lorenz, Dr. Albert Beck, and especially Dr. Larry Tilley, who supplied many of the arrhythmia ECG's.

The exceptional illustrations in Chapters 2 and 3 were done by Mr. Lou Sadler, Medical Illustrator for the Department of Anatomy at the New York State Veterinary College.

Many thanks are extended to Mrs. J. R. McPherson and Mrs. R. E. Hoffer for their invaluable assistance in the preparation of the manuscript.

A final "thank you" is given to Mr. Carroll C. Cann and the entire capable staff of the W. B. Saunders Company, who have created a pleasant atmosphere in which to work.

G. R. B.

CONTENTS

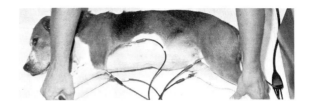

Chapter 1

PRINCIPLES OF ELECTROCARDIOGRAPHY

WHY BUY AN ELECTROCARDIOGRAPH?

Canine electrocardiography has established itself in veterinary medicine as a useful and practical clinical tool. The electrocardiogram is useful in many situations as a diagnostic aid requiring relatively little additional equipment. An electrocardiogram is quickly and easily made and interpreted, and the information obtained is reliable. Electrocardiography adds an additional dimension to the realm of patient evaluation, not only for cardiac diseases but also for those diseases that secondarily affect the heart, such as the metabolic disorders that are discussed later in this chapter.

The electrocardiogram is essential for diagnosis and treatment of cardiac arrhythmias. Diagnosis of arrhythmias must be correct and specific, since treatment is specific and errors may result in fatalities.

The electrocardiogram is no panacea. It does have its limitations, and the electrocardiographic findings must always be correlated with the other findings in each case.

Electrocardiography is easy to learn because it makes sense and can be approached in a systematic manner. As one uses electrocardiography, enthusiasm for the subject grows rapidly.

USES OF THE ELECTROCARDIOGRAM

Table 1–1 summarizes the uses of the electrocardiogram.

Evaluation of Anatomic Cardiac Changes

The electrocardiogram is useful in detecting cardiac enlargement resulting from hypertrophy of the chambers. It can detect enlargement of any of the four cardiac chambers and also gives an indication of the severity of the changes. When evaluating cardiac enlargement, it is best

TABLE 1-1.   USES OF ELECTROCARDIOGRAPHY

Evaluation of Cardiac Diseases
Evaluation of Anatomic Cardiac Changes (Cardiac Enlargement)
Evaluation of Arrhythmias
Evaluation of Therapy
  Drug therapy
  Electrolyte disturbances
  Pericardiocentesis
Evaluation of Prognosis
Evaluation of Progression of Disease

Differentiation of Nonspecific Diseases that Cause Weakness, Fatigue, Fever, Lethargy, Collapse, or Seizures
Metabolic Diseases with Electrolyte Alterations
  Adrenal insufficiency
  Diabetic ketoacidosis
  Severe renal insufficiency
  Eclampsia
  Idiopathic hypokalemia
Cardiac Syncope
  Bradycardias
  Tachycardias
Epilepsy
Endocarditis, Myocarditis, and Cardiac Neoplasia
Systemic Diseases with Toxemias

Monitoring During Anesthesia and Surgery
Monitors Depth of Anesthesia
Monitors Ventilation-oxygenation Changes

Routine Basis
Yearly Physicals (Preventive Medicine)
Evaluation of Dogs that are Scheduled to Have Anesthesia and Surgery
Evaluation of Trauma Cases

Documentation of Data

Sharing Information and Seeking Consultation Service

to compare the electrocardiographic findings with those of the thoracic radiograph. The electrocardiogram may reveal something the x-ray does not, and the radiographs may detect an abnormality that the electrocardiogram did not detect. An evaluation of the lung fields on the chest x-ray is very important in establishing a final cardiac diagnosis.

Evaluation of Cardiac Arrhythmias

Arrhythmias occur frequently. They are usually detected during physical examination either by auscultation of the heart or by palpation of the femoral pulse. Usually a good estimate can be made of which arrhythmia is present, but the electrocardiogram makes the final diagnosis. Treatment should not be initiated unless an electrocardiogram has been taken. For example, if premature beats are auscultated, what type of premature beats are they? If they are supraventricular, then digitalis should be used. If they are ventricular premature beats, quinidine (or one of the other antiarrhythmic agents mentioned in Chapter 4) should be used. If quinidine is given when digitalis is indicated, a fatality could result. The diagnosis of these arrhythmias is dependent on an electrocardiogram and mistakes in treatment are critical.

Evaluation of Cardiac Therapy

The electrocardiogram should be used to monitor the effects of therapy. It is utilized when digitalizing a patient, to look for changes in heart rate, in P-R interval, or to look for the development of arrhythmias. In most instances a dog can be digitalized without making him physically ill if a lead II electrocardiogram is recorded and examined before each dose is given. Antiarrhythmic medications (such as quinidine) can be monitored for effect and toxicity. Successful treatment is signified by a disappearance of the arrhythmia, while toxicity causes atrioventricular block, prolongation of either the QRS complex, the Q-T interval, or the P-R interval, or marked changes in the heart rate (see Chapter 3).

The electrocardiogram is also useful in monitoring changes in electrolyte concentrations during the treatment of metabolic diseases that alter electrolyte balance. This may avoid the necessity of taking serial electrolyte samples, for determining electrolyte levels, and gives the clinician an idea of what the electrolyte situation is like at the cellular level.

The electrocardiogram is also helpful in directing needle placement during diagnostic or therapeutic pericardiocentesis. Arrhythmias will occur if the needle is advanced too far and touches the myocardium.

Evaluation of Prognosis

It is important to forecast a prognosis to the owner. The electrocardiogram helps in this regard by giving an estimate of the amount of cardiac enlargement that has occurred. In general, the more severe the enlargement, the more severe the disease, and the less favorable the prognosis.

Some cardiac arrhythmias carry a more guarded prognosis than others. For instance, ventricular premature beats are worrisome, but can often be controlled with quinidine therapy. Complete atrioventricular heart block, on the other hand, almost never responds to medical treatment and carries a grave prognosis. If atrial fibrillation is diagnosed, in most instances the owner can be told that the dog has about 4 to 6 months to live if medical therapy is adequate, although some dogs have lived for 2 years.

Evaluation of Progression of Disease

The recording of serial electrocardiograms over a period of time is usually more meaningful than the recording of one electrocardiogram. By following the tracings from a dog over a period of time, a trend can be established, and an estimate can be made of the rate at which the disease is progressing. For this reason, each electrocardiogram should be dated and stored in the record for comparison with future electrocardiograms.

Differentiation of Nonspecific Diseases That Cause Weakness, Fatigue, Lethargy, Fever, Collapse, or Seizures

The electrocardiogram may be of help in evaluating and diagnosing some of the diseases that cause vague symptoms of weakness, fatigue, lethargy, fever, collapse, or seizures. Disorders that may be confused when they cause one or all of these signs include metabolic diseases, cardiac diseases, neurologic diseases, and systemic diseases that produce toxemia.

Metabolic diseases usually cause symptoms by altering serum electrolyte concentrations; such disorders include adrenal insufficiency, diabetic ketoacidosis, severe nephropathies, eclampsia, and idiopathic hypokalemia. Symptoms of each disease are similar, and vary from weakness and fatigue to collapse or seizures, and sometimes both. Bradycardia usually occurs and may be detected clinically. The electrocardiogram is sensitive to changes in serum potassium and calcium, and may be the means of detecting these changes more quickly than by having to wait for blood sample test results to be reported.

Cardiac arrhythmias may cause symptoms varying from weakness and fatigue to sudden collapse or seizures, or both. They cause symptoms by causing blood pressure to fall critically. Arrhythmias that can do this include atrioventricular heart block, ventricular tachycardias, supraventricular tachycardias, ventricular fibrillation and, occasionally, sinoatrial arrest. The electrocardiogram indicates the type of arrhythmia that is present, and some of these arrhythmias require emergency treatment.

Epileptic dogs suffer seizures because of a central nervous system lesion. At other times neurologic lesions cause weakness, lethargy, mental confusion, or collapse. Idiopathic epilepsy is generally diagnosed by ruling out all the other causes of seizures. Any animal that experiences seizures, collapses, or has profound weakness should have an electrocardiogram taken as a part of the case evaluation.

Endocarditis, myocarditis, and certain cardiac neoplasms may cause obscure symptoms of weakness, lethargy, persistent or recurring fever, or seizures and collapse. Endocarditis is difficult to diagnose, but if the electrocardiogram detects cardiomegaly of unknown origin or if a murmur suddenly develops with these vague symptoms present, then the disease may be strongly suspected. If the myocardium is involved and myocarditis is present, it is detected by the development of arrhythmias or by S-T segment alterations. Certain neoplasms, such as heart base tumors or hemangiosarcomas, may cause similar clinical signs by causing arrhythmias or pericardial effusion.

Systemic diseases that cause toxemias may also cause signs of weakness, fatigue, lethargy, or collapse. Diseases such as pyometra, intestinal obstruction, pancreatitis, endotoxemia, or uremia may cause "toxic" myocarditis, with the development of arrhythmias. It may be necessary to control the arrhythmia to keep the dog alive long enough to treat the primary disease. The arrhythmia will subside if the toxemia can be corrected.

Monitoring During Anesthesia and Surgery

The electrocardiograph may be taken into the surgical suite to monitor the patient during anesthesia and surgery. This is especially important with critical cases.

The depth of anesthesia is generally evaluated by monitoring heart rate. If the rate begins to fall below baseline levels, or if it ever goes below 70 beats per minute, the animal should be evaluated and the anesthetic depth lightened, if necessary. If the animal is not under deep anesthesia but the heart rate is still slowing, atropine and ventilatory assistance should be given. Isoproterenol may be needed if atropine and forced ventilation fail to increase heart rate.

The electrocardiogram is reliable also in evaluating how well the patient is being oxygenated. The myocardium is very sensitive to hypoxia. Careful observation of the T wave and the S-T segment may warn of early oxygenation problems that can be corrected before serious arrhythmias occur (see Effects of Myocardial Hypoxia on the Electrocardiogram, Chapter 3. p. 71).

Arrhythmias commonly occur during anesthesia. One is often surprised when auscultating a dog after induction of anesthesia; quite often, a dog will be developing ventricular arrhythmias shortly after induction of short-acting barbiturates (Pedersoli and Brown, 1973). These post-induction arrhythmias disappear within minutes, however, and are of little concern if the animal is well ventilated. If they are still present after 5 to 10 minutes, the anesthesia should be kept as light as possible and the animal should be given ventilatory assistance. If they still persist, antiarrhythmic therapy may be needed. If the dog develops arrhythmias during the surgery, the depth of anesthesia is lightened, ventilation is assisted, and an intravenous drip containing 20 meq. of sodium bicarbonate per liter is started. The prevention and treatment of cardiac arrhythmias during anesthesia and surgery has been reported previously (Bolton, 1972). Most of the arrhythmias that occur during anesthesia and surgery can be avoided if the animal is observed closely and the electrocardiogram is monitored.

The Routine Electrocardiogram

Electrocardiograms are indicated as a routine procedure in certain situations. If preventive medicine is to become an effective part of veterinary service, then each year an animal should have a complete physical examination, routine laboratory work, and an electrocardiogram. This is especially true for animals over 5 years of age and animals with known cardiac disease.

Every animal that is to undergo anesthesia for surgery should have a presurgical electrocardiogram taken. Again, this is especially true for older animals.

Every case involving trauma should have an electrocardiogram taken to screen for the development of arrhythmias. An electrocardiogram should also be taken in accident cases, and in surgical cases where recovery is not progressing as well as expected.

Documentation of Data

The electrocardiogram may be saved and stored as a permanent part of the data accumulated while the dog is a patient. Each electrocardiogram should be clearly labeled with the owner's name, the dog's name, and the date it was taken. Notes may be made of any medications given prior to the recording. A chronological series of electrocardiograms is useless unless each electrocardiogram has been labeled and is available to document case findings.

Sharing Information and Seeking Consultation Service

The electrocardiographic tracing folds up and fits easily into an envelope. Since it is so easy to send through the mail, it is very useful for sharing exciting findings and for seeking other opinions.

Professional Status and Referral Cases

As professionals, we should be able to offer specialized services, such as electrocardiography, to our clients, or else be able to refer them to someone who can offer them. It is not possible to master every subject, and if a veterinarian does offer electrocardiography as one of his services, he soon begins to attract referral cases from other veterinarians in the area.

Table 1–2 summarizes the advantages of using electrocardiography

---

TABLE 1–2. ADVANTAGES OF ELECTROCARDIOGRAPHY

Electrocardiography adds a new dimension to the diagnosis and treatment of many disease states.

Electrocardiograms are quickly and easily recorded.

Electrocardiograms are easy to read.

Electrocardiographic results are immediately available.

Electrocardiography is essential in the diagnosis and treatment of cardiac arrhythmias.

Electrocardiography is one of the best ways to evaluate cardiac patients.

Electrocardiograms are useful as visual aids in discussing the problem with the client.

in private practice. It is my hope that this detailed discussion of these advantages will encourage the small animal clinician to explore this field further and implement its use in his practice for the welfare of his patients.

CHOOSING AN ELECTROCARDIOGRAPH

There are many electrocardiographic units on the market. The questions that arise are: What should I look for in a machine? What will I have to pay for one?

Regardless of the type of machine, there is one control that it must have. It must be able to run electrocardiograms at 50 mm./sec. (Fig. 1–1), because canine electrocardiograms should be run at 50 mm./sec. paper speed. Canine heart rates are so rapid that inspecting and measuring the tracing is less accurate at the slower speed (25 mm./sec.). If the machine cannot run at 50 mm./sec. paper speed, then don't buy it.

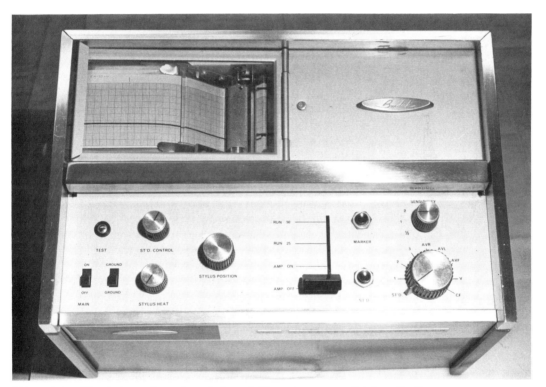

Figure 1–1. The electrocardiograph control panel. The main power switch is on the far left. The ground switch is placed in the position that gives the most steady tracing without electrical interference. The ST'd control knob adjusts the magnitude of the 1 mv. deflection that is produced when the ST'd button is depressed. The stylus heat control is increased to heat the pen and darken the tracing. The paper speed lever can be placed at "run 50" or "run 25" for running at 50 mm./sec. or 25 mm./sec., respectively. The electrocardiographic complexes will be produced at the "amp on" position, but the paper will not run until the lever is advanced to "run 25" or "run 50." At the "amp off" position, the baseline is steady. The marker button is pushed to mark leads or events. The sensitivity switch can either double the height of the complexes or cut them in half. The lead selector switch is left at "ST'd" to standardize the machine, and is advanced to leads 1, 2, 3, aVR, aVL, aVF, and V while the electrocardiograph is running. The CF setting is not used.

A sensitivity control switch is handy but not essential (Fig. 1–1). The sensitivity control switch can cut the complexes to one-half their size if they are too tall, or can double the complexes if they are too small. The switch is usually marked "1/2," "1," "2." Each tracing is started at a sensitivity of "1," with the machine standardized at 1 cm. = 1 mv, (see p. 11). If the complexes are so large that they cannot be kept on the paper, the switch is turned to "1/2." If the complexes are so small that they are difficult to read, the switch may be turned to "2." This will affect only the height of the complexes, not their width. When reading tracings that are recorded at 1/2 sensitivity, the height of the complexes should be doubled to arrive at their correct millivoltage value. If the tracing was recorded at twice the normal sensitivity, then the height of the complexes is divided by 2 to arrive at their true millivoltage.

If the machine does not have a sensitivity control switch, it will have to be restandardized at twice or at half the normal sensitivity, whichever is desired; i.e., at 2 cm. = 1 mv. or at 1/2 cm. = 1 mv. This is not difficult; it is merely less convenient than simply changing a switch.

The other controls are fairly standard from machine to machine. There is an on-off switch, a ground switch, a stylus position control, a lead selector switch and a standardization control knob (Fig. 1–1). There are also an event marker button and a standardization button. Some machines are transistorized and are thus ready to record immediately after the power is turned on. Other machines take a minute or two to warm up before they are ready to record. The ground switch generally has two positions. If electrical interference is a problem, the ground switch is shifted to the position that gives the steadiest, quietest recording. The event marker is used to mark the leads and to mark events that occur. The standardization button consistently delivers 1 mv. to the machine. The height of this 1 mv. deflection is adjusted with the standardization control knob.

Equipment supply houses and electronics manufacturers usually have both new and used machines for sale. A used machine that has been reconditioned is a good investment provided that it has the necessary controls that have just been mentioned. An occasional bargain price may be found. Whether the clinician invests in a new or a used machine is only relative, since the machine will soon pay for itself both financially and in personal satisfaction if it is used properly. The important thing is to purchase a unit, turn it on, and go!

Equipment supply houses and electronics manufacturers also lease electrocardiographs on a monthly or yearly basis. Human hospitals may have used electrocardiographic equipment that they are willing to sell at low cost, but be sure that such equipment has the ability to run at 50 mm./sec. paper speed.

An important consideration when buying a machine is the service representation that is available in your area. When your machine becomes an important part of your practice, breakdowns may cause costly delays, and quick, efficient repairs are an absolute necessity. Important questions to ask your sales representative are how fast the service is, where the parts come from, and whether loaner machines are available while yours is being repaired.

The cost of good chart paper is of little consequence, since the average roll will produce a minimum of 20 to 30 electrocardiograms. The paper is heat sensitive and the tracing is produced when the red hot stylus of the electrocardiograph runs across it and burns the tracing into it. The cheaper papers may burn with more residue and thus cause the stylus to wear out sooner.

Recording and interpreting an electrocardiogram is a professional service. The client of today expects professional service and is willing to pay for your ability to do it.

PRODUCTION OF THE CANINE ELECTROCARDIOGRAM

Positioning the Dog

Whenever the full electrocardiogram is taken, the dog is placed in right lateral recumbency and held with his humeri and femora at right angles to his body and parallel to each other (Ettinger and Suter, 1970) (Fig. 1–2). Most dogs tolerate this position well, especially if they are reassured with a kindly word and a pat on the head. Puppies are the

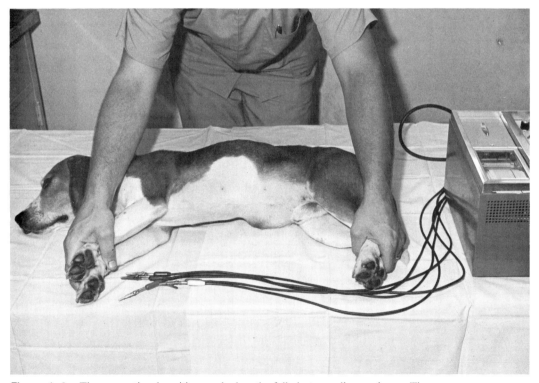

Figure 1–2. The conventional position used when the full electrocardiogram is run. The dog is in right lateral recumbency. The assistant maintains the dog in this position by holding the dog's front legs with his right hand, using his right arm to hold the dog's head. The hind legs and the rump are held with the left hand and arm. The humeri and femora are held at right angles to the body and parallel to each other. The electrode cables are in position and ready to be attached to the dog.

most difficult to restrain, and at first they wiggle and scream. For this reason, it is best to run the puppy's electrocardiogram in the owners' absence, since the puppy's complaints are unduly distressing. If the assistant holds tight and defeats the puppy's first attempts at escape, the dog will usually lie still long enough to complete the tracing quickly.

Attaching the Leads

The leads (electrodes) are labeled right arm (RA), left arm (LA), right leg (RL), and left leg (LL). A fifth lead is the V lead (C), which is an exploring electrode (Fig. 1–3). Alligator clips are used to attach the leads to the dog (Ettinger and Suter, 1970). If the clips are bent out slightly, they are painless to the dog. Even these clips may be uncomfortable to puppies, cats, and thin-skinned dogs. If the animal expresses some discomfort when the leads are applied, the clips may be padded with cotton or with gauze sponge. The arm leads are attached to the appropriate arm just above the elbow, and the leg leads are attached to the appropriate leg just above the stifle (Fig. 1–4). The V lead is attached at various places, depending on which of the exploring leads are to be run (Fig. 1–5) (Detweiler and Patterson, 1965).

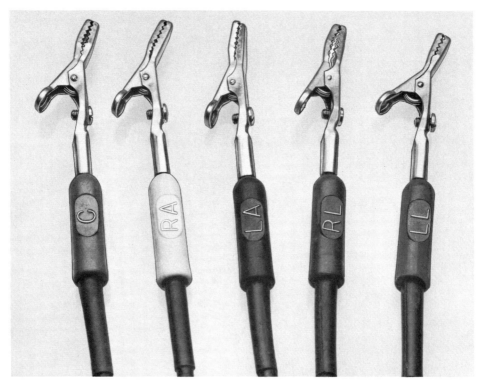

Figure 1–3. Alligator clips, No. 60 size, with the jaws bent slightly, make excellent electrodes when they are clipped to the dog's skin. The alligator clips must be securely fastened to the cable tips. (From Ettinger, S. J., and Suter, P. F. *Canine Cardiology.* W. B. Saunders Co., Philadelphia, 1970.)

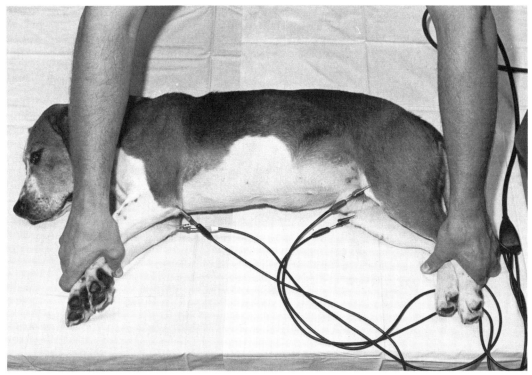

Figure 1–4. The electrocardiograph leads have been attached to the legs. The arm leads are placed just above the elbows, and the leg leads are placed just above the stifles. The standard six-lead electrocardiogram is run using only these four cables. The right hind leg is the ground. Note that the entire cable is placed on the table with the dog to minimize movement artifacts.

Wetting the Clips and Grounding Patient and Machine

The clips should be clean and fit tightly to the leads. The clips and the skin are moistened to establish good clip-to-skin contact and prevent electrical interference (Fig. 1–6). Alcohol works well as a wetting agent, and is not as messy as electrode jellies or pastes. pHisoHex works well, but is also messier and more difficult to remove than alcohol. Wetting the skin is usually adequate, and there is no need to clip the hair or prepare the areas.

The machine is supplied with a ground plug and a ground cord. The ground cord is attached to a nearby water pipe or ground plate. It is preferable to place the dog on an insulated formica table, but this may not be necessary. If electrical interference is a problem, the table may be covered with a rubber sheet or a thick blanket.

Operating the Electrocardiograph

The machine can be standardized before the dog is positioned and the leads are attached. This will minimize the amount of time that the dog must be restrained. The sensitivity switch is positioned at "1," and

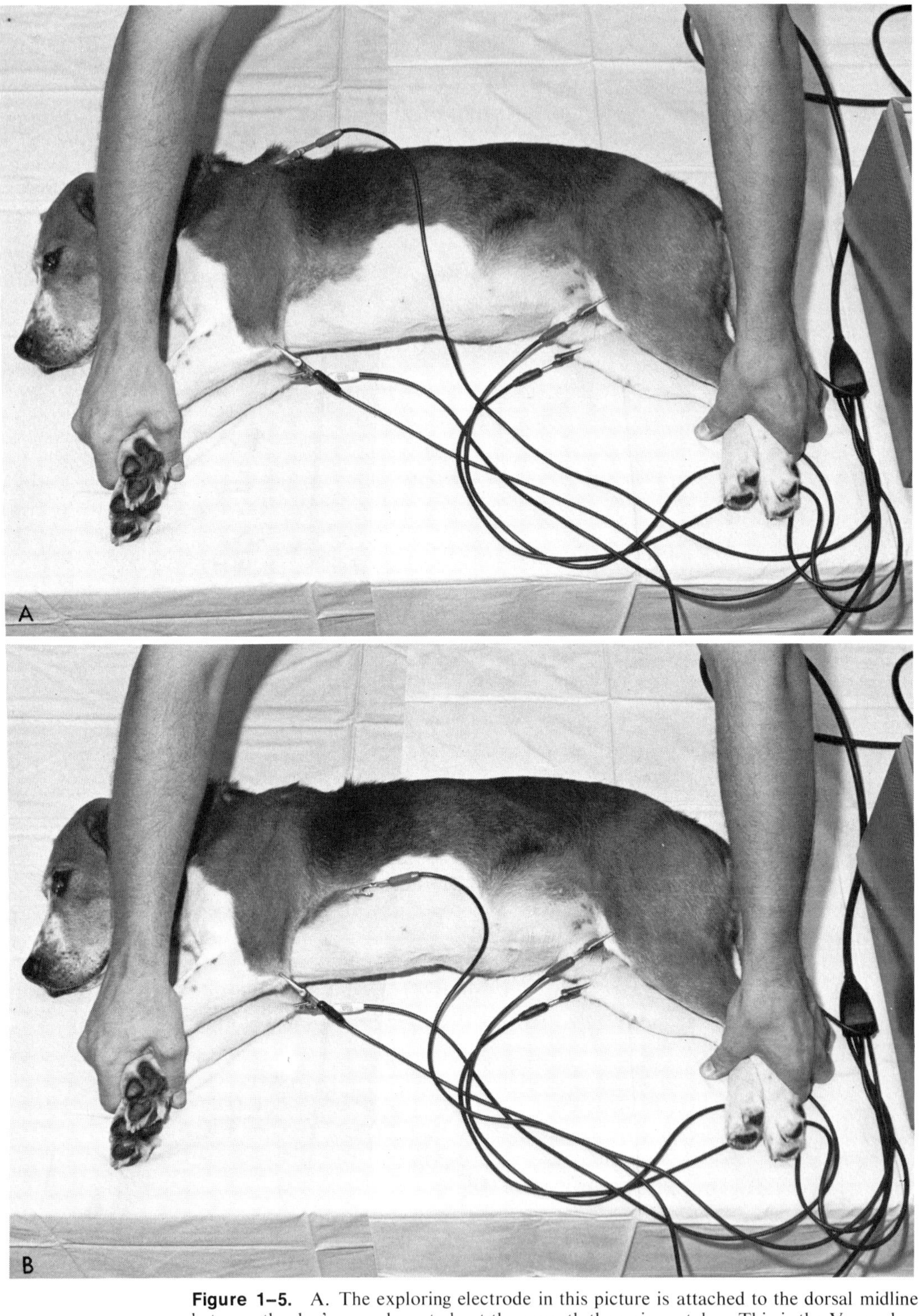

Figure 1–5. A. The exploring electrode in this picture is attached to the dorsal midline between the dog's scapulae, at about the seventh thoracic vertebra. This is the V_{10} exploring lead and is run on the V setting of the electrocardiograph.

B. Another exploring lead (CV_6LU) is produced by moving the exploring lead to a point at the left sixth intercostal space at the costochondral junction. This is also run on the V setting of the electrocardiograph.

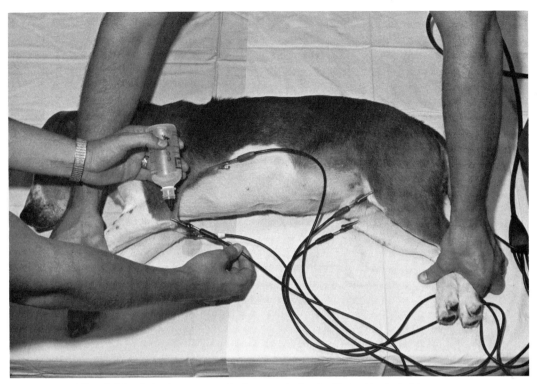

Figure 1-6. The clinician is in the process of using a squirt bottle filled with alcohol to wet the electrodes and establish good skin-to-clip contact.

the standardization control knob is adjusted so that a 1 mv. charge deflects the pen 1 cm., or 10 small boxes. The standardization button will deliver the 1 mv. charge when it is depressed. At this standardization (1 cm. = 1 mv.), each small box is equal to 0.1 mv. Thus, by measuring the height of the complexes in boxes and then multiplying by 0.1, the height of the complexes in millivolts is known. To save paper, the machine is run at 25 mm./sec. while it is being standardized. The machine should be standardized once at the beginning and again at the end of the tracing, and whenever a sensitivity change is made.

Once the machine has been standardized, the dog is in position, and the leads are attached and wetted, the tracing is run. The left hand controls the stylus position knob, and throughout the tracing, the complexes are kept in the center of the paper so that the entire complex can be seen. The right hand starts or stops the paper speed control, changes the lead selector switch to each lead, and marks the leads and events using the marker button (Fig. 1-7).

When everything is ready, the lead selector switch is placed on lead I, and the paper speed control switch is placed on 50 mm./sec. The left hand adjusts the stylus position, so that the complexes of lead I are in the middle of the paper. Two or three good complexes of each lead are all that are necessary. The right hand depresses the marker button once to indicate lead I. Similarly leads II, III, aVR, aVL, and aVF are recorded and marked, while the left hand keeps the complexes of each lead in the center of the paper. The lead selector switch is then returned

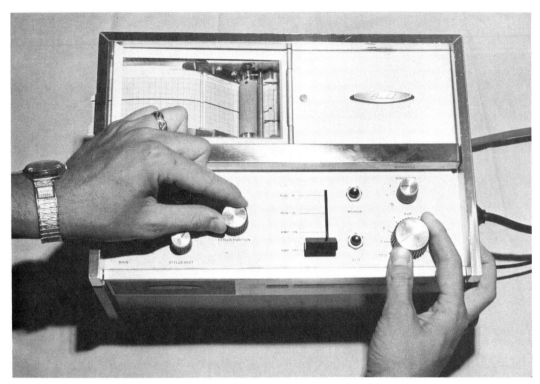

Figure 1–7. This picture illustrates the position of the hands while running the tracing. The left hand remains on the stylus position control and keeps the complexes in the middle of the paper. The right hand starts the paper, dials the lead selector switch, and depresses the marker button to mark lead numbers or events that occur.

to lead II, and 12 to 18 inches of lead II rhythm strip is recorded. If the specialized exploring leads are to be run, the "C" clip is attached to each designated position (see Table 2–1), and wetted. All of the exploring leads are run with the lead selector switch in the V lead position.

If the complexes are too large to fit completely on the paper, the sensitivity control switch is changed to 1/2 sensitivity, or machines that do not have this switch are restandardized so that 1/2 cm. = 1 mv. If the electrocardiographic complexes are very small, they can be doubled in size by changing the sensitivity control switch to "2," or by restandard-izing a machine that lacks this switch to 2 cm. = 1 mv. These changes in sensitivity should be marked so that when the electrocardiogram is read, the reader will remember to adjust the measurements accordingly (p. 8).

The animal is unclipped and released as soon as possible. The completed strip of electrocardiographic recording is generally 2 to 3 feet long and takes less than 2 minutes to do from start to finish.

Daily Monitoring of the Electrocardiogram

The situation often arises in which a dog's electrocardiogram is monitored daily or several times daily. In these instances, heart rate, P-R interval, and heart rhythm are monitored. It is not necessary to run the full electrocardiogram when monitoring these parameters. All that is needed is a foot or two of lead II rhythm strip. Positioning of the dog is not critical in these instances, and the strip may be recorded with the dog standing, sitting, or recumbent on the table, the floor, or even in his cage. The only time that right lateral recumbency is necessary is when the full electrocardiogram is run and complex height and electrical axis are needed. These daily lead II checks are easily done by one person, since restraint is usually not necessary unless the dog happens to have an inborn dislike of medical personnel.

ELECTROCARDIOGRAPHIC TROUBLE SHOOTING

It would be nice if every dog were perfectly calm, every room were free of electrical interference, and our patients would hold their breaths when we told them to do so. Since none of these things are true, there are a few commonplace trouble spots that must occasionally be dealt with if a readable tracing is to be obtained. These trouble areas include 60 cycle electrical interference, respiratory artifacts, and nervous trembling, shaking, and struggling.

60 Cycle Electrical Interference

This electrical artifact commonly causes trouble. An example of 60 cycle interference is shown in Figure 3–42. This can be difficult to remedy, especially when initially trying to get a set-up going in a new room. The following checklist may be helpful in eliminating electrical interference (items are listed in order of importance):

1. Make sure that the clips are clean and attached tightly to the cables. The rust and corrosion that build up on the clips can be removed with sand paper (Ettinger and Suter, 1970). The clips should occasionally be replaced.
2. Check the leads as they are attached to the dog. Try to attach them firmly, with good skin contact. The leads should be wetted adequately, but not excessively, with alcohol. If the leads are wetted too vigorously, the hair may become so wet that electrical contact becomes established between two clips. If this happens, it can be corrected by wadding dry paper towels between the legs to insulate the clips from one another. The table underneath the animal should also be kept as dry as possible to avoid conductivity problems.
3. Make sure that the clips do not touch each other. Paper towels wadded between the legs are also helpful in this regard.
4. Make sure the holder is not touching any of the clips. The body is an excellent conductive medium.
5. Check the ground cord and attach it to various ground contacts.
6. If the machine has a ground switch, flip it back and forth to see which setting is best for producing a smooth, steady tracing. Sometimes turning the plug around in the wall socket helps.
7. Turn out the room lights. Fluorescent lights may be especially troublesome.
8. Place the dog or even the entire table on a rubber mat or a wool blanket for insulation.
9. Unplug any electrical appliances that are connected to the same circuit as the electrocardiograph. (e.g., x-ray view-boxes, centrifuges, radios).
10. Change animal holders. Occasionally some people conduct electricity on certain days, and a change of holders may eliminate the 60 cycle interference.
11. Remove any electric watches from the vicinity. It is best not to wear a watch while doing electrocardiography anyway, since the electrocardiograph has

a powerful electromagnetic field that may eventually cause a watch to malfunction.

12. If all else fails, move to a different room and review the entire checklist. If that fails, move to another state and build a new hospital that has a copper-lined room for doing electrocardiography—but by all means, do electrocardiography!

Respiratory Artifacts

Panting dogs make it difficult to obtain a clear tracing with a steady baseline (Fig. 3–43). Also, large dogs that breathe deeply cause the baseline to fluctuate up and down, making interpretation of the tracing difficult, if not impossible (Fig. 3–46). These abnormal breathing patterns cause the front legs and the front leg electrodes to move up and down or even to bounce wildly, which in turn causes the baseline to shift up and down or bounce wildly. A dog cannot be made to hold his breath for two minutes while the tracing is recorded, but there are things that can be done. The electrode cables should be placed on the table with the dog, and should not be left dangling. Towels or other devices may be wedged between the front legs and the initial portion of the cables to minimize motion caused by chest excursions during respiration. Gentle but firm pressure may be applied to the dog's thorax, using the palm of the hand to decrease respiratory motion and stabilize the legs and cables. These techniques are successful in most instances, but occasionally the dog may need sedation if it can be given safely.

Movement Artifacts

The majority of dogs need no chemical restraint, but tranquilizers and anesthetics can be helpful if they are needed. The timid, trembling, demure little poodle can ruin a tracing just as readily as the wide-eyed, struggling, maniacal German shepherd (or Chihuahua). Most chemical forms of restraint do not significantly alter the electrocardiogram. The real consideration is whether it is safe to administer it to the patient. It is rare that mild tranquilization would be contraindicated to obtain a readable electrocardiogram. Mild sedation will not adversely affect most cardiac patients, and it may even help them. Anesthesia is rarely needed and may not be possible owing to the dog's condition. The electrocardiographic effects of some of the common drugs are discussed in Chapter 3.

REFERENCES

Bolton, G.: Prevention and Treatment of Anesthetic Emergencies During Anesthesia and Surgery. Vet. Clin. of N. Am., 2(2) (1972):411.

Detweiler, D. K., and Patterson, D. F.: The Prevalence and Types of Cardiovascular Disease in Dogs. Ann. N. Y. Acad. Sci., 127 (1965):481.

Ettinger, S. J., and Suter, P. F.: Canine Cardiology. W. B. Saunders Co., Philadelphia, 1970.

Pedersoli, W. M., and Brown, M. K.: A New Approach to the Etiology of Arrhythmogenic Effects of Thiamylal Sodium in Dogs. Vet. Med. Small Anim. Clin., 68 (1973):1286.

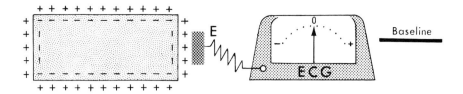

Chapter 2

ELECTROCARDIOGRAPHIC PHYSIOLOGY

The lead II electrocardiogram in Figure 2–1 is a recording of electrical currents generated during the depolarization of a dog's heart. The P wave signifies that the atria have depolarized, causing contraction and ejection of their complement of blood into the ventricles. The P-R segment indicates the short delay that occurs after the atria contract, which allows complete filling of the ventricles before ventricular contraction

Figure 2–1. A normal canine lead II electrocardiographic complex. The electrocardiograph has been standardized at 1 cm. = 1 mv. so that each small box on the vertical axis equals 0.1 millivolt. This tracing is recorded at 50 mm./sec. paper speed so that each small box on the horizontal axis equals 0.02 second.

Atrial depolarization is indicated by the P wave. Following the P wave there is a short delay in the atrioventricular node (P-R segment), after which the ventricles depolarize and produce the QRS complex. The S-T segment and the T wave represent ventricular repolarization.

Measurement of the waves in this lead II complex yields important information, which is discussed and illustrated in Chapter 3. The height and width of the P wave is measured. The P-R interval is measured from the beginning of the P wave to the beginning of the QRS complex. The width of the QRS complex and the height of the R wave from the baseline up are measured. The S-T segment should return to the baseline for a short time before slipping into the T wave, as it does here. The Q-T interval is measured from the beginning of the QRS complex to the end of the T wave. See Table 3–2 for normal values. This complex measures:

P = 0.04 sec. (2 boxes) by 0.3 mv (3 boxes)
P-R int. = 0.09 sec. (4½ boxes)
QRS width = 0.04 sec. (2 boxes) by R wave of 1.8 mv. (18 boxes)
S-T seg. and T wave = normal
Q-T int. = 0.18 sec. (9 boxes)

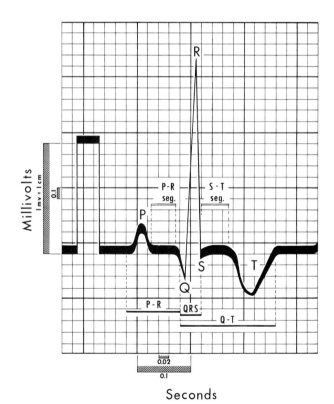

Seconds

occurs. The QRS complex represents ventricular depolarization and contraction with the ejection of blood into the aorta and pulmonary artery. The S-T segment and T wave depict the repolarization of the ventricles.

The electrocardiograph measures these waves of electrical activity and records them on graph paper. The complexes can be measured for height (measured in millivolts) and width (measured in hundredths of seconds). By standardizing the machine to 1 cm. = 1 mv. (as described in Chapter 1), each small box on the vertical axis is 0.1 millivolt (Fig. 2–1). When the electrocardiogram is recorded at 50 mm./sec., each small box on the horizontal axis is 0.02 second (Fig. 2–1). A complex can be measured by counting its height in boxes and multiplying by 0.1 mv., and by counting its width in boxes and multiplying by 0.02 second. These values are then compared with the normal values given in Table 3–2.

When a series of leads is recorded, the direction that the main electrical current is following (electrical axis) can be determined, and can be compared with the normal values in Table 3–2.

This chapter deals with the sequence of cardiac depolarization; how it begins, how it is propagated, why it is in such an orderly sequence, and how it is measured and used for clinical purposes.

CELLULAR PHYSIOLOGY AND THE GENERATION OF ELECTRICAL IMPULSES

Cardiac muscle cell physiology is similar in many ways to that of other muscle cells. In the normal resting state, the cell is said to be polarized. In this polarized state, the inside of the cell is negative with respect to the outside surface (Fig. 2–2A). The polarity is maintained by the distribution and concentration of intracellular and extracellular ions. The cell membrane is mainly responsible for the manner in which these ions are distributed, and several factors are involved.

The cell membrane is nearly impermeable to Na^+, and is partially but poorly permeable to K^+ and Cl^- (Friedberg, 1966). In addition, there is a metabolic cellular "pump" within the cell membrane that actively pumps Na^+ out of the cell and pumps K^+ into the cell (Guyton, 1971). The concentration of Na^+ is much higher extracellularly because of the sodium pump, and because the membrane will not allow sodium to diffuse into the cell. The concentration of K^+ is much higher intracellularly than extracellularly (about 20:1), and this favors the diffusion of K^+ out of the cell through the partially permeable cell membrane (Guyton, 1971). The concentration of Cl^- is greatest extracellularly and this favors the diffusion of Cl^- into the cell (Guyton, 1971).

The net result of all these forces is a greater number of negative charges inside the cell and a greater number of positive charges outside the cell. The relative difference between the charges on each side of the cell membrane can be measured and is called the resting transmembrane potential (RMP) (Fig. 2–3). The resting transmembrane potential is constant and equal to about −90 mv. (Ettinger and Suter, 1970; Guyton, 1971; Winsor, 1968).

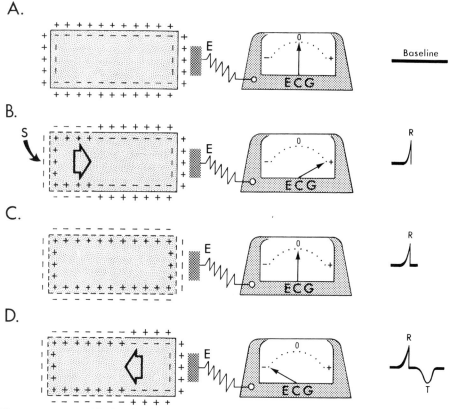

Figure 2–2. A. This drawing illustrates a resting cardiac muscle fiber. The cell is polarized, which means that the outside of the cell is positive with respect to the inside because of the distribution of extracellular and intracellular ions. In this polarized state, there is no electrical activity, and the electrode (E), which is attached to the body surface, records a steady straight baseline.

B. Upon stimulation (S), the fiber begins to depolarize. There is a sudden shift of ions, and the charges reverse themselves. This depolarization process spreads along the entire length of the fiber, the electrode (E) detects a wave of electrical current flowing toward it, and it records a positive deflection (R) on the electrocardiograph.

C. Once the entire fiber has been depolarized, the electrical current no longer flows, and the tracing returns to the baseline.

D. Repolarization begins as the ions gradually return to their original positions. As repolarization of the entire fiber proceeds, another wave of electric current flows. In this instance the current is flowing away from the electrode (E), and a negative deflection occurs (T). In the dog, the T wave can be positive or negative in most leads.

When the cell is polarized and the ions are in their respective places, no electrical activity is produced. If a stimulus is applied to the cell, the membrane suddenly loses its impermeability to Na$^+$ and there is a sudden rush of Na$^+$ into the cell (Guyton, 1971; Friedberg, 1966). This causes a temporary reversal of intracellular charges (Fig. 2–2B). After the cell has been stimulated to depolarize, the depolarization process spreads rapidly for the entire length of the muscle fiber without additional stimulation. This wave of shifting ions produces an electrical current that is measurable (Fig. 2–2B). The magnitude of the electrical forces produced is proportional to the length and diameter of the muscle fiber. It is for this reason that dilatation (lengthening of the muscle fibers) and hypertrophy (thickening of the muscle fibers) will cause an

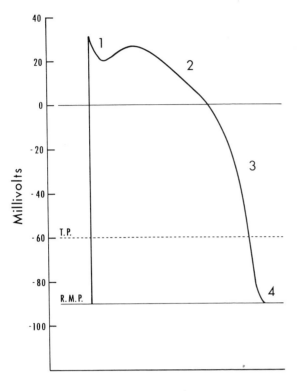

Figure 2–3.   This drawing demonstrates a membrane action potential measured by placing an electrode inside a muscle cell and then recording the changes in electrical potential that occur across the membrane at that point. The resting membrane potential (R.M.P.) indicates that the inside of the resting cell is about 90 mv. more negative than the outside. If the cell is stimulated, an action potential occurs, causing depolarization so that the cell suddenly is more positive intracellularly. During phases 2 and 3 the intracellular electronegativity is gradually restored, and during phase 4 the fiber is again resting. Whenever the threshold potential TP is exceeded, an action potential occurs and causes depolarization of the entire muscle fiber.

increase in electrical forces that can be measured on the electrocardiogram.

Shortly after the cell membrane becomes permeable to Na^+, it becomes much more permeable to K^+, and K^+ begins to leave the cell rapidly (Friedberg, 1966). As the influx of Na^+ slows and the efflux of K^+ accelerates, there is a point at which K^+ loss is greater than Na^+ gain (Friedberg, 1966). At this point, repolarization begins (Fig. 2–2C). Repolarization occurs much more slowly than depolarization. The cell membrane quickly regains its impermeable state, and most of repolarization depends on the gradual removal of Na^+ from the cell by the sodium-potassium pump mechanism. The shifting of ions during repolarization also produces a measurable electrical current (Fig. 2–2D).

The membrane action potential is a recording that is made by placing an electrode inside a cell and then recording the changes in electrical potential that occur across the membrane at that exact point (Fig. 2–3). The depolarization wave starts at that point and continues for the entire length of the muscle fiber. The threshold potential (TP) determines the ease with which a muscle fiber can be stimulated. A stimulatory impulse must be strong enough to exceed the threshold potential before depolarization will begin. Diseases or drugs that alter the threshold potential will alter the sensitivity of the cells. For example, quinidine works by causing an increased threshold potential, making the cells less sensitive to stimulation and less prone to produce arrhythmias (Goodman and Gilman, 1970). When the action potential occurs, muscle contraction is initiated. The mechanism by which the electrical impulse initiates muscle contraction is not known.

Special Physiologic Properties of Cardiac Muscle Cells

The electrical activity in the heart is more organized than that in the brain and most other muscular tissue (Ettinger and Suter, 1970). The electrical excitation of the heart is rhythmic, and occurs rapidly in an orderly sequence. There are several characteristics that cardiac muscle cells possess that allow for such fine coordination. These characteristics include automaticity, conductivity, and excitability.

Certain specialized cardiac tissues have the ability to depolarize automatically, without requiring an outside stimulus. These tissues are called the pacemaker tissues and are said to possess automaticity, or the ability to discharge spontaneously. They possess automaticity because of a difference in their cell membranes' permeability to Na^+, and during phase 4 of the action potential, Na^+ leaks into the cells and raises the electrical potential to the threshold potential (Fig. 2–4). This initiates an action potential, and depolarization begins. The pacemaker tissues are located in the sinoatrial node, junctional fibers (specialized atrial fibers in the area of the atrioventricular node), bundle of His and its branches, and Purkinje fibers. Under extreme conditions other atrial and ventricular muscle fibers are capable of automaticity (Guyton, 1971).

The rate at which each of these pacemaker tissues automatically

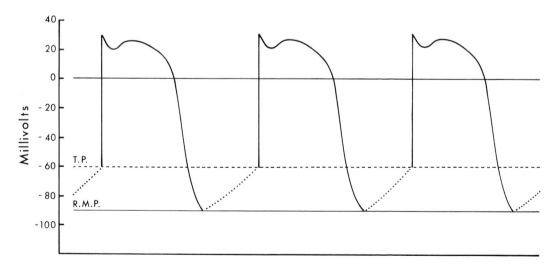

Figure 2–4. Typical action potential of a cardiac pacemaker fiber. Unlike the other fibers, which remain at the resting membrane potential (RMP), the pacemaker tissues have the ability to depolarize themselves automatically. During phase 4 of their action potential, Na^+ gradually leaks into the fiber, and the intracellular space becomes less and less negative until the threshold potential (TP) is reached, an action potential occurs, and the fiber discharges an impulse that is propagated along the conduction pathway to other muscle fibers.

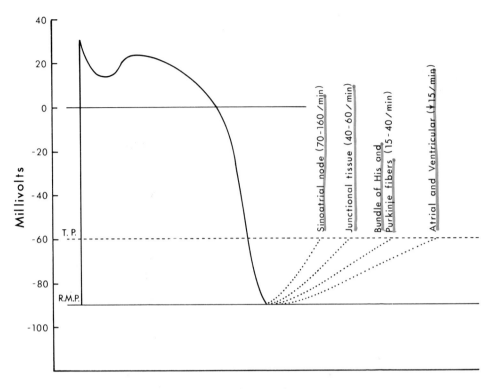

Figure 2-5. The various cardiac pacemaker tissues have different rates of automatic discharge. The sinoatrial node is the usual cardiac pacemaker because it has the most rapid rate of spontaneous depolarization (70 to 160 times per minute). If the sinoatrial node were to become inactive, the junctional tissues in the area of the atrioventricular node would pace the heart at 40 to 60 beats per minute. If both the sinoatrial node and the junctional fibers were to become inactive, the bundle of His or the Purkinje fibers could pace the heart at 15 to 40 times a minute. Under extreme conditions, the atrial and ventricular fibers may discharge at very slow rates, serving as a last-ditch measure to maintain life.

discharges is different. The sinoatrial node normally has the most rapid rate of spontaneous depolarization (70 to 160 times per minute), and it is the usual cardiac pacemaker (Fig. 2–5). If the sinoatrial node were to become inactivated, the junctional tissues would have the next-most-rapid rate of automatic discharge (40 to 60 times per minute), and they would act as the cardiac pacemaker (Fig. 2–5). If both the sinoatrial tissues and the junctional tissues become inactivated, then the bundle of His, its branches, or the Purkinje fibers would pace the heart at 15 to 40 beats per minute (Fig. 2–5). If all the other pacemaker tissues fail, atrial or ventricular fibers can discharge on their own at very slow rates (Fig. 2–5) (Guyton, 1971).

Another important concept of cardiac muscle cell physiology is the functional syncytium principle, or the all-or-none phenomenon. There are two main functional syncytia, the atrial syncytium and the ventricular syncytium. They communicate with each other through the atrioventricular node and the bundle of His. Otherwise, the atrial and ventricular musculature syncytia are separated from each other by fibrous tissue that surrounds and supports the valvular rings (Guyton,

1971). The all-or-none concept means that if one atrial fiber becomes stimulated to depolarize, the impulse will spread and depolarize all the atrial fibers. If the conduction system is intact, the impulse will spread through the atrioventricular node and continue on to discharge the ventricles. As in the case of the atrial fibers, if one ventricular muscle cell depolarizes, all the ventricular muscle cells will depolarize. This is advantageous in producing a single, forceful contraction of the cardiac chambers.

The mechanism by which these cardiac fibers are so conductive, and so easily stimulated, seems to lie in the region of the intercalated discs (Friedberg, 1966). Ordinarily, cell membranes possess high electrical resistance, but the cardiac cell membranes in the region of the intercalated discs are of extremely low resistance (Friedberg, 1966). Thus they are easily stimulated, and the cell-to-cell transfer of electrical current in the cardiac syncytium is facilitated.

The Cardiac Conduction System

The cardiac conduction system is responsible for organizing the sequence of depolarization in the heart. It is composed of specialized tissues that conduct electrical impulses through the heart. Impulses are conducted rapidly, so all the cardiac muscle fibers in the atrial syncytium or in the ventricular syncytium will contract almost simultaneously to produce a forceful contraction. At the same time, a delay is built into the system at the atrioventricular node to allow time for the atria to eject their contents into the ventricles before ventricular contraction occurs. The conduction system consists of the sinoatrial node, the interatrial bundles, the atrioventricular node, the common bundle of His, the right and left branches of the bundle of His, and the Purkinje fibers (Fig. 2–6) (Ettinger and Suter, 1970).

The Sinoatrial Node

The sinoatrial node is a small strip of specialized cardiac muscle located at the junction of the right atrium and the cranial vena cava (Et-

Figure 2–6. The conduction system of the heart includes the sinoatrial node (S-A node), the interatrial bundles, the atrioventricular node (A-V node), the bundle of His and its branches, and the Purkinje fibers. The S-A node lies in the right atrium, and atrial conduction occurs at the rate of 500 to 1000 mm./sec. Conduction through the A-V node is slow (100 mm./sec.), which allows the atria to empty into the ventricles before ventricular contraction occurs. The Purkinje fibers conduct rapidly (2000 mm./sec.) and terminate subendocardially. Muscle cell to muscle cell transmission occurs where the Purkinje fibers terminate, and the conduction across the ventricular muscle cells occurs at the rate of 400 mm./sec.

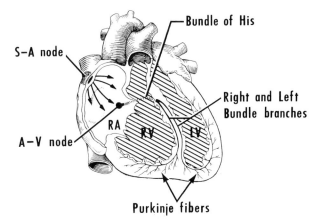

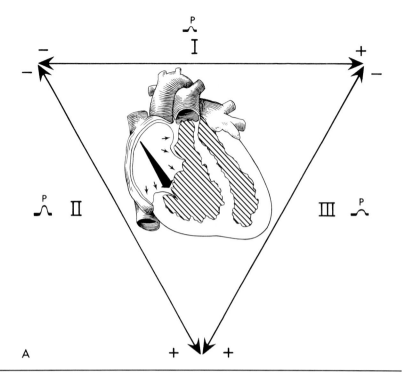

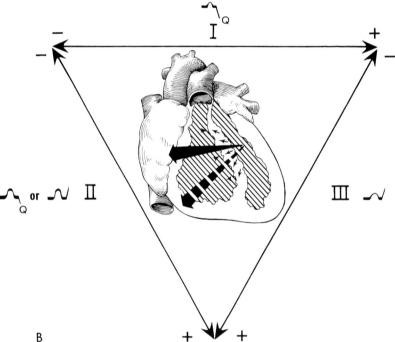

Figure 2–7. A. After the sinoatrial node initiates depolarization, an electrical impulse spreads across the atria to the atrioventricular node, producing the P wave on the electrocardiogram. Leads I, II, and III form an equilateral triangle around the heart (Fig. 2–16), and each lead "sees" the impulse from a different position (Figs. 2–13 and 2–14). After the P wave occurs, the recording returns to the baseline as the P-R segment, indicating the delay in the A-V node just before the ventricles discharge.

B. The first phase of the ventricular activation process is depolarization of the ventricular septum. This produces the Q wave on the electrocardiogram. The Q wave is usually a rather small negative deflection that does not appear consistently on every normal lead II electrocardiogram. Again, each lead sees the impulse from its own position.   (*Illustration continued on opposite page*)

24

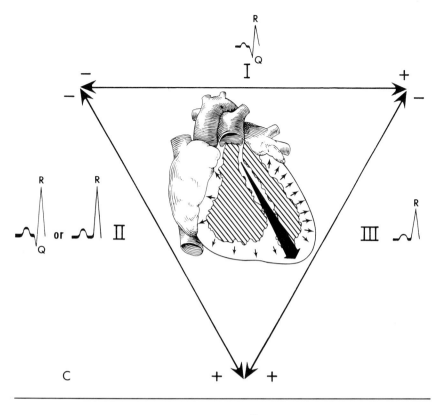

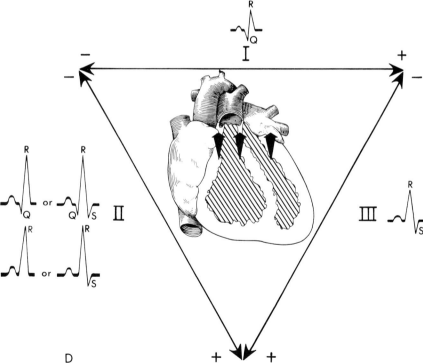

Figure 2–7 Continued. C. The second phase of ventricular activation is depolarization of the left and right ventricular free walls. This produces the R wave on the electrocardiogram, and is the largest force that is produced.

D. The third and last phase of ventricular activation is depolarization of the base of the septum and both ventricles. This produces the S wave on the electrocardiogram. The S wave also occurs variably on the lead II electrocardiogram, and the four possible normal lead II tracings are shown.

(C and D adapted from illustration in *Clinical Symposia,* copyright by CIBA Pharmaceutical Company, Division of CIBA-GEIGY Corporation. All rights reserved.)

tinger and Suter, 1970). It is the usual cardiac pacemaker because it has the most rapid rate of automatic depolarization. The fibers in the sinoatrial node have a low resting transmembrane potential and a high membrane conductance of Na^+, which allows them to depolarize and initiate the cardiac impulse at the normal heart rate of 70 to 160 times per minute.

Atrial Conduction

Once the sinoatrial node initiates depolarization, the electrical impulse spreads across the atria to the atrioventricular node, which produces a P wave on the electrocardiogram (Fig. 2–7A). The P wave represents the sum of all of the electrical forces produced during the depolarization of both atria. Since the sinoatrial node is located in the right atrium, the right atrium begins to depolarize about 0.01 second before the left atrium (Friedberg, 1966). The P wave, then, is a recording of first the right, and 0.01 second later of the left atrial depolarization (Fig. 2–8). This will become important later when atrial hypertrophy patterns are discussed (Chapter 3, p. 53).

The conduction pathways in the atria are mainly muscle to muscle, but there are also interatrial conduction bundles that run more directly from the sinoatrial node to the atrioventricular node, and from the right to the left atrium (Friedberg, 1966). The speed of impulse transmission through the atria is 500 to 1000 mm./sec. (Friedberg, 1966).

The Atrioventricular Node

The atrioventricular node lies in the septal wall of the right atrium, craniodorsal to the septal cusp of the right atrioventricular valve (Ettinger and Suter, 1970). It is composed of specialized tissue very similar to that of the sinoatrial node. As the atrial impulse enters the node, conduction velocity is slowed to 100 mm./sec., preventing the impulse from

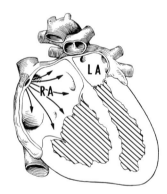

Figure 2–8. The P wave on the electrocardiogram represents the depolarization of first the right, and, 0.01 second later, the left atrium. The normal P wave, then, represents a summation of both the right and left atrial depolarization forces. This will be of importance when atrial hypertrophy patterns are discussed (Fig. 3–17).

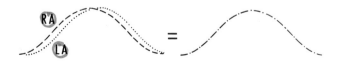

entering the ventricles too soon (Guyton, 1971). This allows the atria time to discharge their complement of blood into the ventricles before ventricular contraction occurs. The delay at the atrioventricular node is recorded electrocardiographically as a straight line (isoelectric period) following the P wave and is called the P-R segment (Fig. 2–7A). The total amount of time required for both atrial depolarization and the delay in the atrioventricular node is measured as the P-R interval (Fig. 2–1).

The Bundle of His and the Purkinje System

The bundle of His leaves the atrioventricular node and courses into the ventricular septum, where it divides into a right and left bundle branch. The bundle branches run just underneath the septal endocardium. The right bundle supplies the right ventricle and the left bundle conducts the impulse to the left ventricle. The Purkinje fibers are the subendocardial terminations of the bundle branches in the walls of the ventricles. Conduction through this portion of the system is rapid (2000 mm./sec.), so that the entire ventricular muscle mass contracts synchronously to produce a forceful beat (Friedberg, 1966). There are three main phases in the usual sequence of ventricular depolarization in the dog. These three phases or waves of electrical activity produce the Q, R, and S deflections on the electrocardiogram (Hamlin and Smith, 1960).

The Q wave is the first negative (downward) deflection on the lead II electrocardiogram. It represents the first phase of ventricular depolarization and is produced by the discharge of the mid and apical portions of the ventricular septum (Fig. 2–7B). The electrical impulse spreads from the left septal surface toward the right, and from the right septal surface toward the left. The electrocardiogram records only the left-to-right forces because they are of so much greater magnitude that they override the right-to-left forces (Hamlin and Smith, 1960).

The R wave is the first positive (upward) deflection on the lead II electrocardiogram. It is produced during the second phase of ventricular depolarization, and is normally the greatest force that is produced (Fig. 2–7C). It occurs as the impulse spreads from the subendocardial terminations of the Purkinje system toward the epicardial surfaces of both ventricles, via conduction from muscle fiber to muscle fiber in the ventricular free walls (Hamlin and Smith, 1960). Even though both the left and right ventricles discharge simultaneously, the electrocardiogram records the deflection as if only the left ventricular forces were present, since they are of much greater magnitude and thus they cancel out the smaller right ventricular electrical forces.

The third phase of ventricular depolarization produces the S wave, which is the first negative (downward) deflection that occurs following the R wave on lead II of the electrocardiogram. This deflection occurs as the muscle fibers at the base of the heart are activated in an apicobasilar direction (Fig. 2–7D) (Hamlin and Smith, 1960).

Thus, although many electrical forces are produced, three major waves of electrical activity are recorded on the electrocardiogram. The Q wave on lead II represents septal activation, the R wave on lead II indicates ventricular free wall myocardial activation, and the S wave on

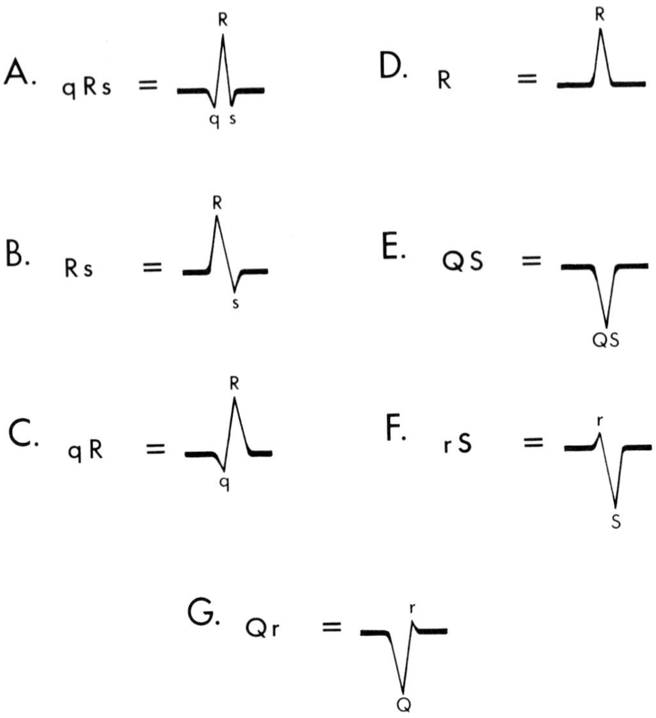

A. qRs =

B. Rs =

C. qR =

D. R =

E. QS =

F. rS =

G. Qr =

Figure 2–9. By definition, the Q wave is the first negative (downward) deflection on the electrocardiogram. The R wave is the first positive (upward) deflection, and the S wave is the first negative deflection following the R wave. This must be kept in mind when determining whether there is a Q, an R, or an S wave present. For labeling purposes, the major deflection is indicated by a capital letter and the minor deflections are indicated by small letters. When discussing QRS morphology with a colleague, it is important to describe the waves in this manner.

A. This complex has all three deflections. There is a small negative q, a large positive R, and a small s wave.

B. There is no Q wave in this complex. A small s wave follows the large positive R wave.

C. There is no S wave in this complex. The small q wave precedes the large R wave.

D. The S and Q waves are missing in this complex; only the R wave is present.

E. When only a negative wave is present, as in this instance, it is considered that both the Q and S waves are present.

F. There is no Q wave in this abnormal complex. Instead, a small r wave precedes a large S wave.

G. There is no S wave in this abnormal complex. A large Q wave precedes the small r wave.

The first four complexes (A, B, C, and D) are normal variations of the lead II electrocardiogram (Fig. 2–7D).

lead II signifies depolarization of the basal septal and ventricular basilar portions of the heart. The direction of the main force (the R wave) varies only slightly, but the Q wave and the S wave are usually quite small deflections that do not appear consistently on lead II in every normal electrocardiogram. There are several QRS configurations that may occur (Fig. 2–9).

Innervation of the Heart

Although the nervous system is not a part of the cardiac conduction system, the heart is generously supplied with both sympathetic and parasympathetic nerves, which do affect the heart rate and the conduction of electrical impulses.

The parasympathetic nerves are distributed mainly to the sinoatrial node, the atrioventricular node, and to some extent the atrial muscle fibers (Guyton, 1971). For practical purposes, the ventricles do not receive parasympathetic innervation (Fig. 2–10). The vagus nerve supplies the parasympathetic innervation of the heart.

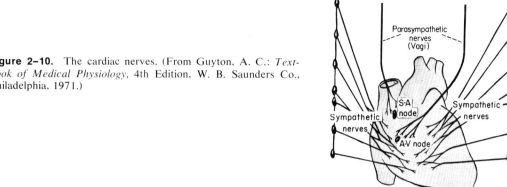

Figure 2-10. The cardiac nerves. (From Guyton, A. C.: *Textbook of Medical Physiology*, 4th Edition, W. B. Saunders Co., Philadelphia, 1971.)

The sympathetic nerves originate from several sources, and their distribution is similar to that of the parasympathetic nerves; also they richly supply the ventricles (Fig. 2-10), (Guyton, 1971).

Stimulation of the vagus nerves increases parasympathetic tone, which decreases the heart rate and slows conduction through the atrioventricular node. Excessive vagal activity can completely stop the rhythmicity of the sinoatrial node, or completely block impulse transmission through the atrioventricular node. These vagal effects are mediated by the release of acetylcholine, which increases cell membrane permeability to K^+. The cells lose K^+, which increases intracellular negativity. The cells are then said to be hyperpolarized, and far greater quantities of Na^+ must enter the cells to reach the threshold potential and thus stimulate depolarization (Guyton, 1971).

Stimulation of the sympathetic nerves causes an increase in both the rate and force of contraction. This is mediated by the release of norepinephrine at the nerve endings. Norepinephrine may increase the permeability of the cell membranes to both Na^+ and Ca^{++} (Guyton, 1971). The rapid entrance of Na^+ into the cells causes the threshold potential to be reached quickly and depolarization to occur more rapidly. The increased availability of Ca^{++} may be responsible for the increased force of contraction.

MEASURING THE ELECTRICAL FORCES WITH THE ELECTROCARDIOGRAPH

The heart is suspended in a conductive medium; the tissues and fluids surrounding it conduct electrical currents easily (Fig. 2-11). During depolarization, current flows from electronegative areas to electropositive areas (Guyton, 1971). The electrocardiogram records only the major waves of electrical activity that occur; these in turn, represent a summation of many smaller forces. Using the arms and legs as electrodes, the electrocardiograph detects, magnifies, and records the major cardiac forces that are conducted to the body surface.

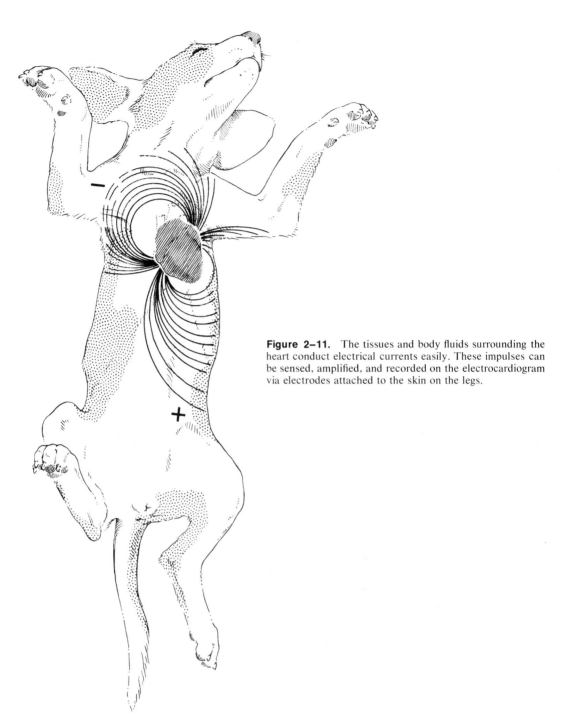

Figure 2–11. The tissues and body fluids surrounding the heart conduct electrical currents easily. These impulses can be sensed, amplified, and recorded on the electrocardiogram via electrodes attached to the skin on the legs.

Cardiac Vectors

Electrical forces possess direction and magnitude, both of which are measurable. A force that has both direction and magnitude is called a vector (Ettinger and Suter, 1970). The cardiac vector can be illustrated by an arrow that represents a summation of many different forces. The cardiac vector has direction (which is indicated by the arrowhead) and

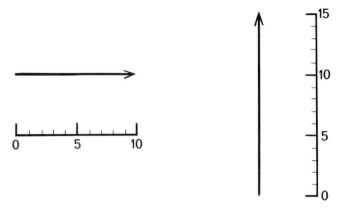

Figure 2–12. The arrow represents the cardiac vector. Its length is proportional to the magnitude of the force, and the direction of the arrow represents the direction of the force from the point of origin. (From Ettinger, S. J., and Suter, P. F.: *Canine Cardiology*. W. B. Saunders Co., Philadelphia, 1970.)

magnitude (which is indicated by the length of the arrow (Fig. 2–12). A series of leads was developed to measure the direction and force of the cardiac vector accurately. Each lead views the vector from a slightly different position (Fig. 2–13). Each lead has a positive and negative pole. If an electrical impulse (vector) is traveling toward the lead's positive pole, a positive (upward) deflection results (Fig. 2–14). If the impulse is traveling in the direction of a lead's negative pole, that lead will record a negative (downward) deflection (Fig. 2–14). If the vector force runs perpendicular to a lead, that lead will record either no deflection or an equal number of positive and negative forces (Fig. 2–14). This is called a zero potential lead, an isopotential lead, or an isoelectric lead. Figure 2–15 shows some examples of leads that are isoelectric.

This information is helpful since if a lead records a positive deflection, that indicates that the cardiac vector is running toward the lead's positive pole. If the lead records a negative deflection, the impulse is traveling toward its negative pole. If the lead is isoelectric, the direction of the impulse is perpendicular to that lead (see Chapter 3, Procedure for Axis Determination).

Figure 2–13. It is apparent that when the cardiac vector is projected within a triangle representing the three standard limb leads, the longest vector will be projected on the lead most nearly parallel to the cardiac vector (lead II in this case). Similarly, the shortest vector will be projected on the lead most nearly perpendicular to the cardiac vector (lead III). (From Ettinger, S. J., and Suter, P. F.: *Canine Cardiology*. W. B. Saunders Co., Philadelphia, 1970.)

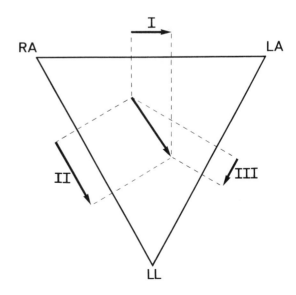

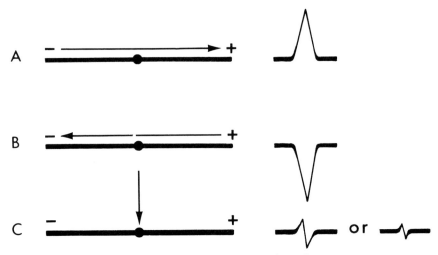

Figure 2–14. Each lead has a positive pole and a negative pole.

A. If the vector (or *impulse*) runs toward the positive pole, a positive (upward) deflection occurs.

B. If the impulse runs toward the negative pole, a negative (downward) deflection results.

C. If the main impulse runs perpendicular to a lead, that lead records an isoelectric deflection, which may be either a very small recording, or a recording showing an equal amount of positive and negative deflection.

Later, when axis is discussed, it will be important to be able to find which lead is isoelectric because the main vector will be running perpendicular to the isoelectric lead (see Chapter 3, pp. 46–52).

Lead Systems

The various lead systems were developed to provide an accurate measurement of the electrical forces produced during cardiac contraction. The most useful system is composed of the basic six-lead electrocardiogram. Table 2–1 lists the various lead systems that are used in canine electrocardiography.

Bailey's Hexaxial Lead System

This lead system is the most widely used one in canine electrocardiography. It combines both the bipolar limb leads and the augmented unipolar limb leads.

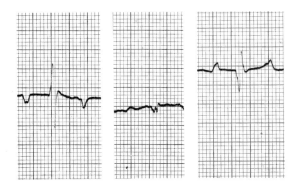

Figure 2–15. A, B, and C are examples of true isoelectric leads since they have an equal number of positive and negative charges.

TABLE 2–1. LEAD SYSTEMS USED IN CANINE ELECTROCARDIOGRAPHY

Bailey's Hexaxial Lead System

Bipolar Limb Leads
Lead I – right arm (−) to the left arm (+)
Lead II – right arm (−) to left leg (+)
Lead III – left arm (−) to left leg (+)

Augmented Unipolar Limb Leads
Lead aVR – right arm (+), compared to left arm and left leg (−)
Lead aVL – left arm (+), compared to the right arm and left leg (−)
Lead aVF – left leg (+), compared to the right and left arms (−)

Unipolar Precordial Leads (Exploring Leads)

Lead V_{10} – over the dorsal spinous process of the seventh thoracic vertebra

Lead CV_6LL – sixth left intercostal space near the edge of the sternum

Lead CV_6LU – sixth left intercostal space at the costochondral junction

Lead CV_5RL – fifth right intercostal space near the edge of the sternum

Orthogonal Lead System

Lead X – sinistrodextral (left-to-right). Equal to lead I

Lead Y – caudocranial (tail-to-head). Equal to lead aVF

Lead Z – dorsoventral (back-to-front). Equal to lead V_{10}

Esophageal Lead

Einthoven's triangle depicts the three bipolar limb leads, leads I, II, and III (Fig. 2–16). The electrodes are attached to the right forelimb (RA), the left forelimb (LA), and the left hindlimb (LL). The right hindlimb (RL) connects the dog to the ground. In lead I, the RA is the negative terminal and LA is the positive terminal (Fig. 2–16). In lead II, RA is the negative terminal and LL is the positive terminal (Fig. 2–16). In lead III, LA is the negative pole and LL is the positive pole (Fig. 2–16).

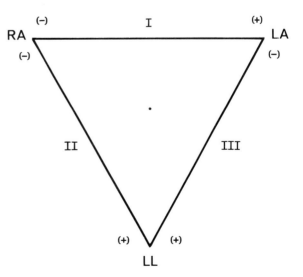

Figure 2–16. The Einthoven triangle. When the three limb leads are connected, the center of the triangle represents the origin of cardiac electrical activity. Lead I is a connection between the positive electrode on the LA and the negative electrode on the RA. Lead II connects the negative RA with the positive LL, and lead III connects the negative LA with the positive LL. (LA = left foreleg; RA = right foreleg; LL = left hindlimb.) (From Ettinger, S. J., and Suter, P. F.: *Canine Cardiology*. W. B. Saunders Co., Philadelphia, 1970.)

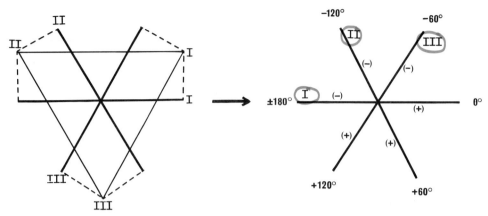

Figure 2–17. Triaxial limb leads. By constructing parallelograms for leads I, II, and III, each lead of the Einthoven triangle can be made to intersect the center of the triangle. The three leads now visualized intersecting the center of the triangle are shown in the drawing on the right. A semicircular portion on one side of lead I is numbered from 0° to 180° in a clockwise direction. On the other side of lead I, the semicircle is numbered from 0° to −180° in a counterclockwise direction. The polarity of the leads is determined by the original position of the positive and negative electrodes on the Einthoven triangle (Fig. 2–16). (From Ettinger, S. J., and Suter, P. F.: *Canine Cardiology.* W. B. Saunders Co., Philadelphia, 1970.)

The three leads form, in theory, an equilateral triangle. The three leads can be redrawn exactly at the same length and polarity by passing each lead through the center point of the triangle (Fig. 2–17). This produces a triaxial lead system, and angle values can be assigned to both the positive and negative pole of each lead (Fig. 2–17).

The augmented unipolar limb leads (aVR, aVL, and aVF), provide three more leads that can be added to make a hexaxial lead system. More angle values can be added for more accurate measurement of the cardiac vector. Basically an augmented unipolar limb lead compares the electrical activity at the reference limb to the sum of the electrical activity at the other two limbs. The machine is wired to do this; all we have to do is dial each lead with the lead selector switch. The "a" stands for augmented; the voltage produced by these leads is small and must be augmented. The "V" stands for vector. The "R" stands for right arm, the "L" stands for the left arm, and the "F" stands for the frontal, and represents the left leg. Thus we have the augmented vector lead of the left arm (aVL), the augmented vector lead of the right arm (aVR), and the augmented vector lead of the frontal plane (aVF). In lead aVR, RA is the positive or reference pole, and the negative pole compares LA and LL (Fig. 2–18). In lead aVL, LA is the positive pole and the negative pole compares RA and LL (Fig. 2–18). In lead aVF, LL is the positive reference point, and RA and LA represent the negative pole (Fig. 2–18). These three leads produce another triaxial lead system (Fig. 2–19). If the two triaxial lead systems are combined, Bailey's six-axis reference system results (Fig. 2–20). Now there are six leads, each with a positive and negative pole, and each pole has an angle value. This six-lead system is used for determining the mean electrical axis (Chapter 3, pp. 46).

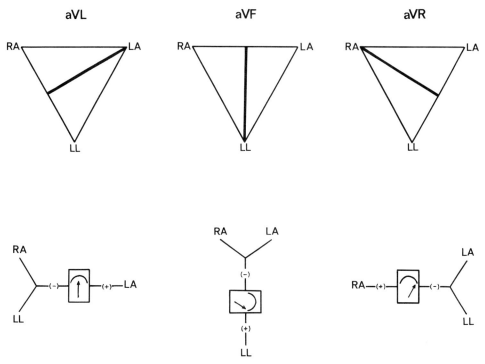

Figure 2–18. Augmented limb leads. Lead aVL compares the positive electrode at the LA position and the mean voltage of the RA and LL electrodes. It may be drawn into the Einthoven triangle as shown. Likewise, the voltage at the positive LL electrode is compared with the mean voltage at the RA and LA electrodes (aVF), and the voltage at the positive RA electrode is compared with the mean voltage at the LA and LL electrodes (aVR). LA = left foreleg; RA = right foreleg; LL = left hindlimb. (From Ettinger, S. J., and Suter, P. F.: Canine Cardiology. W. B. Saunders Co., Philadelphia, 1970.)

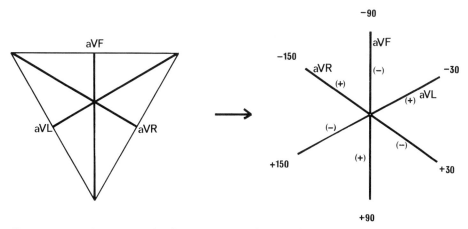

Figure 2–19. The augmented unipolar leads are pictured within the Einthoven triangle (*left*). When the triangle walls are removed, the augmented triaxial leads remain. The outer numbers represent the points of the circle from 0° to 180° and from 0° to −180°. The augmented lead electrode is positive at the point of origin; i.e., aVL is positive on the left forelimb as shown in Figure 2–18. (From Ettinger, S. J., and Suter, P. F.: *Canine Cardiology*. W. B. Saunders Co., Philadelphia, 1970.)

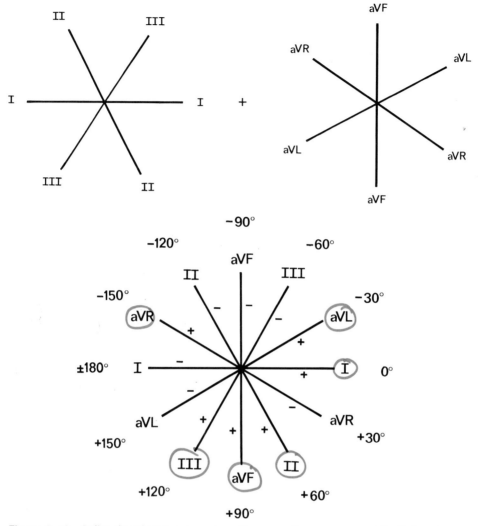

Figure 2–20. Bailey six-axis reference system. The upper diagrams represent the limb and augmented limb triaxial leads after being redrawn through the center of the body. When the two diagrams are combined, the Bailey six-axis reference system for the frontal plane results (bottom). The lead axes are marked in 30° increments from 0° to 180° and from 0° to −180°. The six leads are marked with a + at the positive electrode and a − at the negative electrode. Notice that for leads I, II, III, and aVF the polarity and angle of the leads are positive or negative simultaneously. Leads aVR and aVL are positive at the positions of −150° and −30°, respectively, since the positive electrodes for those leads lie in the negative 0° to −180° zone. (From Ettinger, S. J., and Suter, P. F.: *Canine Cardiology.* W. B. Saunders Co., Philadelphia, 1970.)

Other Lead Systems

UNIPOLAR PRECORDIAL LEADS. The unipolar precordial leads are called the exploring leads, The "C" electrode (Fig. 1–5) is placed in a number of different positions on the dog's body, and all recordings are made using the "V" setting on the electrocardiograph (Chapter 1, pp. 14). The various positions for the electrode are given in Table 2–1. The exploring electrode is the positive pole of each lead, and the electrode is compared with the average voltage across the three standard leads. These leads are not universally used in canine electrocardiography, but may provide additional information on right and left heart enlargment (Detweiler and Patterson, 1965).

ORTHOGONAL LEADS. The orthogonal leads are capable of measuring the cardiac impulse from three planes (see Table 2–1). Lead X measures left-to-right forces, and is roughly equivalent to lead I (Fig. 2–21). Lead Y measures tail-to-head forces, and is roughly equivalent to lead aVF (Fig. 2–21). Lead Z measures back-to-front forces, and is roughly equivalent to lead V_{10} (Fig. 2–21). There are more accurate orthogonal lead systems that produce more accurate X, Y, and Z tracings, but they require expensive, sophisticated equipment and are impractical

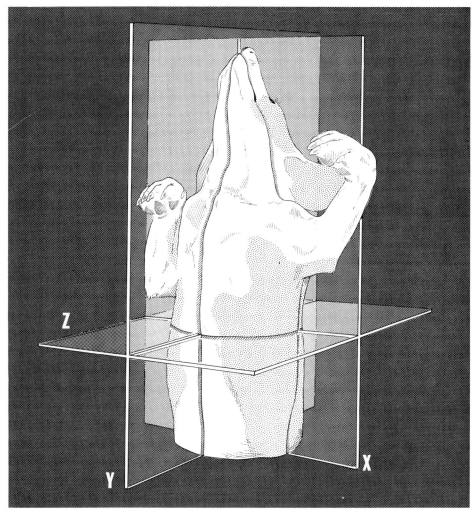

Figure 2–21. The orthogonal lead system bisects the dog's body in three planes. Lead X bisects the dog left-to-right, lead Y bisects the dog tail-to-head, and lead Z bisects the dog back-to-front. Lead X is roughly equivalent to lead I, lead Y is roughly equivalent to lead aVF, and lead Z is approximately equivalent to lead V_{10}.

(Adapted from an illustration in *Clinical Symposia,* copyrighted by CIBA Pharmaceutical Company, Division of CIBA-GEIGY Corporation. All rights reserved.)

in practice. The orthogonal leads have little to add over the basic six lead reference system, and are used only for vectorcardiography.

ESOPHAGEAL LEADS.   An esophageal lead may be used on rare occasions to differentiate the presence of P waves when there is doubt whether the P wave is present or not (Ettinger and Suter, 1970). The lead looks like a flexible catheter and is placed in the esophagus with the tip lying over the base of the heart. The end opposite the tip is connected to the left arm (LA) electrode, and the electrocardiograph is run on lead I. It is preferable to compare the bizarre esophageal lead deflections with those of a standard lead that produces a more recognizable pattern. The two leads should be recorded simultaneously, but this requires multichannel equipment (Ettinger and Suter, 1970).

REFERENCES

Detweiler, D. K., and Patterson, D. F.: The Prevalence and Types of Cardiovascular Disease in Dogs. Ann. N. Y. Acad. Sci., 127 (1965):481.

Ettinger, S. J., and Suter, P. F.: Canine Cardiology. W. B. Saunders Co., Philadelphia, 1970.

Friedberg, C. K.: Diseases of the Heart. 3rd ed. W. B. Saunders Co., Philadelphia, 1966.

Goodman, L. S., and Gilman, A.: The Pharmacological Basis of Therapeutics. 4th ed. The MacMillan Co., New York, 1970.

Guyton, A. C.: Textbook of Medical Physiology. 4th ed. W. B. Saunders Co., Philadelphia, 1971.

Hamlin, R. L., and Smith, C. R.: Anatomical and Physiological Basis for Interpretation of the Electrocardiogram. Amer. J. Vet. Res., 21 (1960):701.

Winsor, T.: The Electrocardiogram in Myocardial Infarction. In *Clinical Symposia*, CIBA, Vol. 20, No. 4, Oct.-Nov.-Dec., CIBA Corp., Summit, New Jersey, 1968.

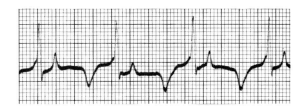

Chapter 3

INTERPRETING THE ELECTROCARDIOGRAM

Electrocardiograms are read in a systematic manner. There are five steps in the process of interpreting an electrocardiogram, and each tracing is read in the same way. Table 3–1 lists the steps in the system. In each instance the rate, rhythm, and axis are determined, the complexes are measured for both width and height, and finally, the tracing is examined for miscellaneous criteria. The values obtained are compared to the normal values that are given in Table 3–2, and any abnormalities are recorded as the electrocardiographic diagnosis. With practice, reading electrocardiograms soon becomes a matter of routine.

DETERMINATION OF HEART RATE

There are two ways to use the lead II rhythm strip at the end of the tracing to determine heart rate.

All recording paper has a series of marks at the top or bottom of the paper (Fig. 3–1). These marks are spaced so that at 50 mm./sec. paper speed they are 1½ seconds apart. To estimate the heart rate per minute, count the number of complexes that occur in three seconds and multiply by 20 (Fig. 3–2).

TABLE 3–1. THE SYSTEMATIC APPROACH TO ELECTROCARDIOGRAPHY

1. Determine heart rate.
2. Determine heart rhythm.
3. Determine mean electrical axis.
4. Measure and multiply.
5. Apply miscellaneous criteria.

TABLE 3–2. CRITERIA FOR THE NORMAL CANINE ELECTROCARDIOGRAM*

Normal Heart Rates
70 to 160 beats per minute in adult dogs
Up to 180 beats per minute in toy breeds
Up to 220 beats per minute in puppies

Normal Heart Rhythms
Normal sinus rhythm (NSR)
Sinus arrhythmia
Wandering pacemaker

Normal Heart Axis
+40° to +100° in all dogs
+40° to +90° in toy breeds

Normal Measurements**
P wave—measured from the beginning to the end of the P wave, and from the top to the bottom (baseline)
   Width: maximum 0.04 second (2 boxes wide)
   Height: maximum 0.4 mv. (4 boxes tall)
P-R interval—measured from the beginning of the P wave to the beginning of the QRS complex
   Width: 0.06 to 0.13 second (3 to 6½ boxes)
QRS complex—measured from beginning to end of QRS complex, and measured from baseline to top of the R wave
   Width:
      Maximum 0.05 second (2½ boxes) in toy breeds
      Maximum 0.06 second (3 boxes) in larger breeds
  Height of R wave:
      Maximum 2.5 mv. (25 boxes) in toy breeds
      Maximum 3.0 mv. (30 boxes) in larger breeds
S-T segment—between the end of the S wave and the beginning of the T wave
   Runs along the baseline before going into the T wave (no S-T slurring)
   No S-T depression
      Should not lie more than 0.2 mv (2 boxes) below the baseline in lead II
      Not depressed more than 0.1 to 0.2 mv. (1 to 2 boxes) in lead III
   No S-T elevation
      Should not lie more than 0.15 mv. (1½ boxes) above the baseline in lead II or lead III
T wave—very few requirements in the canine
   Can be positive or negative or biphasic in most leads
   Should be negative in lead V_{10} (except in Chihuahuas)
   Generally not higher than one-fourth the amplitude of the R wave (requires judgment)
Q-T interval—measured from the beginning of the Q wave to the end of the T wave
   Width: 0.14 second to 0.22 second (7 to 11 boxes).
   Varies with heart rate. Slower heart rates have longer Q-T intervals

---

   *Obtained through personal observations and from Ettinger and Suter (1970), and sources that are summarized by Ettinger and Suter (1970).
   **All measurements are taken on lead II except where indicated otherwise. Width measurements in seconds and in numbers of boxes are derived from electrocardiograms recorded at 50 mm./sec. and standardized at 1 cm. = 1 mv.

A second method of determining heart rate per minute is to count the number of small boxes from R wave to R wave and divide into 3000 (Fig. 3–3). There are 3000 small boxes per minute at 50 mm./sec. paper speed, and by dividing the number of boxes per R-R interval into 3000, the heart rate per minute is obtained. This method is more accurate, and

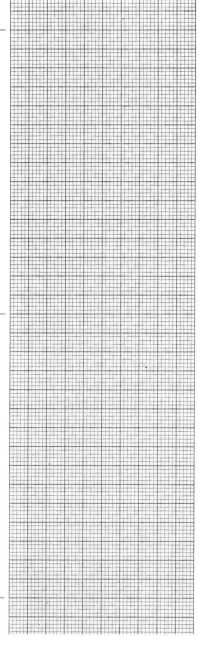

Figure 3–1. Along the top of this ECG recording paper are marks that are seen at regular intervals (three of them are shown here). When the paper is run at 50 mm./sec., the time between the marks is 1 1/2 seconds. To estimate heart rate, count the complexes that occur in 3 seconds, and multiply by 20.

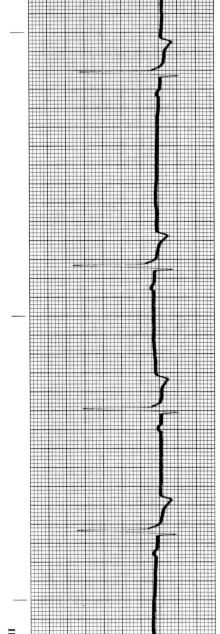

Figure 3–2. In this tracing, there are four complexes that occur in 3 seconds. Therefore, this dog's heart rate is 80 beats per minute.

Paper speed = 50 mm./sec., 1 cm. = 1 mv.

II

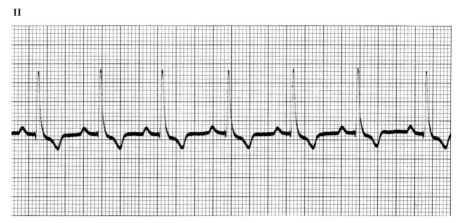

Figure 3–3. In this tracing heart rate can be determined by counting the number of small boxes in each R-R interval and dividing into 3000. The distance from R wave to R wave here averages about 16 to 18 boxes, so the heart rate is 166 to 187 beats per minute. This is a slightly more accurate way of determining heart rate, but is more time consuming than the paper mark method.

Paper speed = 50 mm./sec., 1 cm. = 1 mv.

several R-R intervals may be checked if the heart rhythm is irregular (Fig. 3–3).

The normal heart rate in the dog is 70 to 160 beats per minute (see Table 3–2). If the heart rate is above normal, the dog has tachycardia. If the heart rate falls below normal, he has bradycardia. The significance of tachyarrhythmias and bradyarrhythmias is discussed in the next chapter.

DETERMINATION OF HEART RHYTHM

A system should also be used when evaluating the heart rhythm. If everything is normal, each complex should occur with a P wave, followed by a short pause (P-R interval), then a QRS complex, and finally a T wave. The components of each complex should also be in definite relationship to one another. When evaluating heart rhythm, the following questions are considered:

1. Is the heart rate normal or abnormal?
2. Is the rhythm regular or irregular?
3. Is there a P wave for every QRS complex, and a QRS complex for every P wave?
4. Are the P waves related to the QRS complexes?
5. Do all the P waves and all the QRS complexes look alike?

To evaluate heart rhythm, the lead II rhythm strip is used. The heart rate determines whether tachycardia or bradycardia is present, and the strip can be quickly surveyed to tell whether the rhythm is regular or irregular. Gross irregularities are obvious, and smaller irregularities can be evaluated by measuring the R-R intervals to see if they vary. The P waves should be related to the QRS complexes. This can be verified by checking to see that all the P-R intervals are the same. The normal rhythm in the dog is sinus in origin (meaning that P waves are present for every QRS complex). If there is a sinus rhythm that is perfectly reg-

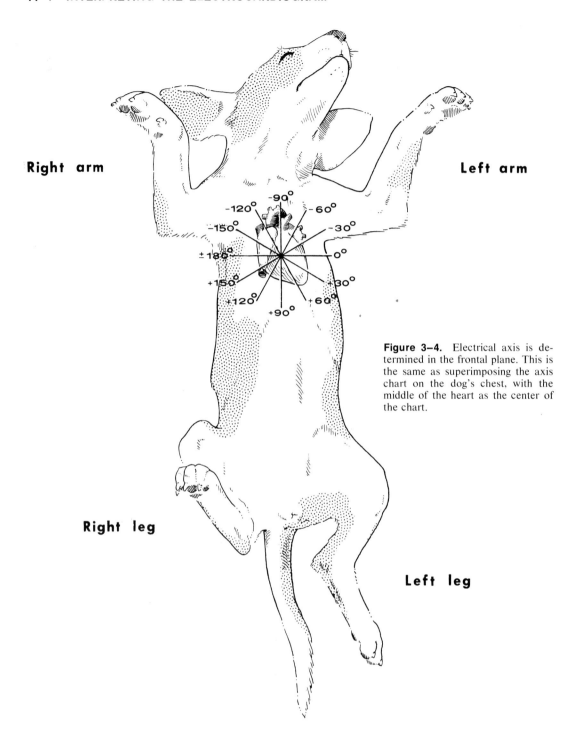

Right arm

Left arm

Right leg

Left leg

Figure 3–4. Electrical axis is determined in the frontal plane. This is the same as superimposing the axis chart on the dog's chest, with the middle of the heart as the center of the chart.

ular, it is called normal sinus rhythm (NSR). If there is a sinus rhythm that has some irregularity, it is called a sinus arrhythmia (a normal rhythm for the dog). Wandering pacemaker is another normal variation in the dog. These rhythms are discussed and illustrated in the next chapter.

DETERMINATION OF MEAN ELECTRICAL AXIS

Significance of Axis

When determining the heart axis, or mean electrical axis, the mean wave of electrical activity (cardiac vector) that occurs when the ventricles depolarize is measured. The mean electrical axis is a measurement of the direction that the force is traveling, and is determined by examining the QRS complexes in each of the six basic leads of the Bailey's hexaxial lead system (Figs. 2–20 and 3–29). The other lead systems are not used for determining the mean electrical axis; this is done in the frontal plane, which is the same as standing the dog up on his hind legs, and looking straight at his chest (Fig. 3–4). Normally, the mean electrical axis in the dog is between +40° and +100° (Fig. 3–5). If the direction of the axis becomes less than +40°, it has shifted toward the animal's left arm; this is called left axis deviation. Left axis deviation indicates left ventricular hypertrophy (Fig. 3–6A). If the axis shifts and becomes greater than +100°, it has shifted toward the dog's right arm; this is called right axis deviation. Right axis deviation indicates right

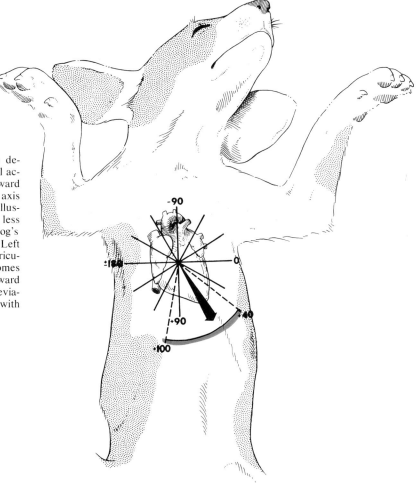

Figure 3–5. When the ventricles depolarize, the main wave of electrical activity (axis) travels downward toward the left rear leg. The dog's normal axis is between +40° and +100°, as illustrated here. If the axis deviates to less than +40°, it is shifted toward the dog's left arm, and is a left axis deviation. Left axis deviation is caused by left ventricular hypertrophy. If the axis becomes more than +100° it is deviated toward the right arm and is a right axis deviation. Right axis deviation occurs with right ventricular hypertrophy.

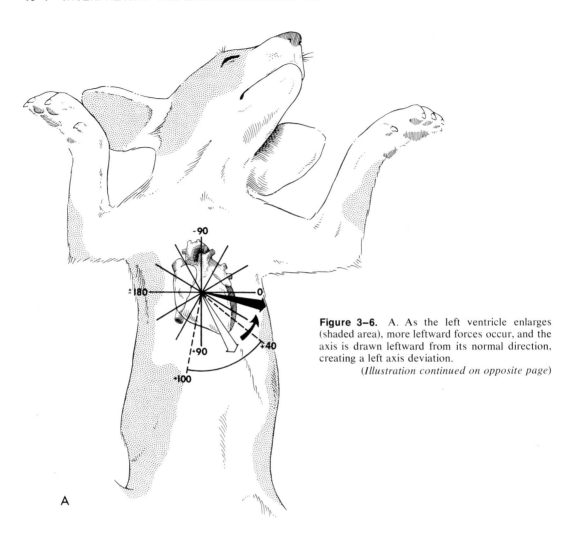

Figure 3–6. A. As the left ventricle enlarges (shaded area), more leftward forces occur, and the axis is drawn leftward from its normal direction, creating a left axis deviation.

(Illustration continued on opposite page)

A

ventricular hypertrophy (Fig. 3–6B). The left axis range includes from +40° to approximately −90°, and the right axis range includes from +100° rightward to −90°. The axis is rarely if ever −90°, but whenever it is, it is most likely because of right ventricular hypertrophy. Left ventricular hypertrophy rarely causes the axis to deviate beyond −60°.

Usually, if both ventricles are hypertrophied the axis remains normal; so if other criteria indicate hypertrophy of one ventricle but the axis remains normal, biventricular hypertrophy should be suspected.

Procedure

The procedure for determining axis is easy. There are three steps:

1. Find an isoelectric lead (see Figures 2–14 and 2–15).

2. Use the 6-axis reference chart (Figs. 2–20 and 3–29), and find which lead is perpendicular to the isoelectric lead.

3. Find out if the perpendicular lead is positive or negative on the tracing that is being examined.

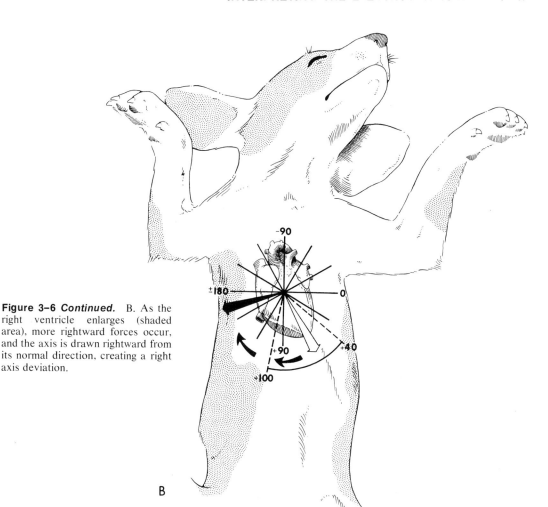

Figure 3–6 *Continued*. B. As the right ventricle enlarges (shaded area), more rightward forces occur, and the axis is drawn rightward from its normal direction, creating a right axis deviation.

It was stated that if a lead is isoelectric, then the mean electrical impulse (axis) would run perpendicular to it (Fig. 2–14). For example, if lead aVL was the isoelectric lead, then the axis lies along the lead that is perpendicular to lead aVL. By inspecting the six-axis reference chart (Figs. 2–20 and 3–29), it can be seen that lead II is perpendicular to lead aVL. This means that the axis lies along lead II. It can also be seen on the chart that lead II has a positive pole at +60° and a negative pole at −120°. Now it is necessary to know if the axis is running toward the positive pole or the negative pole, since +60° is normal but −120° is a right axis deviation. It was also stated in Chapter 2 that if the impulse runs toward a lead's positive pole, then a positive (upward) deflection occurs, and if the impulse runs toward the lead's negative pole, a negative (downward) deflection will result (Fig. 2–14). To tell whether the axis is running toward lead II's positive or negative pole, examine lead II. If the axis is running toward +60° (lead II's positive pole), lead II will show a positive deflection. If the axis is running toward −120° (lead II's negative pole), lead II would be a negative deflection. Now given

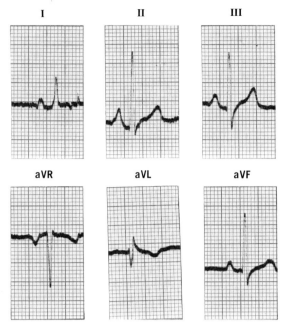

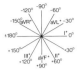

Figure 3–7. Of the six basic leads in this electrocardiogram, lead aVL is isoelectric. The lead perpendicular to aVL (consult the axis chart) is lead II. Lead II on this tracing is positive. This puts the axis at lead II's positive pole, or +60° (see chart). An axis of +60° is normal.

Paper speed = 50 mm./sec., 1 cm. = 1 mv.

the circumstances that aVL is isoelectric and that lead II is positive, then the dog's axis is +60° (Fig. 3–7), which is within normal limits.

What would be the interpretation if lead I were isoelectric? The axis chart shows that the perpendicular to lead I is lead aVF. If lead aVF is positive, then the dog's axis is +90° (lead aVF's positive pole), which is also normal (Fig. 3–8). Figure 3–9 shows an example of right axis deviation (right ventricular hypertrophy), and Figure 3–10 shows an example of left axis deviation (left ventricular hypertrophy).

It is not always possible to find a lead that is perfectly isoelectric. In these instances the lead that is the closest to isoelectric is used (Figs. 3–

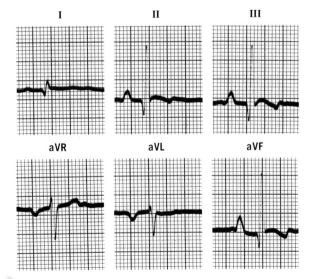

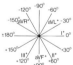

Figure 3–8. In this electrocardiogram, lead I is isoelectric. On the axis chart, lead aVF is perpendicular to lead I. Since lead aVF is positive on this tracing, the axis runs toward aVF's positive pole, or +90°. An axis of +90° is normal.

Paper speed = 50 mm./sec., 1 cm. = 1 mv.

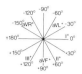

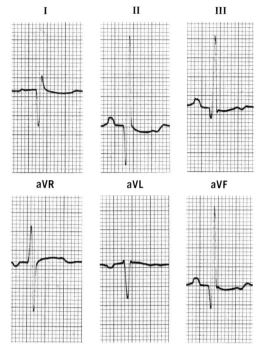

Figure 3–9. When there is no lead that is perfectly isoelectric, the one most nearly so is used; in this tracing, lead aVR is closest to isoelectric. The perpendicular to lead aVR is lead III (see axis chart). On this tracing, lead III is positive. Lead III's positive pole is at +120°. Since +120° is greater than +100°, this is a right axis deviation, and means that the dog has right ventricular hypertrophy.

Paper speed = 50 mm./sec., 1 cm. = 1 mv.

9 and 3–11). If two leads are isoelectric, either one may be used (Fig. 3–12). Occasionally, all the leads will appear to be isoelectric. When this happens, it is termed an electrically vertical heart, and axis cannot be determined (Fig. 3–13).

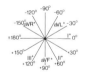

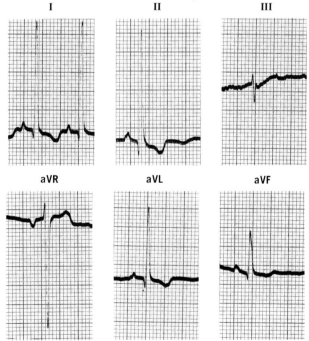

Figure 3–10. The isoelectric lead in this tracing is lead III. The perpendicular to lead III (see chart) is lead aVR. Lead aVR on this tracing is negative, which means that the axis runs toward the negative pole of aVR, or toward +30°. Since +30° is less than +40°, this dog has a left axis deviation, indicating left ventricular hypertrophy.

Paper speed = 50 mm./sec., 1 cm. = 1 mv.

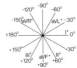

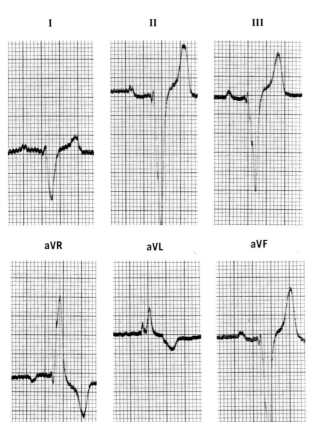

Figure 3–11. In this electrocardiogram, as in Figure 3–9, it is not possible to find a lead that is perfectly isoelectric, so the one most nearly so in this tracing, lead aVL, is used. Lead II is perpendicular to lead aVL and is negative. Lead II's negative pole is at −120° (see chart). This is a severe right axis deviation, and indicates severe right ventricular hypertrophy.

Another indication of right ventricular hypertrophy is the presence of an S wave in leads I, II, and III. This is called the S_1, S_2, S_3 pattern, and also indicates right ventricular hypertrophy (see page 60).

Paper speed = 50 mm./sec., 1 cm. = 1 mv.

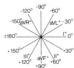

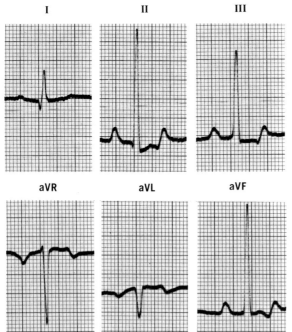

Figure 3–12. In this tracing, no lead is perfectly isoelectric, but lead I and lead aVL are both equally close. If lead I is used, the perpendicular is aVF, and since aVF is positive the axis would be +90° (normal). If lead aVL is used as isoelectric, lead II is perpendicular and is positive, indicating a +60° axis, which is also normal. If the two are averaged, the result is +75°. Either way, the axis is still normal.

Paper speed = 50 mm./sec., 1 cm. = 1 mv.

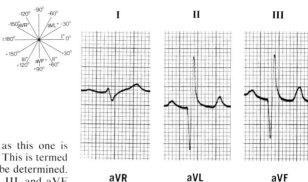

Figure 3–13. Occasionally a tracing such as this one is recorded in which all the leads are isoelectric. This is termed an electrically vertical heart, and axis cannot be determined. The presence of a deep Q wave in leads II, III, and aVF would suggest right ventricular hypertrophy (see page 61), although this criterion is somewhat tenuous in larger dogs.
Paper speed = 50 mm./sec., 1 cm. = 1 mv.

When the isoelectric lead is not perfectly isoelectric, as in Figures 3–9, 3–11 and 3–12, a more precise estimate of the axis can be made by adding a fourth step to the procedure. The fourth step is to return to the isoelectric lead. For instance, in Figure 3–12 we said that, although no lead was perfectly isoelectric, lead I was close. Lead aVF is perpendicular to lead I, and since lead aVF was positive, we said the axis was +90°. But, since lead I was not perfectly isoelectric, then the axis is not exactly +90°. By adding the fourth step and going back to inspect lead I more closely, it can be seen that lead I is more positive than negative. This means that the axis should be shifted a little from +90° toward the positive pole of lead I; call it +80°. We said that lead aVL was close, also. Lead II is perpendicular to aVL and is positive, so, using aVL as isoelectric, the axis would be about +60°. But again, by returning to the isoelectric lead (aVL), we see that it is more negative than positive, so shift the axis a little from +60° toward lead aVL's negative pole, or call it +70°. This fourth step is a little more accurate when the isoelectric lead is not perfect, but, as stated earlier, using the lead that is closest to isoelectric still allows the electrical axis to be established with an acceptable degree of accuracy.

Another point should be clarified. Occasionally confusion may result because of the angle values that are assigned to the poles of each lead on the axis chart. By inspecting the axis chart it can be seen that the positive pole of lead aVR is located at −150°, and that the positive pole of lead aVL is located at −30°. These are the only two leads whose positive poles are at negative angle values. To illustrate the point, if lead III were isoelectric, then lead aVR would be the perpendicular lead. If lead aVR were positive, then the dog's axis would be −150° (lead aVR's positive pole). This would be a right axis deviation, indicating right ventricular hypertrophy.

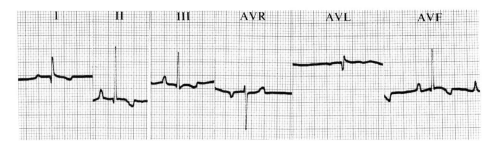

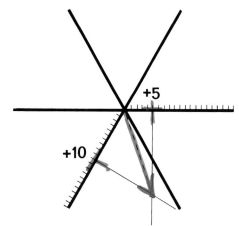

Figure 3–14. Mean electrical axis (MEA). *Above,* The six limb leads from a normal dog recorded at paper speed of 50 mm./sec. and standard amplitude of 1 mv. *Below,* Choosing any two of the limb leads (I and III), the positive and negative deflections for each lead are added (I = +5; III = +10). Using the three- or six-axis reference system, perpendicular lines are drawn from the positive or negative point determined for each lead. The perpendicular lines are extended until they meet, and the dotted line drawn from the origin of the reference axis system to the site of their intersection is the mean electrical axis. The mean electrical axis in the frontal plane in this recording from a normal dog is +70°. (From Ettinger, S. J., and Suter, P. F.: *Canine Cardiology.* W. B. Saunders Co., Philadelphia, 1970.)

Another method for determining mean electrical axis involves selecting any two limb leads (I, II, or III) and adding up the total number of positive and negative charges on each of the two leads that are selected (Ettinger and Suter, 1970) (Fig. 3–14). The summated value achieved is plotted on each lead and a perpendicular is drawn from each lead (Fig. 3–14). A line drawn from the center of the axis chart to the point at which the two perpendicular lines meet will run toward the dog's true electrical axis (Fig. 3–14). This method is more time consuming, and offers no advantage over the inspection method.

The electrical axis is a very dependable and accurate assessment of ventricular hypertrophy, and the magnitude of the axis deviation consistently varies in accord with the severity of the hypertrophy of the ventricle.

MEASURING AND MULTIPLYING

Much information can be obtained by measuring the complexes and the intervals on the lead II rhythm strip. All the measurements are on lead II unless otherwise indicated. Measurements include the height and width of the P wave, the length of the P-R interval, the width of the QRS complex, the height of the R wave, the S-T segment and T wave, and the Q-T interval.

Measuring the P Wave

The P wave on the electrocardiogram indicates atrial depolarization. By measuring the height and width of the P wave, the size of both right and left atria can be assessed (Fig. 3–17).

Right Atrial Hypertrophy. When the right atrium hypertrophies, the P waves become tall and peaked but remain normal in width (Fig. 3–15). This is called "P pulmonale" and indicates right atrial hypertrophy (Ettinger and Suter, 1970). By definition, P pulmonale is present whenever the P wave is consistently taller than 0.4 mv. (4 boxes) on lead II of the electrocardiogram (Table 3–3). The normal atrial depolarization is shown in Figure 2–8, and Figure 3–17 illustrates the mechanism by which tall P waves occur with right atrial hypertrophy.

Another less frequent manifestation of right atrial hypertrophy is the "T_a" (T sub a) wave (Fig. 3–18). This is a depression of the P–R segment caused by large right atrial repolarization forces (Ettinger and Suter, 1970).

Left Atrial Hypertrophy. When the left atrium enlarges, the P waves become wide and notched (Fig. 3–16). This is termed "P mitrale," and indicates left atrial hypertrophy (Ettinger and Suter, 1970). By definition, P mitrale is present whenever the P waves are consistently wider than 0.04 second (2 boxes), on lead II of the electrocardiogram (Table 3–3). Figure 3–17 also depicts the mechanism by which wide P waves occur with left atrial hypertrophy. A notched P wave is not significant unless it is also too wide.

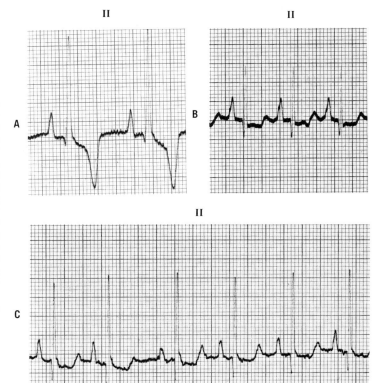

Figure 3–15. Shown are three different examples of "P pulmonale," indicating right atrial hypertrophy. In each of the three tracings, the P waves are consistently taller than 0.4 mv. (4 boxes). When they become tall they tend to become peaked. In strip C, the variation in P wave height is called "wandering pacemaker," but the average height of the P waves is too tall. If the average height of the P waves had been less than 0.4 mv. in strip C, with only an occasional one being too tall, it would not have been "P pulmonale."

Paper speed = 50 mm./sec., 1 cm. = 1 mv.

TABLE 3-3. CRITERIA FOR HYPERTROPHY OF THE CARDIAC CHAMBERS*

Atrial Hypertrophy
Right atrial hypertrophy (P pulmonale)
  P wave is taller than 0.4 mv. (4 boxes) in lead II
  P wave becomes tall and peaked
  "T_a" wave may appear
Left atrial hypertrophy (P mitrale)
  P wave is wider than 0.04 second (2 boxes) in lead II
  P wave becomes notched
  May prolong the P-R interval

Ventricular hypertrophy
Right ventricular hypertrophy (RVH)
  Right axis deviation—axis greater than +100° (+90° in toy breeds).
  S_1, S_2, S_3 pattern—S wave present in leads I, II and III.
  Deep Q in II, III, and aVF—Q wave deeper than 0.5 mv. (5 boxes) in leads II, III, and aVF.
  Deep S wave in CV_6LU—S wave deeper than 0.7 mv. in lead CV_6LU.
  T wave positive in lead V_{10}—except in Chihuahuas.
  P pulmonale—may accompany RVH
Left ventricular hypertrophy (LVH)
  Left axis deviation—axis less than +40°
  QRS complex wider than 0.06 second (3 boxes) in all dogs, or 0.05 second (2½ boxes) in toy breeds
  R wave taller than 3.0 mv. (30 boxes) in all dogs, or 2.5 mv. (25 boxes) in toy breeds
  S-T segment changes (repolarization changes)
    S-T slurring
    S-T depression
  P mitrale—may accompany LVH
Biventricular hypertrophy
  Axis usually normal
  Tall R waves
  Wide QRS complexes
  Deep Q waves
  P mitrale, P pulmonale, or both

---

*Obtained from personal observations, and from Ettinger and Suter (1970), and from sources summarized by Ettinger and Suter (1970). All measurements are based on a paper speed of 50 mm./sec., and standardized at 1 cm. = 1 mv.

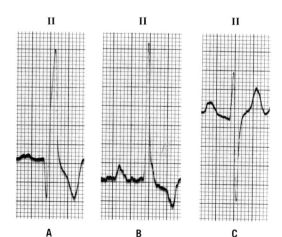

II   II   II

A   B   C

Figure 3-16. Shown are three examples of "P mitrale" recorded from three different dogs, indicating left atrial hypertrophy. In each of the three tracings, the P wave is wider than 0.04 second (two boxes). When the P wave becomes wide, it usually has a notch in it, as in these three examples. A notched P wave is not significant unless it is also too wide.
    Paper speed = 50 mm./sec., 1 cm. = 1 mv.

A **Normal**

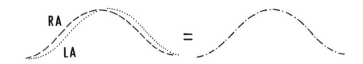

B **Left Atrium** ↑

P Mitrale

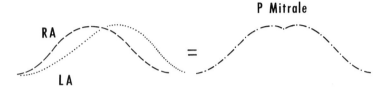

C **Right Atrium** ↑

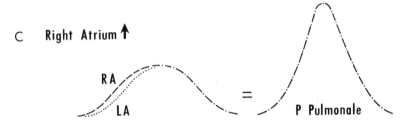

P Pulmonale

Figure 3–17. A. The normal P wave is produced by depolarization of the right, and 0.01 second later of the left, atrium.

B. When the left atrium hypertrophies, the impulse takes longer to traverse it, and the left atrial forces are prolonged. This produces a wide P wave with a notch in it, called "P mitrale."

C. When the right atrium hypertrophies, the impulse takes longer to traverse it, and the right atrial forces are prolonged. This causes a summation of the right and left atrial forces, since they now occur more nearly simultaneously, and a larger millivoltage (taller P wave) is produced. This tall, peaked P wave is called "P pulmonale."

In summary, the P waves cannot be taller than 0.4 mv. (4 boxes), nor can they be wider than 0.04 second (2 boxes) on lead II. If they are too tall, right atrial hypertrophy is indicated, and if they are too wide, left atrial hypertrophy is indicated. If the P waves are too wide and too tall, biatrial hypertrophy is diagnosed (Figs. 3–17 and 3–18).

The P-R Interval

The P-R interval is measured from the beginning of the P wave to the beginning of the QRS complex. The normal value in the dog is 0.06 to 0.13 second (3 to 6½ boxes wide). The P-R interval is a measurement that is helpful when digitalizing a dog. One of the consistent effects of oral digitalis glycosides is a prolongation of the P-R interval. If the P-R interval is prolonged 0.02 to 0.03 second (1 to 1½ boxes), the desired effect of digitalis has been obtained. In most instances this happens

II

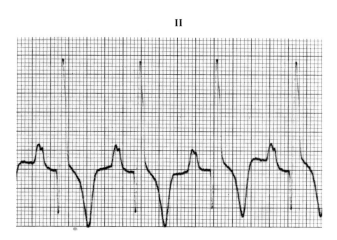

Figure 3–18. This lead II tracing demonstrates biatrial hypertrophy. The P waves are both too tall and too wide. They are 0.5 to 0.6 mv. tall (5 to 6 boxes), and 0.06 second wide (3 boxes). They are also notched. The electrocardiographic diagnosis is P pulmonale and P mitrale (biatrial hypertrophy).

A less frequent manifestation of right atrial hypertrophy is also present. Following the P wave, the baseline dips below the original baseline, and the P-R segment is depressed. This is called a "T_a" (T sub a) wave, and is caused by the large right atrial repolarization forces.

Left ventricular hypertrophy is also demonstrated by the wide QRS and the presence of S-T slurring. The QRS is 0.07 second (3½ boxes) wide and the S-T segment slurs into the T wave without straightening out along the baseline. The deep Q waves should arouse suspicion that there is also right ventricular hypertrophy.

Paper speed = 50 mm./sec., 1 cm. = 1 mv.

before the onset of physical signs of digitalis intoxication. If the P-R interval is monitored before each dose of digitalis, the dog can often be digitalized without making him physically ill. First degree heart block is diagnosed if the P-R interval becomes prolonged beyond 0.13 second (see Figure 4–49).

The P-R interval is also used when evaluating a dog's cardiac rhythm. Usually, the P-R intervals are almost exactly the same from beat to beat, which proves that the P waves are related to the QRS complexes. If the P-R intervals vary greatly from beat to beat, a serious arrhythmia or conduction disturbance may be suspected (see next chapter). The P-R interval usually varies inversely with the heart rate, and it is generally shorter when the heart rate is rapid (Ettinger and Suter, 1970).

The QRS Complexes

Two measurements are made on the QRS complex. The width is measured from the beginning of the Q wave to the end of the S wave.

II   II

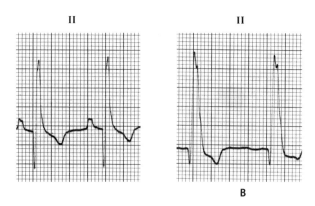

B

Figure 3–19. In these two examples of left ventricular hypertrophy the QRS complexes are too wide. In A, the QRS is 0.06 to 0.07 second (3 to 3½ boxes) wide. In B, the QRS is 0.09 second (4½ boxes) wide. The dog from which strip A was recorded was a miniature poodle, and the dog in strip B was a Doberman. A small dog like the poodle should not have a QRS complex wider than 0.05 second (2½ boxes) and the larger dog's QRS complex should not exceed 0.06 second (3 boxes). Since each dog's QRS complex is too wide, left ventricular hypertrophy is diagnosed in both cases. The Doberman has no P waves because he is in atrial fibrillation, which will be discussed in Chapter 4.

Paper speed = 50 mm./sec., 1 cm. = 1 mv.

II

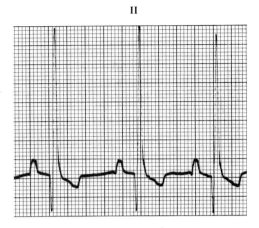

Figure 3–20. In this tracing the R wave averages 3.8 mv. (38 boxes). The R wave should not be taller than 3.0 mv. (30 boxes) in any dog. A tall R wave indicates left ventricular hypertrophy. The measurement is made from the baseline (not from the bottom of the Q wave) to the top of the R wave.

Two other criteria that indicate left ventricular hypertrophy are present. The QRS complex is 0.07 second (3 1/2 boxes) wide, and S-T slurring is present, since the S-T segment moves into the T wave without straightening out along the baseline.

Paper speed = 50 mm./sec., 1 cm. = 1 mv.

The second measurement is the height of the R wave, which is measured from the baseline to the top of the R wave. In the normal dog, the QRS complex should not be wider than 0.06 second, or 3 boxes (Table 3–2). Dogs of smaller breeds should not have QRS complexes wider than 0.05 second, or 2 1/2 boxes. If the QRS complex is too wide, it indicates left ventricular hypertrophy (Fig. 3–19), as noted in Table 3–3.

The R wave should not be taller than 3.0 mv. or 30 boxes in any dog, and should not be taller than 2.5 mv. (25 boxes) in smaller dogs (Table 3–3). An R wave that is too tall also indicates left ventricular hypertrophy (Fig. 3–20).

The S-T Segment

The S-T segment lies between the end of the S wave and the beginning of the T wave. It should run along the baseline and then slip into

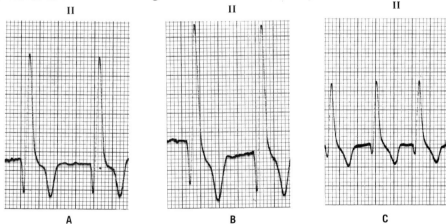

A   B   C

Figure 3–21. A. The S-T segment in this tracing is normal. Notice that it straightens out along the baseline before dropping into the T wave. The QRS, however, is 0.09 second (4 1/2 boxes), indicating that left ventricular hypertrophy is present. The S-T segment lies below the baseline, but looks more depressed than it really is because the baseline is shifting downward a bit because of movement of the animal.

B and C. These two tracings demonstrate S-T repolarization changes called S-T slurring. This slurring of the S-T segment into the T wave indicates left ventricular hypertrophy. In both of these tracings, the QRS is also too wide, which also indicates left ventricular hypertrophy.

Paper speed = 50 mm./sec., 1 cm. = 1 mv.

the T wave (Fig. 3–21A). If the S-T segment slurs directly into the T wave without first straightening out along the baseline it is called S-T slurring and indicates left ventricular hypertrophy (Fig. 3–21B, C).

The S-T segment is also abnormal if it lies above or below the baseline. When the S-T segment lies below the baseline, it is called S-T depression (see Table 3–3). When it lies above the baseline, the S-T segment is elevated (see Table 3–3). S-T segment depression may result from several causes, including left ventricular hypertrophy, myocardial hypoxia, myocarditis, or electrolyte disturbances such as hypocalcemia (Fig. 3–22). S-T segment elevation is not as common, but when it does occur it is most often associated with myocardial hypoxia or myocarditis (Fig. 3–23). It may also occur with hypercalcemia (see Figure 3–37).

The T Wave

In the dog, there are very few restrictions placed on the T wave. The T wave can be almost anything it pleases to be. It may be positive, or negative, or biphasic in most leads. It should be negative in lead V_{10}, but Chihuahuas may normally have a positive T wave in this lead (Detweiler and Patterson, 1965).

It is said that the T wave should not be larger than ¼ the height of the R wave (Ettinger and Suter, 1970). This requires judgment, however, since if the R wave is not very tall, the T wave may falsely appear to be too large. In general, as the ventricles hypertrophy and the QRS

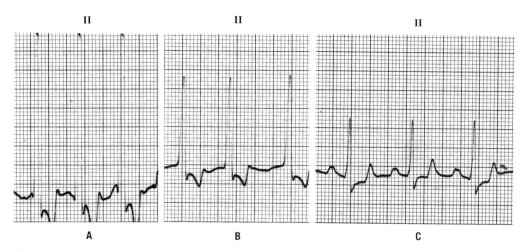

Figure 3–22. A. This dog's tracing demonstrates that he has left ventricular hypertrophy as indicated by the tall R waves and the S-T segment depression. The R waves are 4.3 mv. (43 boxes) tall. The S-T segment lies 0.4 mv. (4 boxes) below the baseline. The S-T segment depression of left ventricular hypertrophy almost always is accompanied by the tall R wave.

Paper speed = 50 mm./sec., 1 cm. = 1 mv.

B. This is the same dog recorded at one-half sensitivity, so that the entire tracing can be gotten on the paper. At one-half sensitivity, all height measurements must be doubled. Width measurements do not change.

Paper speed = 50 mm./sec., 1/2 cm. = 1 mv.

C. The S-T depression in this dog was thought to be due to hypoxia. The dog had been hit by a car and was in respiratory distress due to traumatic lung syndrome. As the lungs and the breathing improved, the S-T segment changes returned to normal.

Paper speed = 50 mm./sec., 1 cm. = 1 mv.

II

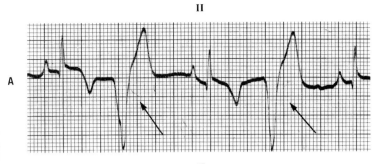

A

Figure 3–23. A. This electrocardiogram was recorded from a
dog with traumatic myocarditis
that had been hit by a car. Two
ventricular premature beats are
present (arrows). The three normal PQRST complexes show elevation of the S-T segment above
the baseline.

B. The next day the premature beats are gone, but the S-T
segment elevation persists as a
result of the myocarditis.

C. One week later, the S-T
segment elevation has returned to
normal, since the myocarditis has
resolved itself.

Paper speed = 50 mm./sec.,
1 cm. = 1 mv.

II

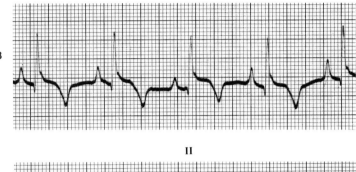

B

II

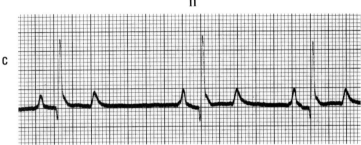

C

complexes become larger, the T waves may also appear larger. It is
mainly a judgment call when speculating on the size of the T waves.

There are times when it is possible to recognize that the T wave is
abnormal. One way this can be done is by observing changes in the T
wave on serial electrocardiograms, or while monitoring a patient under
anesthesia. If the T wave reverses its polarity in a lead, this is abnormal.
For instance, if lead II is being monitored during anesthesia and the T
reverses itself from negative to positive, that must be taken as a warning
sign of myocardial hypoxia, and the ventilatory status of the patient
should be evaluated (Fig. 3–38).

As with changes in polarity, changes in configuration of the T wave
must be investigated. Again, using the same example, if the lead II tracing were being monitored during anesthesia and the T wave were to
become larger and larger, that would also have to be regarded as a warning sign of myocardial hypoxia, and the depth of anesthesia or the
ventilation of the patient would have to be evaluated (see Figure 3–38).

T wave changes may also be observed in association with electrolyte changes such as hyperkalemia or hypokalemia. Classically, T waves
become large and spiked with hyperkalemia, and they become small and
biphasic with hypokalemia (see Figures 3–32 and 3–34).

In general, it can be said that the T wave in the dog is not often judged to be abnormal, but changes may occur as a result of ventricular hypertrophy, myocardial oxygen deficits, and electrolyte disturbances. Changes in a dog's normal T wave polarity or in T wave configuration are significant.

The Q-T Interval

The Q-T interval is measured from the beginning of the Q wave to the end of the T wave. The normal Q-T interval in the dog is from 0.14 to 0.22 second (7 to 11 boxes) and varies inversely with the heart rate. The more rapid heart rates have shorter Q-T intervals, and slow heart rates have longer ones.

The Q-T interval is significant in electrolyte changes. Hypokalemia consistently prolongs the Q-T interval beyond 0.22 second (see Figure 3–34). The Q-T interval may also be prolonged owing to hypocalcemia or hyperkalemia (see Figures 3–32 and 3–35). Hypercalcemia may shorten the Q-T interval, but it is usually not significantly shorter (Friedberg, 1966).

MISCELLANEOUS CRITERIA

The fifth and final step in the examination of the electrocardiogram is examining the tracing for miscellaneous criteria that were not observed in the first four steps. These miscellaneous criteria include the S_1, S_2, S_3 pattern, the deep Q in II, III, and aVF pattern, a deep S wave in CV_6LU, and the positive T wave in lead V_{10}. If any of these criteria is present, right ventricular hypertrophy is indicated.

S_1, S_2, S_3 Pattern

If there is an S wave present in leads I, II and III, it indicates right ventricular hypertrophy (Figs. 3–11 and 3–24). Normally there is no S

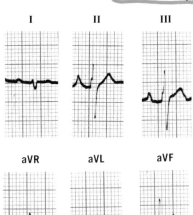

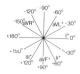

Figure 3–24. In this tracing there is an S wave present in leads I, II, and III, indicating right ventricular hypertrophy. Lead I shows a tiny R wave followed by a slightly larger S wave, and leads II and III have quite large S waves. Leads III and aVL are almost perfectly isoelectric, which places the axis between −150° and −120°. This is a severe right axis deviation, and also indicates right ventricular hypertrophy.
Paper speed = 50 mm./sec., 1 cm. = 1 mv.

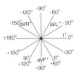

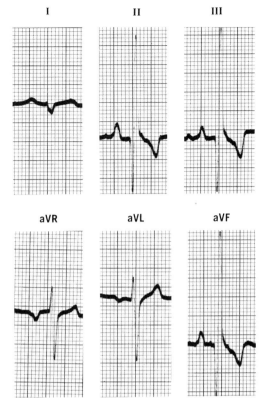

| I | II | III |

| aVR | aVL | aVF |

Figure 3–25. This tracing is recorded from an older Miniature Poodle. It indicates right ventricular hypertrophy as shown by Q waves in leads II, III, and aVF that are deeper than 0.5 mv. (5 boxes). When the Q wave is this deep in lead II, it usually will be deep also in leads III and aVF. The R wave in lead II is 2.8 mv. (28 boxes) tall, which exceeds the normal limit of 2.5 mv. (25 boxes) in this type of dog. This finding indicates that left ventricular hypertrophy is also present. The axis remains normal at roughly +90°, as it usually does when both ventricles hypertrophy.

Paper speed = 50 mm./sec., 1 cm. = 1 mv.

wave in lead I, the S wave is variably present in lead II, and it is often present in Lead III. When all three leads have an S wave, right ventricular hypertrophy is diagnosed.

Deep Q in II, III, and aVF

Q waves deeper than 0.5 mv. (5 boxes) in leads II, III, and aVF are suggestive of right ventricular hypertrophy (Fig. 3–25). This criterion is valid in the small breeds, but is somewhat tenuous in larger dogs, especially large thin dogs. For example, a good percentage of pointers may normally have deep Q waves in these leads.

Deep S in CV₆LU

The presence of an S wave deeper than 0.7 mv. (7 boxes) in the special exploring lead CV₆LU also indicates right ventricular hypertrophy (Fig. 3–26). This lead is not usually run, but it will occasionally be abnormal when the other leads are normal. This has been the case in a surprising number of dogs with heartworm disease, and for this reason it is suggested that this lead be recorded whenever this condition is suspected.

Positive T Wave In Lead V₁₀

Lead V_{10} is another of the exploring leads. The T wave in lead V_{10} should be negative. A positive T wave in lead V_{10} indicates right ven-

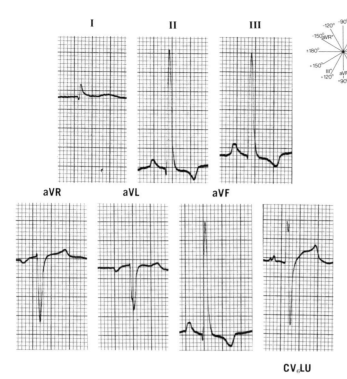

Figure 3–26. This electrocardiogram demonstrates that the S wave in lead CV₆LU is deeper than 0.7 mv. (7 boxes). This finding indicates right ventricular hypertrophy. The R wave in lead II is 3.1 mv. (31 boxes) tall, pointing to left ventricular hypertrophy. The axis is roughly +90°, which is normal, suggesting biventricular hypertrophy.

Paper speed = 50 mm./sec., 1 cm. = 1 mv.

tricular hypertrophy (Fig. 3–27). The Chihuahua may be an exception to this rule (Detweiler and Patterson, 1965). This abnormality is not very common, and lead V₁₀ is not universally used.

Biventricular Hypertrophy

When biventricular hypertrophy occurs, the electrical axis usually remains normal. The P wave may show signs of right, left, or biatrial hypertrophy, and the QRS complex is wide and has deep Q waves and tall R waves. S-T slurring is usually present (Fig. 3–28).

Even though several criteria are given for right and left ventricular hypertrophy, the electrocardiogram has to demonstrate only one of them. It does not have to satisfy all the criteria to be meaningful.

RECORDING ELECTROCARDIOGRAPHIC FINDINGS

When all five steps have been completed, the abnormal findings are listed, and the electrocardiographic diagnosis is made. It is helpful to have a small form made up that can be filled out and kept with the dog's record (Fig. 3–29). Of the following two tracings (Figs. 3–30 and 3–31), one is normal and the other is abnormal. Please read them using the five-step approach. Compare your findings with those listed in the legend.

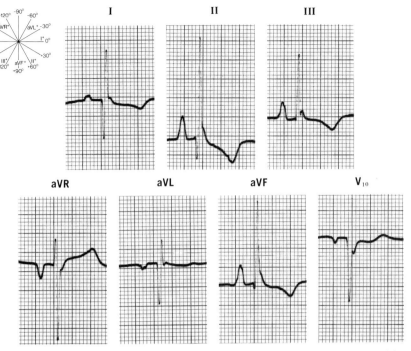

Figure 3-27. The positive T wave in lead V_{10} demonstrates that this dog has right ventricular hypertrophy. The tall peaked P wave is 0.6 mv. (6 boxes) high, indicating that right atrial hypertrophy is also present ("P pulmonale"). The P wave is also 0.06 second (3 boxes) wide, indicating left atrial hypertrophy ("P mitrale"). Left ventricular hypertrophy may be suspected since the axis remains normal (+90°). The Q-T interval in lead II is 0.26 second (13 boxes) wide (normal is up to 0.22 second). This would indicate that the dog's serum K^+ and Ca^{++} levels should be checked, since the Q-T prolongation may also be caused by hypokalemia, hyperkalemia, or hypocalcemia.

Paper speed = 50 mm./sec., 1 cm. = 1 mv.

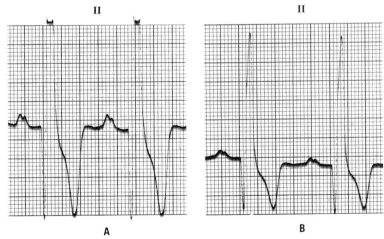

Figure 3-28. Biventricular hypertrophy is characterized by a wide QRS complex, tall R waves, and deep Q waves. The S-T segment usually is slurred, and the P wave often indicates hypertrophy of one or both of the atria. In this lead II tracing, A is run at full sensitivity and B is the same electrocardiogram at 1/2 sensitivity. In A, the R waves are so tall and the Q waves are so deep that the tracing cannot fit on the paper. Even at 1/2 sensitivity (B), the complex fills the paper. The P wave is wide (0.06 second, or 3 boxes) and notched, indicating "P mitrale," or left atrial hypertrophy. The P-R segment is depressed ("T sub a" wave), suggesting right atrial hypertrophy. The Q waves are 2.8 mv. deep (double the measurement in strip B) suggesting right ventricular hypertrophy. The R waves are too tall (6.6 mv. or 66 boxes), the QRS complexes are too wide (0.10 second, or 5 boxes), and the S-T segment is slurred; all three abnormalities indicate left ventricular hypertrophy.

Two conditions must be suspected when the electrocardiographic complexes are this large: severe mitral insufficiency, and patent ductus arteriosus. This was a postoperative tracing recorded after surgical correction of a patent ductus arteriosus.

Strip A: Paper speed = 50 mm./sec., 1 cm. = 1 mv.
Strip B: Paper speed = 50 mm./sec., 1/2 cm. = 1 mv.

ELECTROCARDIOGRAPHY

CLIENT_____ CASE NO. _____

SPECIES_____ BREED_____

AGE_____SEX_____

C.V. EXAM:

    1. HEART _____

    _____

    2. LUNGS _____

    _____

HEART RATE_____

RHYTHM_____

P _____

P–R_____

QRS_____

ST–T_____

QT_____

AXIS_____

OTHER:_____

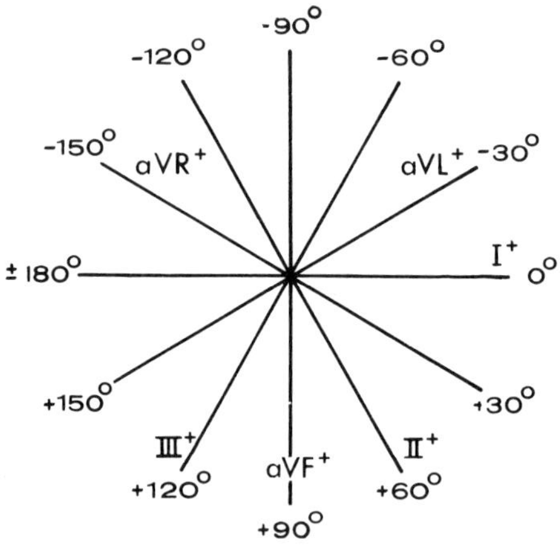

ECG DIAGNOSIS:_____

_____

_____

DIAGNOSTIC IMPRESSION: _____

_____

_____

_____

_____

_____

_____

Figure 3–29. A form such as this one can be designed for recording the electrocardiographic findings. Findings on physical examination can be recorded, and a case summary including chest x-ray findings can be written under "diagnostic impression." This form can be stored in the animal's record.

Figure 3-30 *PRACTICE ELEC-TROCARDIOGRAM.*

1. Heart Rate = 176 (R-R interval is 17 boxes, divided into 3000). See page 40.

2. Rhythm = normal sinus rhythm (NSR). See page 44.

3. Axis = + 90°. See page 48.

4. Measure and multiply:

> P = 0.04 second (2 boxes) by 0.3 mv. (3 boxes). See page 53.
> P-R = 0.10 second (5 boxes). See page 55.
> QRS = 0.04 second (2 boxes) by 1.9 mv. (19 boxes). See page 56.
> ST segment and T wave = normal. See page 57.
> Q-T = 0.16 second (8 boxes). See page 60.

5. Miscellaneous criteria = none

> Electrocardiographic diagnosis = normal

> Paper Speed = 50 mm./sec., 1 cm. = 1 mv.

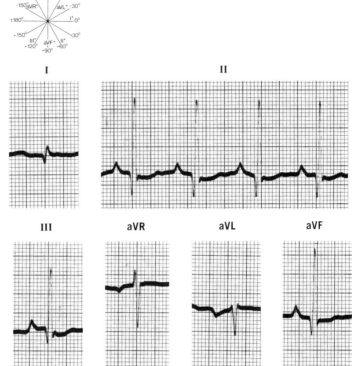

EFFECTS OF ELECTROLYTE DISTURBANCES ON THE ELECTROCARDIOGRAM

The electrocardiogram is sensitive to changes in serum potassium and calcium levels. This is fortunate, since in many instances therapy can be instituted before laboratory tests are returned. This is important, for example, in cases of acute adrenal insufficiency, in which the dog would probably die before the serum sodium and potassium values could be returned from the laboratory. The electrocardiogram can also be monitored to judge improvement during treatment.

Hyperkalemia

The electrocardiogram in most instances is sensitive to detecting hyperkalemic states. Mild elevations in serum potassium level (6.0 to 6.5 meq./l.) cause the T waves to become tall and peaked, but the heart rate and the P waves usually remain normal (Fig. 3-32A). At moderate elevations (6.5 to 7.0 meq./l.), the heart rate begins to slow, the P waves begin to flatten, and the T waves are usually still large (Fig. 3-32B). Figure 3-33 illustrates a marked effect on the P waves. The P-R interval and QRS complex may be prolonged. At high elevations of serum potassium (7.5 meq./l. or higher), the heart rate becomes very slow (usually below 60/min.), atrial standstill may occur, the Q-T interval may or may not be prolonged, and the T wave may or may not be large (Fig. 3-32C).

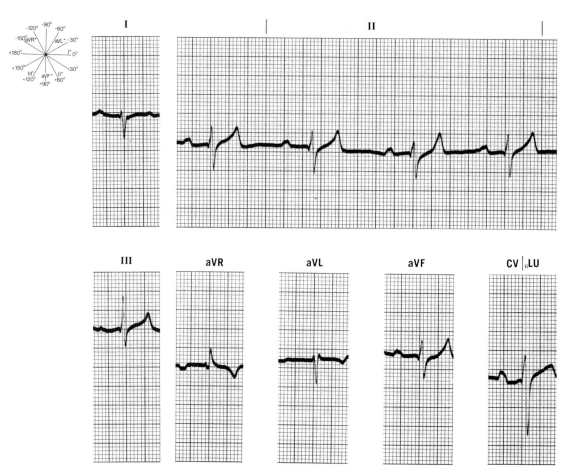

Figure 3–31 *PRACTICE ELECTROCARDIOGRAM.*

1. Heart rate = 111 to 120 (shortest R–R is 25 boxes, longest is 27 boxes).

2. Rhythm = sinus arrhythmia (R–R varies slightly.)

3. Axis = +150 (if II is used as isoelectric), ±180 (if aVF is used as isoelectric). It may be averaged at +165°.

4. Measure and multiply:

   P = 0.04 second (2 boxes) by 0.2 mv. (2 boxes)
   P–R = 0.13 to 0.14 second
   QRS = 0.05 second (2½ boxes) by 0.5 mv. (5 boxes)
   ST segment and T wave = normal
   Q–T = 0.18 second (9 boxes)

5. Miscellaneous:
   S_1, S_2, S_3 pattern (S waves present in leads I, II, and III)
   Deep S wave in CV_6LU (S wave deeper than 0.7 mv. in lead CV_6LU)

Electrocardiographic diagnosis:

1. Right axis deviation ⎫
2. S_1, S_2, S_3 pattern   ⎬ — Right ventricular hypertrophy
3. Deep S in CV_6LU ⎭

Clinical diagnosis: pulmonic stenosis

Paper speed = 50 mm./sec., 1 cm. = 1 mv.

When the serum potassium reaches 9.5 meq./l. or higher, cardiac arrest can occur at any time. If hyperkalemia is diagnosed in time, response to treatment is dramatic (Fig. 3–32D). Hyperkalemia may occasionally cause complete heart block. The treatment of hyperkalemia has been reported (Lorenz, 1972; Bolton, 1974).

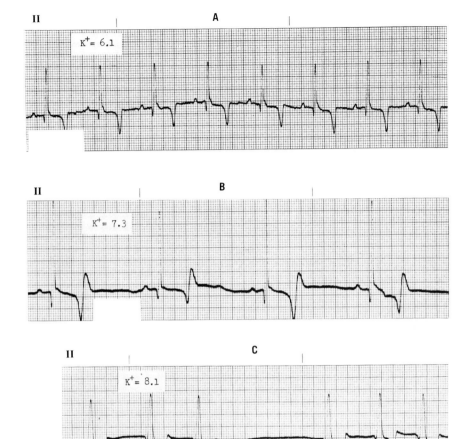

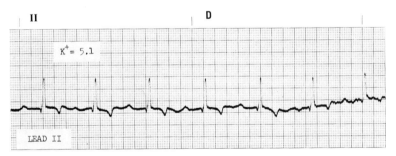

Figure 3–32. A. With mild elevations of serum potassium levels, the first effect noted on the electrocardiogram is the presence of large, peaked T waves.

B. As the serum potassium levels increase, the heart rate begins to slow, and the P waves begin to flatten. At moderate elevations, such as seen here, the T waves are usually still large.

C. As the serum potassium elevation becomes severe, the P wave is lost and atrial standstill occurs. A slow, irregular idioventricular rhythm is present here, with no P waves and a straight steady baseline. The T waves may or may not be large when the elevation is severe, and the Q-T interval may or may not be prolonged.

D. Response to treatment can be dramatic. This strip was recorded just one hour after the previous one. Treatment with intravenous hydrocortisone, dextrose and saline, and DOCA intramuscularly made the dramatic difference. This dog eventually died several days later of renal insufficiency.

Paper speed = 50 mm./sec., 1 cm. = 1 mv.

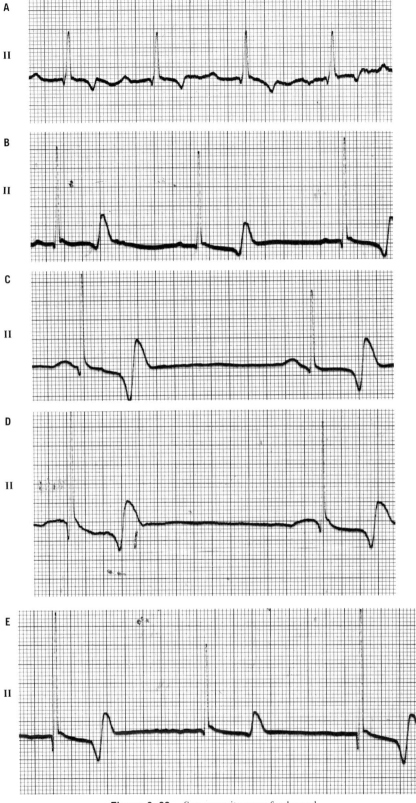

Figure 3–33. See opposite page for legend.

A

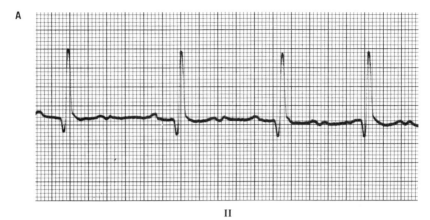

II

B

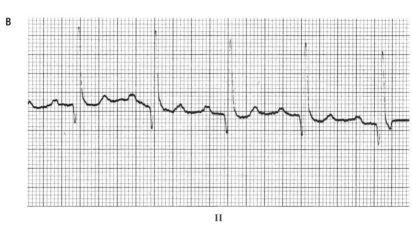

II

Figure 3–34. Strip A is a lead II electrocardiogram recorded from a St. Bernard that had hypokalemia of undetermined origin. His only clinical sign was profound weakness and inability to rise. His serum K+ was 2.8 meq./l. The significant changes on the electrocardiogram were the prolongation of the Q-T interval to 0.28 sec. (14 boxes) and the small biphasic T waves. Strip B was recorded after 2 days of intravenous potassium replacement therapy. The serum K+ was 4.2 meq./l. at the time of this recording. The dog could stand and walk with good strength. Two such cases have been diagnosed as idiopathic hypokalemia in our clinic. Neither dog has had a reoccurrence of the condition.

Paper speed = 50 mm./sec., 1 cm. = 1 mv.

Hypokalemia

Low serum levels of potassium occur less frequently but may be caused by excessive diuretic therapy, severe vomiting and diarrhea, or occasionally idiopathic hypokalemia may be diagnosed. Electrocardiographic changes due to hypokalemia include bradycardia, prolonged Q-T

Figure 3–33. This dog is being given potassium chloride in an intravenous drip to show the effect of hyperkalemia. Strip A was recorded before K+ was given. Strips B, C, D, and E are taken as K+ is being infused. In strip B, the rate has slowed, the P waves are becoming flattened, the T waves are larger, and the Q-T interval is prolonged. Strip C shows an even slower heart rate, and now the P waves and P-R intervals are becoming prolonged. The T waves are even larger and the Q-T interval is prolonged even more. In strip D, the P waves are wide and flat, the heart rate is 44 beats per minute, the T waves are large and the Q-T interval is grossly prolonged. In the final tracing, the P waves have disappeared and atrial standstill has occurred. The QRS complexes are ventricular in origin.

Paper speed = 50 mm./sec., 1 cm. = 1 mv.

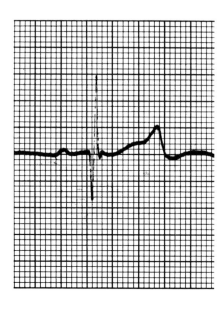

Figure 3–35. The dog from which this electrocardiogram was recorded had a serum Ca^{++} of 8.0 meq./l. His other serum electrolytes were normal (phosphorus was not done). The striking abnormality in this lead II tracing is the prolongation of the Q-T interval to 0.50 second (25 boxes). The T wave is also broad and quite tall.

Paper speed = 50 mm./sec., 1 cm. = 1 mv.

interval, and small biphasic T waves (Fig. 3–34A). Changes may occur when serum potassium level falls below approximately 3.0 meq./l., and a level of 2.0 meq./l. or less is severe. The treatment is potassium replacement, intravenously or orally (Bolton, 1974); the results of potassium therapy may be rewarding (Fig. 3–34B).

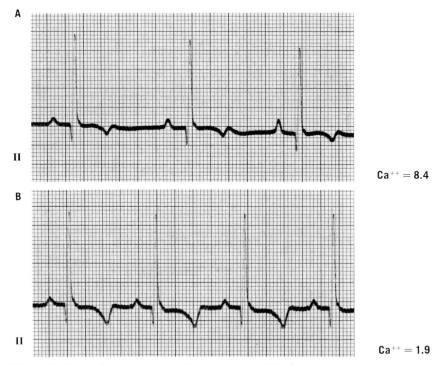

Figure 3–36. In this tracing hypocalcemia was caused by the intravenous administration of EDTA. The first strip was taken prior to treatment, and the second strip after EDTA was administered. Even though there is a profound drop in serum Ca^{++} levels, the only changes on the electrocardiogram are a nonspecific change in T wave configuration, a slight prolongation of the Q-T interval, and a moderate increase in heart rate.

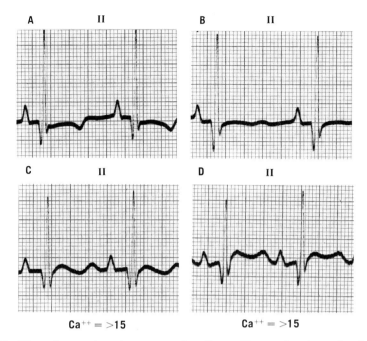

Ca^{++} = >15   Ca^{++} = >15

Figure 3–37. These four tracings demonstrate the effects of hypercalcemia on the electrocardiogram. This was caused by the intravenous administration of calcium gluconate. Strip A is pretreatment, strip B is taken after a slight elevation of the serum calcium level, and in strip C and D, when the elevations are severe, the S-T segment becomes elevated. Shortening of the Q-T interval, as reported in human medicine, is not seen.

Paper speed = 50 mm./sec., 1 cm. = 1 mv.

Hypocalcemia and Hypercalcemia

The electrocardiographic effects of hypocalcemia and hypercalcemia are not well established. These conditions are infrequently seen in small animals.

The hypocalcemic electrocardiogram may mimic one caused by hypokalemia, with the most consistent change being a prolonged Q-T interval (Figs. 3–35 and 3–36). The most consistent change with hypercalcemia in dogs seems to be elevation of the S-T segment (Fig. 3–37). In man, shortening of the Q-T interval is consistently reported with hypercalcemia (Bernreiter, 1963; Friedberg, 1966).

EFFECTS OF MYOCARDIAL HYPOXIA ON THE ELECTROCARDIOGRAM

The myocardium is sensitive to changes in arterial blood oxygen concentration. The electrocardiogram can detect even small discrepancies in myocardial oxygenation. This is of the utmost practical importance in the anesthetic management of the surgical patient, although severe pulmonary problems (such as the traumatic lung syndrome, severe pneumonia, diaphragmatic hernia, or pulmonary edema) can also cause hypoxic electrocardiographic changes. If the patient is not being properly ventilated, the lead II electrocardiogram can detect early changes caused by myocardial hypoxia. These early electrocardiographic abnormalities should be regarded as warning signs of impending disasters such as severe arrhythmias, cardiac arrest, and death. If black blood in the surgical site is the only sign that one relies on to warn him-

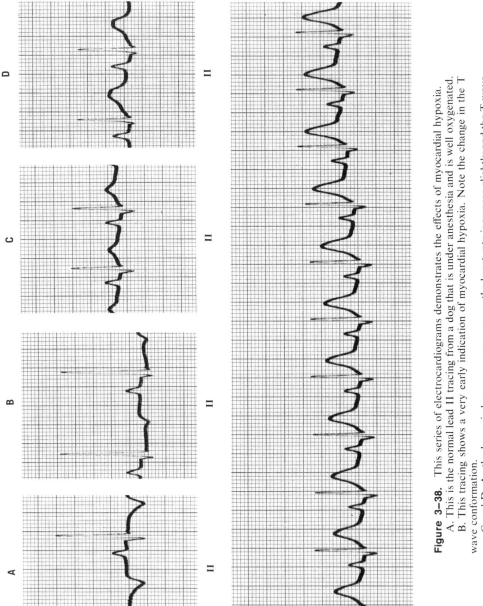

Figure 3–38. This series of electrocardiograms demonstrates the effects of myocardial hypoxia.

A. This is the normal lead II tracing from a dog that is under anesthesia and is well oxygenated.

B. This tracing shows a very early indication of myocardial hypoxia. Note the change in the T wave conformation.

C and D. As the hypoxia becomes more severe, the heart rate increases slightly and the T wave actually reverses polarity and becomes positive.

E. Now the hypoxia is very severe. The heart rate begins to increase rapidly and the T waves become very tall. If the hypoxia were allowed to persist, arrhythmias and cardiac arrest would occur.

Paper speed = 50 mm./sec., 1 cm. = 1 mv.

self of anesthetic problems, then none of these problem cases will be saved. When monitoring the anesthetic patient with the lead II electrocardiogram, the heart rate is noted, the S-T segment and the T wave are watched closely, and the recording is examined for the presence of arrhythmias. An initial tracing is recorded early in the anesthetic procedure so that changes will be noticed when they occur.

One of the earliest changes that occur in the electrocardiogram is a change in the heart rate. If the anesthetic depth is too great, there will be a sudden or a gradual decrease in heart rate. If the heart rate has been holding steady and begins to fall, the patient should be re-evaluated, the anesthetic concentration should be decreased if possible, and the animal's ventilation should be assisted until the heart rate is steady again. If the heart rate falls below 70/min., it is cause for concern. When myocardial oxygenation is severely compromised and the animal is becoming hypoxic, the heart rate increases (Fig. 3-38). If the heart rate begins to climb rapidly, steps to correct the hypoxia must be taken immediately.

Changes in the S-T segment and the T wave also occur early, and if they are observed and corrected, more severe difficulties can be avoided. An early sign of myocardial hypoxia is an elevation or depression of the S-T segment (see Figures 3-22 and 3-23). Therefore the S-T segment should be closely observed and compared to the animal's normal one. Like the changes in the heart rate, the appearance of elevation or depression of the S-T segment warns of worse things to come (the arrhythmias), and the animal is re-evaluated, anesthetic concentration is decreased if possible, and respiration is assisted until the S-T segment changes are resolved.

The T wave should be observed for changes in configuration. Changes in the shape or the polarity of the T wave are early warning signs of myocardial hypoxia and warn of impending disaster (Fig. 3-38). If the T wave is being observed and it suddenly goes from negative to positive or from positive to negative, or it suddenly begins to grow larger and larger, watch out (Fig. 3-38)! It is a sign of serious trouble, and a fatal arrhythmia may occur. Again, re-evaluate the patient for anesthetic depth, color of mucous membranes, capillary refill time, respiration, pulse, heart rate, and S-T segment changes; decrease the anesthetic depth if possible, and ventilate the animal mechanically until the T wave returns to normal.

The development of an arrhythmia is the most advanced and most serious sign that the anesthetic course is traveling a bumpy road. Usually, by the time an arrhythmia appears, the animal has already been hypoxic for awhile, and the early signs of it have been missed. The most common arrhythmias that occur are ventricular premature beats (see Chapter 4, the Arrhythmias). It is possible, however, for almost any arrhythmia to occur. Ventricular tachycardia, ventricular fibrillation, and cardiac arrest or standstill are by far the most serious and most advanced signs that the animal is not doing well. When ventricular fibrillation and cardiac arrest or standstill occur, the blood turns dark in the surgical field. If this is the first sign that is noticed, then it is usually too late.

If arrhythmias continue to be a problem even though the anesthetic depth is kept to a minimum and the patient is kept well ventilated, then an intravenous drip of sodium bicarbonate (15 to 20 meq./500 cc.)

should be given. When hypoxia and acidosis are severe, as much as 3 to 9 meq./kg. of sodium bicarbonate can immediately be given intravenously. If the arrhythmias are still persistent and severe, antiarrhythmic therapy may be needed (see Chapter 4), and the anesthetic procedure may need to be discontinued. See Bolton (1972) for management of the surgical patient under anesthesia.

The electrocardiogram, then, may be put to good use for monitoring patients in which a problem might be anticipated. Ideally, it would be nice to monitor every surgical patient with the electrocardiogram. This is why a monitoring device of some sort would be worth the money in the surgical suite or intensive care unit. The philosophy to keep in mind is that when a heart stops, everything stops.

EFFECTS OF DRUGS ON THE ELECTROCARDIOGRAM

Digitalis

In addition to increasing the force of myocardial contraction, digitalis has other effects that can be seen on the electrocardiogram. Digitalis slows the heart rate by both vagal and extravagal means (Friedberg, 1966; Ettinger and Suter, 1970; Smith, 1973). One of the ways that digitalis controls the heart rate is by its effect of slowing conduction through the atrioventricular node. This effect is seen clinically as a prolongation of the P-R interval on the electrocardiogram. When digitalizing a patient, if his normal P-R interval is prolonged 0.02 to 0.03 second (1 to 1½ boxes) one should consider him to be digitalized even if he is not physically ill from the drug. It is usually possible to digitalize a dog without making him ill if the P-R interval is measured before each dose. The P-R interval prolongation does not always occur first, however, and vomiting, anorexia, diarrhea, or lethargy may occur without any prolongation of the P-R interval. For this reason, the dog as well as his electrocardiogram should be monitored before each dose of digitalis during the digitalization process. Changes in the S-T segment and T wave may also occur, and sinus arrhythmia may be exaggerated (Ettinger and Suter, 1970). In ventricular muscle cells digitalis effects a more rapid recovery by shortening the action potential. This may be seen on the electrocardiogram as a shortening of the Q-T interval (Smith, 1973).

When digitalis is given in toxic doses, arrhythmias occur. First degree heart block is a common result of digitalis toxicity. Second degree heart block, junctional premature beats and junctional rhythms, third degree heart block, ventricular premature beats, and ventricular tachycardia may also develop. Digitalis can cause any arrhythmia ever reported. Unlike the oral forms, intravenous digitalis can produce arrhythmias such as ventricular premature beats, ventricular tachycardia, and ventricular fibrillation before changes in the P-R interval occur (Ettinger and Suter, 1970).

Quinidine and Procainamide

Quinidine and procainamide similarly affect the heart and may alter the electrocardiogram. They depress myocardial contractility and excitability, they slow conduction velocity, and they have anticholinergic and antivagal effects (Ettinger and Suter, 1970). They are used clinically to suppress ectopic arrhythmias. An increase in heart rate may be seen secondary to their antivagal and anticholinergic effects (Ettinger and Suter, 1970). Prolongation of the P-R interval may occur as a result of delayed conduction through the atrioventricular node. Another result of the depression of conduction velocity is prolongation of the QRS complexes (Ettinger and Suter, 1970).

At high dosage, prolongation of the P wave, the P-R interval, the QRS complex, and the Q-T interval may occur, as well as S-T segment alterations. Prolongation of the QRS complex by 25 per cent or more should be regarded as a sign of drug intoxication, and the drug should be discontinued. If severe intoxication occurs, atrioventricular heart block, atrial standstill, ventricular tachycardia, or ventricular fibrillation may develop (Ettinger and Suter, 1970).

Other Antiarrhythmic Agents

Other antiarrhythmic agents, such as propranolol, also have the effect of decreasing conduction velocity, and toxic doses of these agents may also produce prolongation of the complexes and intervals as quinidine and procainamide do. Propranolol has a profound effect on myocardial contractility and conduction velocity and should be used with care.

Dilantin is one antiarrhythmic agent that has special qualities. It may actually enhance conduction through the atrioventricular node and may be a useful drug for incomplete heart block (Damato, 1966; Helfant, et al., 1967; Mason, et al., 1973).

Tranquilizers and Sedatives

Most tranquilizers and sedatives do not significantly alter the electrocardiogram. They do tend to cause bradycardia (Figs. 3–39 and 3–40), which may be prevented by the simultaneous use of atropine (Fig. 3–40). The author has observed ventricular premature beats when phenothiazine derivative tranquilizers were used (Figs. 3–39 and 3–40), but they were never clinically significant. Atropine also alleviates these arrhythmias (Fig. 3–40). The mean electrical axis and the measurements are not changed by tranquilization (the P-R interval and Q-T interval may be slightly prolonged secondary to the bradycardia that occurs).

Xylazine (Rompun) has caused serious bradycardia and conduction disturbances (Fig. 4–51), which may not be completely reversed by atropine. The use of this drug for cardiac patients should be questioned.

Anesthetic Agents

The arrhythmogenic effects of anesthetic agents are well recognized (Ettinger and Suter, 1970; Pedersoli and Brown, 1973; Weirich, 1974). In one study 85 per cent of the dogs anesthetized with thiamylal sodium developed arrhythmias (Pedersoli and Brown, 1973). These tend to be temporary, but should be carefully watched. Other intravenous barbiturates also cause arrhythmias (Weirich, 1974). Pentobarbital is one intravenous barbiturate that does not have this effect (Weirich, 1974). Inhalation anesthetics such as methoxyflurane and halothane are known

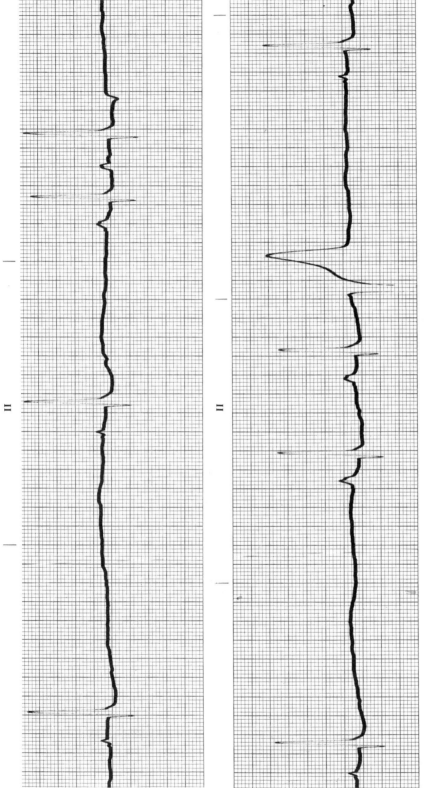

Figure 3–39. This electrocardiogram was recorded from an 8-month-old mixed breed dog, 4 months after the correction of a patent ductus arteriosus. She was given acepromazine without atropine to sedate her. Prior to administration of the tranquilizer, her heart rate was 180 beats per minute and steady. These lead II recordings were taken 15 minutes after the tranquilizer was given intravenously.

A. This tracing demonstrates marked bradycardia due to sinus arrest.

B. In addition to sinus arrest and bradycardia, an occasional ventricular premature beat occurs (bizarre beat second from right). These arrhythmias were corrected by administering 0.02 mg./lb. of atropine intravenously.

Paper speed = 50 mm./sec., 1 cm. = 1 mv.

to be arrhythmogenic (Ettinger and Suter, 1970; White, 1971). Figure 3–41 demonstrates ventricular premature beats that occurred in a dog when both halothane and then methoxyflurane anesthesia were used. One study (Pedersoli and Brown, 1973) provided good evidence that the thiamylal sodium–induced arrhythmias were due to a release of epinephrine from the adrenal medulla by the anesthetic. Other than through their arrhythmogenic effects, anesthetic agents will not alter the electrocardiogram.

DETECTION OF ELECTROCARDIOGRAPHIC ARTIFACTS

Artifacts due to errors in recording can make the interpretation of the electrocardiogram difficult if not impossible. Such artifacts include 60 cycle electrical interference, movement artifacts, improper patient positioning, and electrode placement errors.

60 Cycle Electrical Interference

Electrical interference occurs when the patient is not properly grounded. When electrical interference is a problem, a series of possible causes must be checked. The 60 cycle interference appears as a regular saw-toothed pattern that makes the baseline look jagged rather than smooth (Fig. 3–42). This artifact makes taking the measurements difficult.

Chapter 1 gives a checklist for eliminating 60 cycle interference from the tracing (page 15).

Movement Artifacts

A nervous, trembling animal causes the baseline to tremble because of the shaking and muscle tremors. This appears as a jagged baseline that is not as regular or as rapid as the 60 cycle artifacts (Fig. 3–43). A struggling animal causes the stylus to jump wildly, which makes it impossible to record a tracing (Fig. 3–44). A periodic muscle twitch can look like a premature beat on the electrocardiogram (Fig. 3–45).

Respiratory movements such as panting, deep respiration, or coughing will cause the baseline to vacillate up and down (Fig. 3–46).

Chapter 1 explains how to minimize movement artifacts (page 16).

Patient Positioning Artifacts

Changes in the dog's position cause changes in the electrocardiogram. Even in right lateral recumbency, minor changes in forelimb position will produce significant changes on the electrocardiogram (Cagan and Barta, 1959; Detweiler and Patterson, 1965; Hill, 1968). Measurement intervals involving complex width do not change, but complex height and axis do change with alterations in position of the animal (Fig. 3–47).

Text continued on page 86.

A

II

B

II

Illustration continued on opposite page.

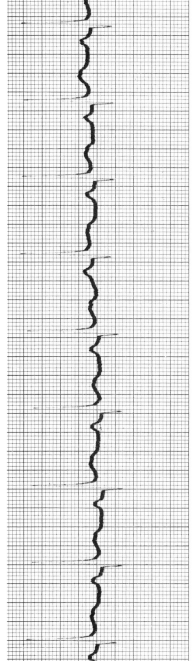

Figure 3–40. The two tracings on the opposite page were recorded from a 1-year-old mixed breed dog that had pulmonic stenosis. He was given piperacetazine (Psymod), 1 mg./20 lb. body weight intramuscularly for sedation and strips A and B were recorded 15 minutes later. No atropine was given.

A. In this tracing the heart rate averages 60 beats per minute, and sinus arrhythmia is present.

B. A ventricular premature beat (second from left) occurred occasionally, as demonstrated here.

C. The dog was given atropine intravenously at 0.02 mg./lb., and this tracing was recorded 5 minutes later. Now the heart rate is 150 per minute, and the ventricular premature beats are gone.

Paper speed = 50 mm./sec., 1 cm. = 1 mv.

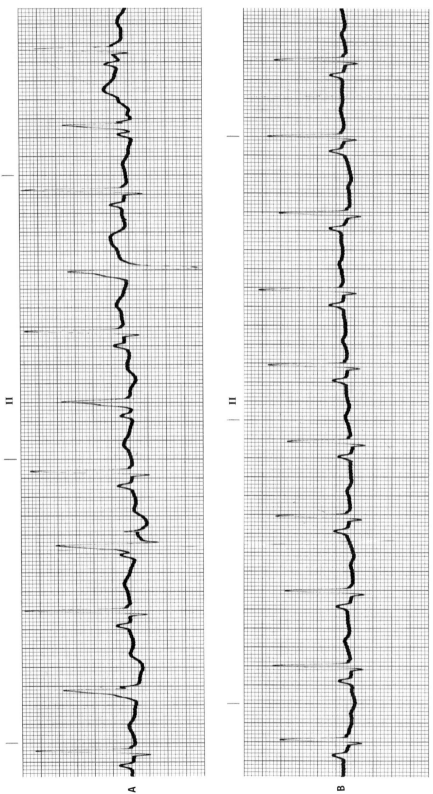

Figure 3–41. A. This electrocardiogram was recorded from a dog that had been hit by a car one day previously, and had sustained a humeral fracture. He was under halothane anesthesia for radiography, and an arrhythmia was auscultated. In this tracing, every other beat is a ventricular premature beat–such beats (second, fourth, sixth, eighth, and tenth, beats from left) are seen to occur early, to be followed by a pause, to have an abnormal conformation, and to be unassociated with a P wave. These premature beats are also of multifocal origin (this will be discussed in Chapter 4).

B. Halothane anesthesia was stopped and the dog was maintained on nitrous oxide and O_2. This strip was recorded moments later. All the beats are normal now. Whenever halothane was resumed, the arrhythmias reoccurred and persisted.

Illustration continued on opposite page.

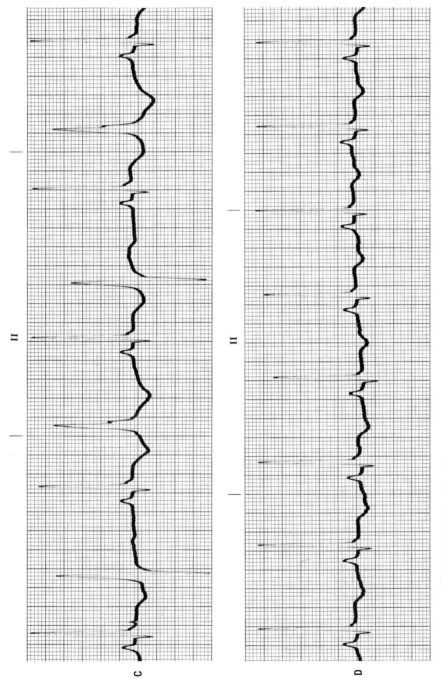

Figure 3–41 *Continued*

C. The dog was switched to methoxyflurane anesthesia, which also caused the arrhythmias to reoccur. Here again every other beat is a ventricular premature beat (second, fourth, sixth, and eighth beats from left).

D. All anesthesia attempts were discontinued and the tracing returned to normal, as demonstrated here. The dog was allowed to rest for 4 days, and at that time anesthesia and radiography were performed without difficulty. It was thought that the myocardium may have been traumatized as a result of the accident, and thus became especially sensitive to the anesthetics.

Paper speed = 50 mm./sec., 1 cm. = 1 mv.

II

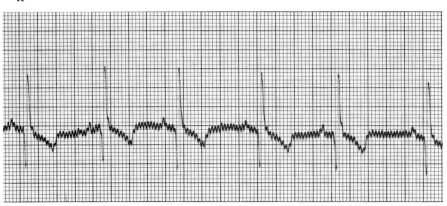

Figure 3–42. When this lead II electrocardiogram was recorded the dog was not properly grounded, and the regular saw-toothed artifact of 60 cycle electrical interference is seen. Such an error makes measurements and observations difficult. Here it is hard to measure the P wave or to see if an S wave is present. Chapter 1, page 15 has a checklist for avoiding this pesky artifact.

Paper speed = 50 mm./sec., 1 cm. = 1 mv.

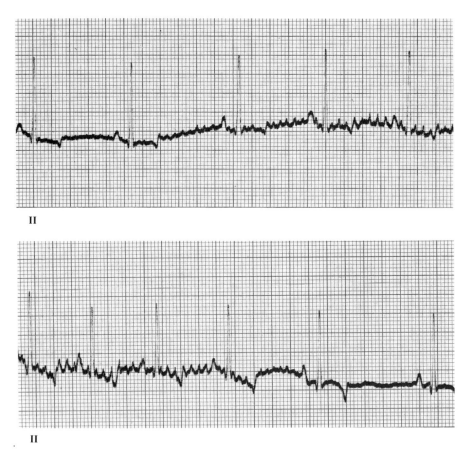

II

II

Figure 3–43. These two strips are a continuous lead II tracing recorded from a nervous poodle that would alternately tremble, relax, tremble, and so forth. Notice that, early in the top strip, the baseline is fairly smooth, but as he begins to tremble, the baseline becomes jagged, and atrial flutter could be falsely diagnosed. Note that the jagged tracing is not as rapid or regular as the 60 cycle interference in Figure 3–42. Toward the end of the bottom strip he relaxes again.

Paper speed = 50 mm./sec., 1 cm. = 1 mv.

82

II

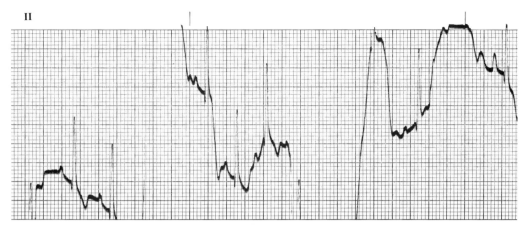

Figure 3–44. This tracing was made while wrestling with an uncooperative German Shepherd. The struggling of the animal makes it impossible to keep the stylus on the paper. To correct this, the dog is tranquilized and the tracing can be completed when everyone concerned is calm, cool, and collected.

Paper speed = 50 mm./sec., 1 cm. = 1 mv.

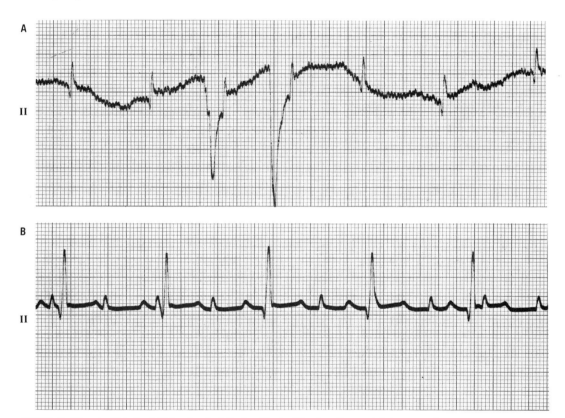

Figure 3–45. A. This lead II tracing is full of artifacts. The baseline undulates up and down because of respiratory artifact, there is 60 cycle interference, and the two bizarre looking deflections that occur could be mistaken for ventricular premature contractions. What really happened is that the dog jerked one leg twice and created the two beat artifacts.

B. In this lead II tracing it appears that there are extra P waves that occur. It can be seen, however, that they occur without relation either to the QRS complexes or to the P waves. They were artifacts caused by a muscle twitch from the dog.

When movement artifacts are noted while taking the tracing, the lead marker button can be pushed several times as a reminder when reading the tracing.

Paper speed = 50 mm./sec., 1 cm. = 1 mv.

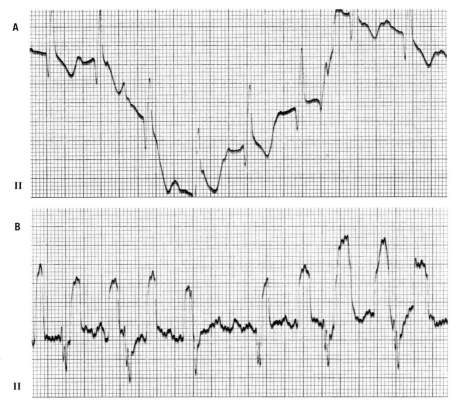

Figure 3–46. These two lead II strips are examples of respiratory artifacts.

A. Each time this dog took a breath, the tracing would shift downward, making it impossible to keep the complexes on the paper.

B. This dog was panting, which caused the baseline to jump with each breath. This gives a false impression of abnormal beats.

Paper speed = 50 mm./sec., 1 cm. = 1 mv.

Figure 3–47. The electrocardiograms in A, B, C, and D demonstrate the effects of placing the patient in various positions. All tracings should be run in the standard right lateral position to avoid these position alterations. All four tracings were run on the same dog.

A. This tracing was run with the dog in the normal right lateral position.

B. This tracing was taken with the dog in left lateral recumbency. Note the difference in the height of the complexes. This makes his millivoltage measurements invalid. The axis has also changed from +60° in strip A to about +75° in this tracing.

C. This tracing was recorded with the dog in sternal recumbency. Again, the height of the complexes varies from normal in strip A, and the axis in this position is +80° to +85°.

D. The dog is standing up for this recording. The height measurements are more erroneous than in any of the previous tracings. The axis now is +50°.

These variations point out the need for running every electrocardiogram with the dog in the correct position. When only the rhythm is being monitored and measurements are not important, any position is adequate.

If a dog is in such severe difficulty that placing him in right lateral recumbency would compromise his respiration, a preliminary lead II recording can be obtained in any position he feels comfortable, and the full electrocardiogram can be recorded later when he is in better condition.

Paper speed = 50 mm./sec., 1 cm. = 1 mv.

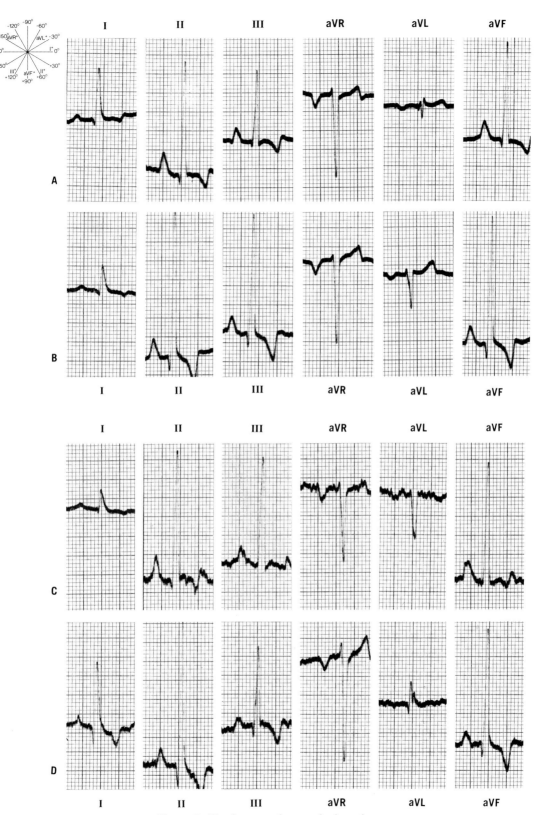

Figure 3-47. See opposite page for legend.

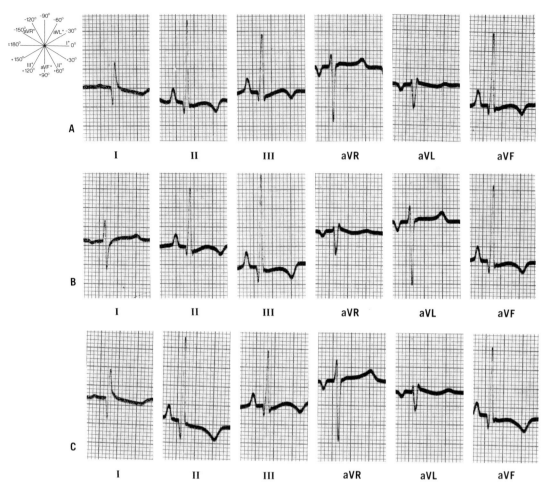

Figure 3–48. All three of these electrocardiograms were recorded from the same dog, to demonstrate the effects of improper electrode placement.

A. This is the dog's normal electrocardiogram.

B. In this tracing the front leg electrodes have been reversed. Note that this reverses leads II and III, and also reverses leads aVR and aVL compared to strip A. It also reverses the polarity of lead I.

C. The hindleg electrodes have been reversed for this tracing and the foreleg electrodes are in their proper position. Note that the reversal of the hindleg electrodes does not alter the tracing, as compared to strip A.

Paper speed = 50 mm./sec., 1 cm. = 1 mv.

Electrode Placement Errors

A common mistake is made by attaching the electrodes to the wrong legs. If the foreleg electrodes are reversed, lead II is really lead III, and leads aVR and aVL are also reversed (Fig. 3–48). The polarity of the P wave and the QRST complex in lead I will also be reversed (Fig. 3–48). Reversing the hind limb electrodes does not markedly affect the electrocardiogram (Fig. 3–48). When a forelimb electrode is accidentally reversed with a hind leg electrode, one of the leads may record only a baseline.

SUMMARY

It is hoped that applying this systematic approach to electrocardiography will allow each electrocardiogram to be carefully dissected and evaluated to obtain the maximum possible information. The electrocardiogram is merely a clinical tool and, like all other clinical aids, must be evaluated in relation to the other clinical findings.

REFERENCES

Bernreiter, M.: Electrocardiography. 2nd ed. J. B. Lippincott, Philadelphia, 1963.

Bolton, G. R.: Prevention and Treatment of Cardiovascular Emergencies During Anesthesia and Surgery. Vet. Clin. N. Am., 2 (1972):411.

Bolton, G. R.: Secondary Cardiac Diseases. In *Current Veterinary Therapy V*. Edited by Kirk, R. W. W. B. Saunders Co., Philadelphia, 1974, p. 308.

Cagan, S., and Barta, E.: Bedingungen des konstanten Elektrokardiogramms beim Hunde. Z. Kreislaufforsch., 48 (1959):1101.

Damato, A. N.: Diphenylhydantoin: Pharmacological and Clinical Use. Progr. Cardiovasc. Dis., 8 (1966):364.

Detweiler, D. K., and Patterson, D. F.: The Prevalence and Types of Cardiovascular Disease in Dogs. Ann. N. Y. Acad. Sci., 127 (1965):481.

Ettinger, S. J., and Sutter, P. F.: Canine Cardiology. W. B. Saunders Co., Philadelphia, 1970.

Friedberg, C. K.: Diseases of the Heart. 3rd ed. W. B. Saunders Co., Philadelphia, 1966.

Hill, J. D.: The Significance of the Foreleg Position in the Interpretation of Electrocardiograms and Vectorcardiograms from Research Animals. Amer. Heart J., 75 (1968):518.

Lorenz, M. D.: Metabolic Emergencies. In Vet. Clin. N. Am., 2 (1972):331.

Mason, D. T., Amsterdam, E. A., Massumi, R. A., Mansour, E. J., Hughes, J. L., and Zelis, R.: Combined Actions of Antiarrhythmic Drugs: Electrophysiologic and Therpeutic Considerations. In *Cardiac Arrhythmias*. Edited by Dreifus, L. S., and Likoff, W. The Twenty-Fifth Hahnemann Symposium. Grune and Stratton, New York, 1973, p. 531.

Pedersoli, W. M., and Brown, M. K.: A New Approach to the Etiology of Arrhythmogenic Effects of Thiamylal Sodium in Dogs. Vet. Med. Small Anim. Clin., 68 (1973):1286.

Smith, T. W.: Drug Therapy. Digitalis Glycosides (First of Two Parts). N. Eng. J. Med., 288, 14 (1973).

Weirich, W. E.: Electrocardiographic Monitoring of the Surgical Patient. In *1974 Scientific Presentations and Seminar Synopses*, A.A.H.A., 41st Annual Meeting, A.A.H.A., South Bend, Ind., 1974, p. 82.

White, R. J.: Cardiac Arrhythmias During Anesthesia. In *Textbook of Veterinary Anesthesia*. Edited by Soma, L. R. Williams and Wilkins, Baltimore, 1971, p. 580.

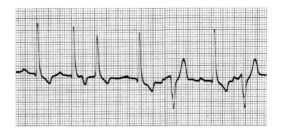

Chapter 4

THE
ARRHYTHMIAS

The excitement and challenge of electrocardiography lie in the discovery, diagnosis, and successful treatment of an arrhythmia. The electrocardiographic changes and clinical signs can be spectacular, and the results of therapy can be equally remarkable and rewarding. Most arrhythmias respond quickly when the diagnosis and treatment are correct. Some of the arrhythmias cause catastrophic clinical signs, while others are of little concern. The often fatal results of inappropriate management of the arrhythmias make them challenging.

Arrhythmias are common and occur weekly, if not daily, in every small animal hospital. It is reported that arrhythmias occur in 85 per cent of dogs given thiamylal sodium anesthesia (Pedersoli and Brown, 1973). Arrhythmias may be secondary to, and complicate, such widely diversified disease conditions as diabetes mellitus, adrenocortical insufficiency, renal insufficiency, pyometra, trauma, hemangiosarcoma, mitral insufficiency, aortic stenosis, idiopathic cardiomyopathy, endocarditis, intestinal obstructions, septicemias, toxemias, heat-stroke, eclampsia and electric cord bites, among many other causes (Bolton, 1974; Ettinger and Suter, 1970).

Some of the normal variations of the natural canine rhythm can be remarkably irregular. These normal variations must be recognized as normal, and they require differentiation from other more serious arrhythmias.

When the arrhythmias become significant, a number of clinical signs may occur. Milder ones include weakness, fatigue, lethargy, and intolerance to exercise. More severe manifestations are profound weakness, ataxia, and mental confusion. Collapse, seizure, coma, and sudden death are the catastrophic results of the more serious arrhythmias.

Although these signs are not pathognomonic for cardiac arrhythmias, any animal that shows vague signs of weakness, fatigue, loss of stamina, seizures, or collapsing episodes, or any animal that is presented in a state of coma or collapse, should be screened for the presence of an arrhythmia (see Chapter 1).

The arrhythmias cause these clinical signs by causing a decrease in cardiac output. Tachycardia, bradycardia, and irregular rhythms all cause the cardiac output to decrease. When cerebral and peripheral perfusion is compromised significantly by the resulting low blood pressure, clinical signs develop.

Tachycardia can be either beneficial or detrimental, depending on the magnitude of the rate increase. At rates up to about 180 beats per minute, an increase in heart rate will increase the cardiac output (Friedberg, 1966). At rates above 180 beats per minute in adult dogs, cardiac output begins to fall, because the pause between beats is so short that the ventricles beat before they can fill completely with blood. This decreases the stroke output and, consequently, cardiac output. If the heart rate exceeds 220 beats per minute, cardiac output falls drastically. If the tachycardia is prolonged, congestive heart failure can result owing to the prolonged drop in cardiac output.

The same mechanism occurs in the case of premature beats. When the premature beat discharges the ventricles too quickly, they are forced to contract before they fill adequately with blood, and blood pressure drops (Fig. 4–1). Their effect on blood pressure does not become clinically significant until they begin to occur frequently.

Bradycardia affects cardiac output because the heart does not beat often enough to maintain the mean arterial blood pressure at an acceptable level. The cardiac output is equal to the output per beat times the number of beats per minute. At slow heart rates the heart compensates by pumping more blood with each beat because of the long filling time, but blood pressure is often fixed at a low level (Bellet, 1972). The blood pressure may be adequate at rest but inadequate during exercise. The clinical signs, then, are aggravated by exercise or excitement, or may occur only upon exertion.

The realization that an arrhythmia is occurring begins during the physical examination. Tachycardia, bradycardia, or irregular heart beat is noticed during auscultation of the heart, or during palpation of the femoral pulse. When such an abnormality is detected, three clinical observations should be made.

First, an attempt is made to correlate the arrhythmia with respiration. Respiratory influences on vagal tone may cause the heart rate to increase during inspiration and decrease during expiration. If fluctuations in the heart rate can be positively correlated with the respiratory movements, it is a sinus arrhythmia, which is a normal variation of the canine cardiac rhythm.

Next, the heart rate and the femoral pulse are compared simultaneously. Normally, a femoral pulse occurs after each heart beat. Some arrhythmias, such as premature beats or atrial fibrillation, cause a pulse deficit in which there are more heart beats than femoral pulses. A pulse deficit is a sign of a severe arrhythmia (Fig. 4–1).

A third observation that may provide a helpful clue in the physical examination of an animal with an arrhythmia is the presence of a jugular pulse. Arrhythmias such as ventricular premature beats, ventricular tachycardia, and complete heart block cause a jugular pulse. These arrhythmias cause the ventricles to contract before the atria. By the

II

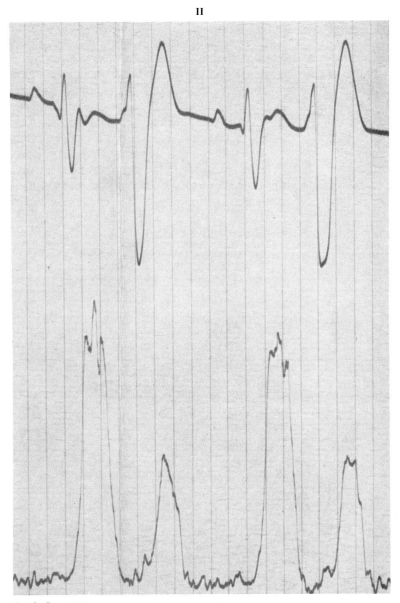

Aortic Pressure

Figure 4–1. The top tracing is a dog's lead II electrocardiogram. The bottom is a recording of his aortic pressure. The first and third beats are the dog's normal sinoatrial beats. The second and fourth beats are ventricular premature beats. Note the precipitous drop in blood pressure when the premature beats occur. The pulse pressure produced by these premature beats would not be adequate to produce a femoral pulse, and a pulse deficit would be present.

Paper speed = 100 mm./sec., 1 cm. = 2 mv.

time the atria contract, the atrioventricular valves have already closed, and instead of pushing blood down into the ventricles, atrial contraction pumps the blood backward. This backward flow of blood is transmitted to the jugular vein, producing a jugular pulse. This type of jugular pulse is called a cannon "a" wave (Ettinger and Suter, 1970). Dogs in atrial fibrillation have a jugular pulse because they are in right-sided heart failure.

The electrocardiogram provides the only way to identify positively an arrhythmia. A thorough history and physical examination allow the clinician to make an educated guess of which arrhythmia is present, but a good guess is not enough. The different types of arrhythmias are distinctly different in many respects, including treatment. Mistakes in diagnosis and treatment may be fatal, and the arrhythmias are one area in which the electrocardiogram is indispensable.

It is the objective of this chapter to develop a logical approach to the electrocardiographic diagnosis of the arrhythmias. Clinical signs and physical examination are stressed, because it is useful to know the type of animal, to identify all his problems, and to know the situations in which each arrhythmia tends to occur. Treatment of each arrhythmia is also discussed.

CLASSIFICATION OF THE ARRHYTHMIAS

Arrhythmias are often classified in such a way that nobody can understand them. There are two schemes that do help one to understand

---

TABLE 4–1. THE ANATOMICAL AND PHYSIOLOGICAL CLASSIFICATION OF THE CARDIAC ARRHYTHMIAS

Sinoatrial Arrhythmias
 Sinus arrhythmia
 Sinus arrest and sinoatrial block
 Wandering pacemaker
 Sinus tachycardia
 Sinus bradycardia

Ectopic Arrhythmias
 SUPRAVENTRICULAR ARRHYTHMIAS
  Atrial premature beats
  Junctional premature beats
  Atrial tachycardia
  Atrial fibrillation
  Atrial flutter
  Junctional tachycardia
 VENTRICULAR ARRHYTHMIAS
  Ventricular premature beats
  Ventricular tachycardia and atrioventricular dissociation
  Ventricular fibrillation
 ESCAPE RHYTHMS
  Junctional escape beats and rhythms
  Ventricular escape beats and rhythms

Conduction Disturbances
 HEART BLOCK (A-V BLOCK)
  First degree heart block
  Second degree heart block
  Third degree (complete) heart block
 SINOATRIAL STANDSTILL
 BUNDLE BRANCH BLOCK
  Right bundle branch block (RBBB)
  Left bundle branch block (LBBB)
 WOLFF-PARKINSON-WHITE SYNDROME (WPW)

TABLE 4–2. CLASSIFICATION OF CARDIAC ARRHYTHMIAS BY HEART RATE

Tachycardias
- Sinus tachycardia
- Atrial tachycardia
- Atrial fibrillation
- Junctional (nodal) tachycardia (sometimes)
- Atrial flutter
- Ventricular tachycardia (sometimes)

Bradycardias
- Sinus bradycardia
- Sinoatrial standstill
- Ventricular escape rhythms
- Junctional (nodal) escape rhythms
- Complete heart block
- Advanced second degree heart block
- Sinus arrest (sometimes)

Arrhythmias With Normal Rates
- Sinus arrhythmia
- Sinus arrest (usually)
- Atrial premature beats
- Junctional (nodal) premature beats
- Ventricular premature beats
- Junctional (nodal) tachycardia (usually)
- Ventricular tachycardia (usually)
- First degree heart block
- Second degree heart block (usually)
- Bundle branch blocks
- Wolff-Parkinson-White syndrome (W-P-W)

---

them better. Table 4–1 classifies them physiologically and anatomically. Table 4–2 classifies them on the basis of heart rate.

Table 4–1 classifies arrhythmias in three main groups: those that involve the sinoatrial node; those that are ectopic, which means that they arise from somewhere other than the sinoatrial node; and those in which the cardiac impulse is either blocked or conducted at an abnormal rate. Table 4–2 classifies them according to heart rate, which may also aid in differential diagnosis.

In general, sinoatrial arrhythmias require no specific treatment. Ectopic arrhythmias of the supraventricular type are usually treated with digitalis, while those of ventricular origin are treated with quinidine (or other antiarrhythmic agents). The conduction disturbances, if they are clinically significant, are usually treated with atropine or isoproterenol to increase heart rate. Table 4–3 lists the drugs used to treat arrhythmias, their special considerations, and some dosages. In summary: supraventricular—think digitalis; ventricular—think quinidine; heart block—think atropine or isoproterenol. There are few exceptions.

One drug that deserves special mention is digitalis. Digitalis can cause every arrhythmia that has ever been reported. *Any arrhythmia that develops while an animal is receiving digitalis therapy must be considered to be a sign of digitalis intoxication until proved otherwise.*

TABLE 4-3. DRUGS USED TO TREAT ARRHYTHMIAS

Digitalis Glycosides
INDICATIONS
  Supraventricular premature beats and tachycardia
  Ventricular premature beats and tachycardia *only* if due to myocardial hypoxia
    from severe congestive heart failure
CONTRAINDICATIONS
  Atrioventricular heart block
  Ventricular premature beats or ventricular tachycardia (usually), including atrio-
    ventricular dissociation
NONINDICATIONS
  Sinus tachycardia due to fever, nervousness, or excitement
  Shock
PREPARATIONS AND DOSAGES
  See Ettinger and Suter (1970).
WARNING
  Digitalis can cause any arrhythmia ever reported; therefore, caution should be
    exercised in its use.

Antiarrhythmic Agents
INDICATIONS
  Ventricular premature beats and ventricular tachycardia
  Atrial fibrillation, but only after the heart rate and congestive heart failure are under
    control with digitalis
CONTRAINDICATIONS
  Atrioventricular heart block
  Congestive heart failure
  Idiosyncratic reactions
DRUGS AND DOSAGES
  Quinidine preparations
    Cardioquin (Purdue Frederick) — 3 gr. tablets every 8 to 12 hours
    Quinaglut Duratabs (Cooper) — 5 gr. tablets every 8 to 12 hours
    Quinidine Gluconate Injectable (Lilly) — 80 mg./cc. every 6 to 8 hours
    Quinidine Sulfate — 3 gr. tablets every 4 to 6 hours
    Dosage: 3 to 10 mg./lb. q6–8 hours orally or intramuscularly. Long acting tablets
      are given every 8 to 12 hours.
  Procainamide (Pronestyl — Squibb)
    Procainamide — 250 mg. capsules
    Procainamide — 100 mg./cc. injectable
    Special indications:
      Acts similarly to quinidine
      Can be used in combination with quinidine, at lower dosages of each
    Dosage:
      *5–10 mg./lb. every 3 to 6 hours, intramuscularly
      *100 mg./min. intravenously until intoxication or conversion
      125–500 mg. every 4 to 6 hours orally
      *For ventricular tachycardia only

(Table continued on opposite page)

THE SYSTEMATIC APPROACH TO THE ARRHYTHMIAS

The heart rhythm is evaluated using the lead II rhythm strip. Each time a series of questions should be asked:

1. Is the heart rate normal or abnormal?

2. Is the rhythm regular or irregular?

3. Is there a P wave for every QRS complex and a QRS complex for every P wave?

4. Are the P waves and QRS complexes related? (Check the P-R intervals.)

TABLE 4-3. DRUGS USED TO TREAT ARRHYTHMIAS (*Continued*)

Lidocaine (2 per cent, without epinephrine)
  For intravenous emergency therapy
  Acts within seconds, lasts 15 to 20 minutes at most
  Dosage:
    2 to 4 mg./lb. by intravenous bolus, over 1 to 2 minutes
    2 mg./cc. intravenous drip of 5% dextrose in water, as needed
Diphenylhydantoin (Dilantin—Parke, Davis)
  Capsules: 30 mg., 100 mg.
  Special property: increases conduction time through the atrioventricular node
  Useful only for ventricular arrhythmias.
  Dosage:
    2 to 4 mg./lb. orally three times daily
Propranolol (Inderal—Ayerst)
  Tablets: 10 mg.
  Injection: 1 mg./cc.
  Very potent: can cause congestive heart failure
  Special indication: supraventricular arrhythmias caused by digitalis intoxication
  Dosage:
    10 to 40 mg. orally three times daily
    1 to 3 mg. slowly intravenously with electrocardiographic monitoring

Positive Chronotropic Agents
INDICATION
  Bradycardia
CONTRAINDICATIONS
  Congestive heart failure
  Isoproterenol is arrhythmogenic (ectopic arrhythmias).
DRUGS AVAILABLE
  Isoproterenol
    Injection: 0.2 mg./cc. (Isuprel—Winthrop)
    Tablets: 15 mg., 30 mg. (Proternol—Key)
    Dosage:
      15 to 30 mg. orally every 4 to 6 hours
      0.1 to 0.2 mg. subcutaneously or intramuscularly every 4 to 6 hours
      1 mg./250–500 cc. fluids given intravenously as needed
  Atropine
    Injection: 1/120 gr. (0.5 mg.)/cc.
    Tablets: 1/200 grain atropine sulfate
    Dosage:
      Injection: 0.02 mg./lb., intravenously, intramuscularly, or subcutaneously every
        4 to 6 hours
      Tablets: 0.02 mg./lb. every 6 to 8 hours
        (tablets are too small to break, so come as close as possible)

5. Are all the P waves similar in configuration, and are all the QRS complexes similar?

Is the Heart Rate Normal or Abnormal?

By determining the heart rate and using Table 4–2, many of the arrhythmias can be ruled out.

Is the Rhythm Regular or Irregular?

It is easy to see whether the rhythm is grossly irregular (Fig. 4–2). Smaller irregularities are harder to see, but can be determined by measur-

II

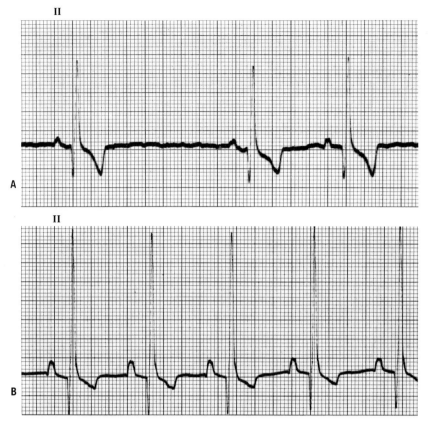

A

II

B

Figure 4–2. When checking for irregularity, the R-R intervals are examined. It is easy to see whether the rhythm is grossly irregular (as in strip A). In strip B, the irregularity is more subtle, and the distances from R wave to R wave must be counted to see that they are slightly irregular. Both these strips are examples of sinus arrhythmia.

Paper speed = 50 mm./sec., 1 cm. = 1 mv.

ing the distance from R wave to R wave (R-R interval) for several of the beats (Fig. 4–2).

Is There a P Wave for Every QRS Complex and a QRS Complex for Every P Wave?

Every beat should have a P wave, followed at a regular interval by a QRS complex. If this orderly sequence is broken, an arrhythmia is present. If a P wave occurs without a QRS, or a QRS occurs without a P wave, it is abnormal.

Are the P Waves and QRS Complexes Related?

Each P wave should have a definite relationship to its accompanying QRS complex. This is evaluated by checking the P-R intervals. Ideally, every P-R interval should be the same. It does vary slightly with the heart rate, being slightly longer with slower heart rates. The P-R interval seldom varies more than ½ to 1 box (0.01 to 0.02 sec.). If a complex has an obviously different P-R interval than the other complexes, it signifies that that P wave and QRS complex are unrelated. If the P-R interval varies so much that no consistent correlation can be shown between any of the P waves and the QRS complexes, then the atria and ventricles are beating independently of one another and a serious arrhythmia exists.

Are All the P Waves Similar in Configuration, and Are All the QRS Complexes Alike?

Normally, each impulse follows an identical pathway across the atria, through the atrioventricular node, and into the ventricles. All the P waves, then, are identical, as are all the QRS complexes. If the impulse originates from an abnormal site, or is conducted via an abnormal pathway, the complex will be altered. Atrial premature beats are an example of this. When an ectopic atrial impulse arises from a source other than the usual place (i.e., the sinoatrial node), the shape of the P wave is altered (Fig. 4–13). Likewise, if a ventricular ectopic beat arises, it alters the shape of the QRS complex (Fig. 4–24). When bundle branch block occurs the QRS complexes are altered, because the normal ventricular conduction pathway is blocked, and depolarization occurs in an aberrant manner (Fig. 4–54).

The Sinoatrial Arrhythmias

Normal sinus rhythm, sinus arrhythmia, sinus arrest, and wandering pacemaker are all normal variations of the canine cardiac rhythm. Since some of these normal arrhythmias can be remarkably irregular they must be recognized as such and differentiated from the rhythmic disorders indicating heart disease.

Normal Sinus Rhythm

ASSOCIATIONS. This is the perfect normal canine rhythm.

PHYSICAL EXAMINATION. Upon auscultation of the heart, the heart rate is normal, and the rhythm is perfectly regular. There is no pulse deficit.

ELECTROCARDIOGRAPHIC DIAGNOSIS

1. The heart rate is normal.
2. *The rhythm is perfectly regular (all R-R intervals are exactly alike).*
3. There is a P wave for every QRS complex and a QRS complex for every P wave.
4. The P waves and QRS complexes are related (all P-R intervals are constant).
5. All the PQRST complexes are identical.

Most dogs have some degree of sinus arrhythmia. In order to diagnose normal sinus rhythm (NSR), all the R-R intervals must be identical

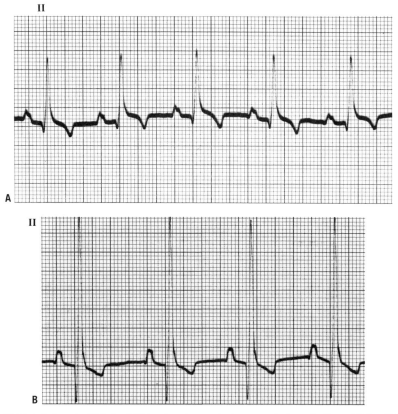

Figure 4-3. A. This lead II tracing demonstrates normal sinus rhythm. All the R-R intervals are exactly the same.

B. Even though this tracing looks quite regular, the R-R intervals can be seen to vary if they are measured. When even the slightest variation occurs in the R-R interval of a sinus rhythm, sinus arrhythmia is present. Most dogs have some sinus arrhythmia.

Paper speed = 50 mm./sec., 1 cm. = 1 mv.

(Fig. 4–3A). If the R-R intervals vary even slightly, sinus arrhythmia is diagnosed (Fig. 4–3B).

TREATMENT. No treatment is required.

The Vagal Arrhythmias: Sinus Arrhythmia, Sinus Arrest (Sinoatrial Block), and Wandering Pacemaker

ASSOCIATIONS. Sinus arrhythmia, sinus arrest, and wandering pacemaker all result from respiratory influences on vagal tone. As the dog inhales, vagal tone diminishes and the heart rate accelerates. As he exhales, vagal tone increases and the heart rate decreases. Since respiration is regular, these arrhythmias are characterized by being "regularly irregular."

Sinus arrest is for all practical purposes an exaggerated sinus arrhythmia, and wandering pacemaker is seen in conjunction with both arrhythmias. Usually these arrhythmias are of no clinical importance, but occasionally sinus arrest pauses may be long enough to cause bradycardia. This usually occurs in brachycephalic breeds of dogs. In these breeds, stertorous respiration constantly irritates the pharynx, causing reflex hypertonia of the vagus nerve. This causes syncope during exercise or exertion, because the exaggerated vagal tone will not allow the heart rate to increase even though the dog is exercising. As a result, cardiac output is insufficient during exercise, and these dogs experience syncopal episodes. This diagnosis should be considered whenever a brachycephalic dog is experiencing episodic syncope.

Cervical or thoracic masses can also cause reflex vagal bradycardia by putting pressure on the vagus nerve or reflexly stimulating it. Examples are thyroid carcinoma, carotid body tumors, or thoracic neoplasms impinging on the vagus nerve. If atropine-responsive bradycardia of unknown origin is diagnosed, the neck should be carefully palpated, and the chest should be x-rayed.

PHYSICAL EXAMINATION. Unlike other arrhythmias, the vagal arrhythmias are "regularly irregular" and can be positively correlated with respiration. There is no pulse deficit.

ELECTROCARDIOGRAPHIC DIAGNOSIS

1. Heart rate is usually normal (occasionally bradycardia occurs).

2. The rhythm is irregular. *In cases of sinus arrhythmia, the pauses are shorter than twice the normal R-R interval, while in cases of sinus arrest, the pauses are longer, and are twice or greater than twice the normal R-R interval.*

3. There is a P wave for every QRS complex and a QRS complex for every P wave.

4. The P waves and QRS complexes are related (the P-R intervals are constant).

5. The P waves vary in height, and may even become negative if wandering pacemaker is present. The QRS complexes are all identical.

Figure 4–4 demonstrates a mild sinus arrhythmia, while Figure 4–5 demonstrates a more exaggerated one. In Figure 4–5, wandering pacemaker is evidenced by the fluctuation in the height of the P waves.

II

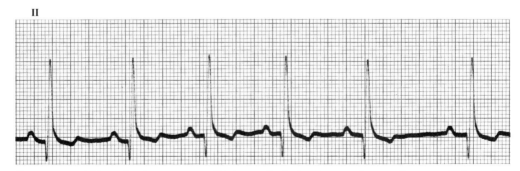

Figure 4–4. This tracing demonstrates mild sinus arrhythmia. There are P waves for every QRS complex and the P waves are related to the QRS complexes, which make this a sinus rhythm. It can also be seen that the R-R intervals vary. An irregular sinus rhythm is a sinus arrhythmia. If the animal were watched, the heart rate would speed up as he inhaled and slow down as he exhaled.

Paper speed = 50 mm./sec., 1 cm. = 1 mv.

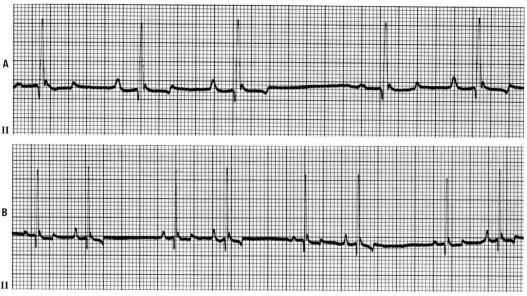

Figure 4–5. This tracing demonstrates a more exaggerated sinus arrhythmia. It is a sinus rhythm, and it is grossly irregular. If the pauses are measured, they are less than twice the normal R-R interval, which differentiates this from sinus arrest. The bottom tracing was recorded at 25 mm./sec. to demonstrate that the rhythm is "regularly irregular." This is a clue that it is associated with respirations, which are regular, and it is thus a hallmark of sinus arrhythmia. If the dog were watched, it would be seen that on inspiration two beats occur, and during expiration, the pauses occur.

This tracing also demonstrates wandering pacemaker. It can be ssen that the P waves vary in height. They become smaller after the pauses, and larger as the heart rate accelerates.

    A. Paper speed = 50 mm./sec., 1 cm. = 1 mv.

    B. Paper speed = 25 mm./sec., 1 cm. = 1 mv.

Usually, as the heart slows down, the P waves become smaller, and, as the heart speeds up, the P waves grow taller (Fig. 4–5). Wandering pacemaker occurs because vagal tone inhibits the sinoatrial node and causes a shifting of the pacemaker site within the atrium, which causes the P wave to look different. Figure 4–6 also demonstrates sinus arrhythmia and wandering pacemaker. Occasionally, the pacemaker site can shift all the way down in the atria to the region of the atrioventricular node; in these instances, the P wave actually becomes negative as the impulse travels backward through the atria (Fig. 4–7B). If the pacemaker site shifts about halfway down the atria, the P wave may become biphasic (isoelectric), as in Figure 4–7A. When the P wave does become isoelectric it can be hard to see, but if all the leads are checked, the P wave may be more easily seen in one of the other leads (Fig. 4–8).

The differentiation between sinus arrhythmia and sinus arrest is made electrocardiographically. This is usually of more academic than clinical importance. Two normal R-R intervals are measured. If the pauses in the rhythm are shorter than twice the normal R-R interval, sinus arrhythmia is present (Figs. 4–5, and 4–6). If the pauses are equal to or greater than twice the normal R-R interval, sinus arrest is diagnosed (Fig. 4–9). In some tracings, sinus arrhythmia, sinus arrest, and wandering pacemaker may all be present.

Text continued on page 104.

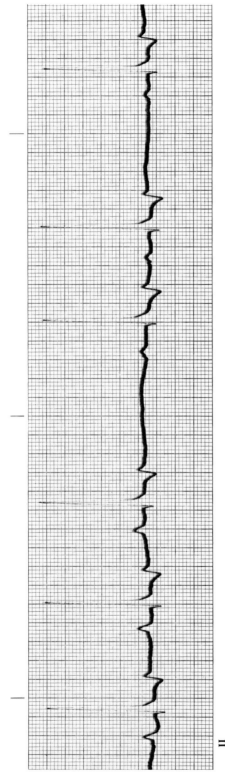

Figure 4–6. This is another tracing demonstrating sinus arrhythmia and wandering pacemaker. The P waves initiate the rhythm, showing it to be a sinus rhythm, and the irregularity is obvious. If the first two R-R intervals are taken as two normal R-R intervals, it can be seen that the pauses are less than two normal R-R intervals, which differentiates this from sinus arrest. Wandering pacemaker is evidenced by the variation in the height of the P waves.

Paper speed = 50 mm./sec., 1 cm. = 1 mv.

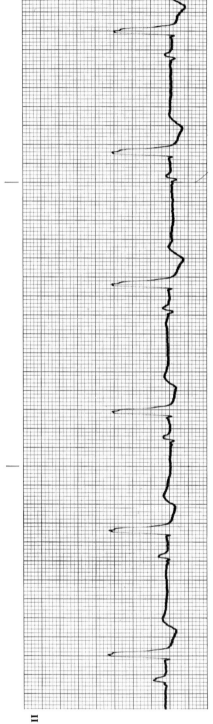

Figure 4–7. A. This tracing demonstrates wandering pacemaker in which the P waves actually become biphasic toward the end of the tracing, as the pacemaker site shifts about halfway down into the atria. Mild sinus arrhythmia is present, since the R-R intervals vary slightly.

Paper speed = 50 mm./sec., 1 cm. = 1 mv.

Illustration continued on opposite page.

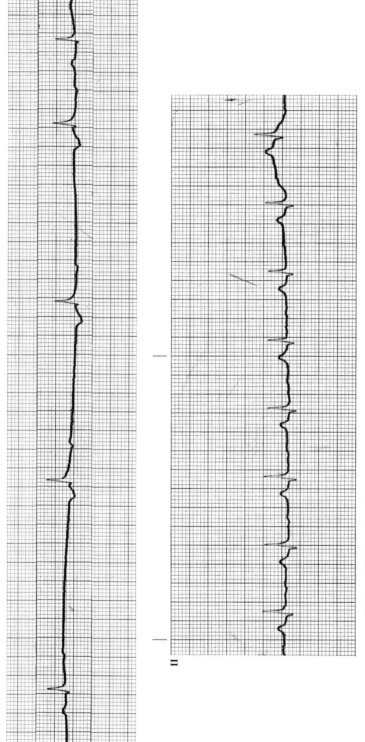

Figure 4–7B *Continued.*

B. In the above tracing, wandering pacemaker is so exaggerated that the P waves even become negative, since the pacemaker site shifts all the way down to the area of the atrioventricular node (junctional area). The lower tracing was recorded after the administration of atropine, which proves that the arrhythmia was vagally induced, since atropine abolished it.

Paper speed = 50 mm./sec., 1 cm. = mv.

II

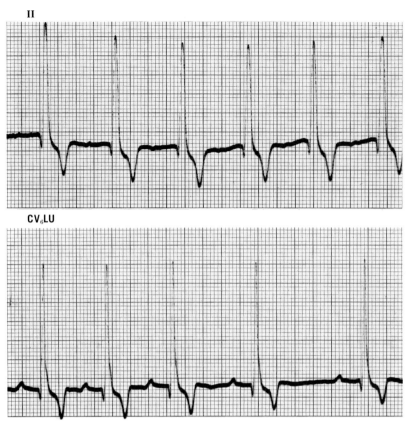

CV$_6$LU

Figure 4–8. In the top tracing, the P waves are hard to see because they are nearly isoelectric. By measuring one P-R interval and comparing it to the other beats, it can be seen that the small waves that are P waves all occur at the same interval from the QRS complexes. When the P waves are difficult to see in one lead, they may show up much better in another lead. In this case, when lead CV$_6$LU was recorded (bottom tracing), the P waves were much easier to see than in lead II.

Paper speed = 50 mm./sec., 1 cm. = 1 mv.

Sinoatrial (SA) block is a term that is sometimes seen in the literature. This really cannot be differentiated from sinus arrest on the electrocardiogram. Usually, with sinoatrial block, the pauses are exactly twice the normal R-R interval, while with sinus arrest the pauses are more than twice the normal R-R interval. For our purposes, sinus arrest and sinoatrial block will be considered as one and the same entity.

TREATMENT. If no clinical signs are present no treatment is required, as is usually the case. If syncope occurs in a brachycephalic dog and vagal arrhythmias are suspected to be the cause, atropine will suppress the vagal influence and improve the clinical signs.

Occasionally, the irregularity of the heart beat is so spectacular that atropine may be given to convince oneself that vagal tone is truly the cause (Fig. 4–10).

Sinus Tachycardia

ASSOCIATIONS. Sinus tachycardia is the most frequent arrhythmia of the dog, and its most frequent cause is nervousness. It is not usually

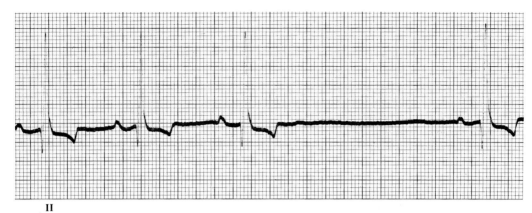

II

Figure 4–9. This lead II electrocardiogram demonstrates sinus arrest. It is a sinus rhythm because the P waves and the QRS complexes are related, and the tracing is grossly irregular. If the first two R-R intervals are used as the normals, it can be seen that the pause is longer than two of the normal R-R intervals, which makes this sinus arrest rather than sinus arrhythmia. A minor degree of wandering pacemaker is also present, as indicated by the slight fluctuation in the height of the P waves.

Paper speed = 50 mm./sec., 1 cm. = 1 mv.

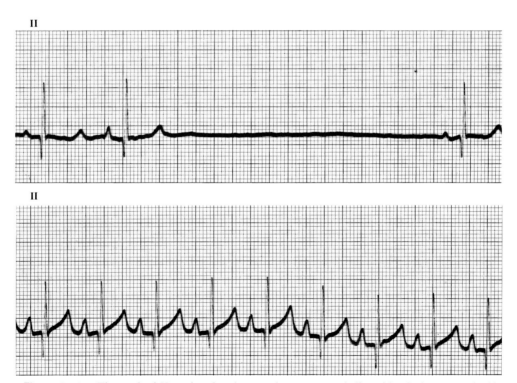

II

II

Figure 4–10. The top lead II tracing also shows a sinus arrest, as indicated by the long pause in this sinus rhythm, which is obviously longer than twice the normal R-R interval. A slight degree of wandering pacemaker is also present. The bottom strip was recorded after the administration of atropine, which proves that the arrhythmia was vagally induced.

Paper speed = 50 mm./sec., 1 cm. = 1 mv.

too surprising to discover that little Fifi has a heart rate of 200 beats per minute after she has been grabbed and wrestled to the table, and an electrocardiogram has been taken of her against her will. Sinus tachycardia also occurs secondary to a host of other disease states such as congestive heart failure, pneumonia, fever, anemia, hyperthyroidism, shock, or hexachlorophene poisoning, or after the dog has bitten an electric cord (Ettinger and Suter, 1970).

Clinical signs, when present, are usually referable to the primary disease, and sinus tachycardia is only another manifestation of the disease process.

PHYSICAL EXAMINATION. On physical examination, a continuous, rapid, usually regular heart beat is observed. There is no pulse deficit. The entire patient is evaluated to make a primary diagnosis. Usually the signs of the primary disease are noticed first, and the tachycardia is a secondary observation.

ELECTROCARDIOGRAPHIC DIAGNOSIS

1. The heart rate exceeds 160 beats per minute (180 beats per minute in toy breeds).

2. The rhythm is regular (there is usually a slight variation in the R-R intervals as a result of sinus arrhythmia).

3. There is a P wave for every QRS complex and a QRS complex for every P wave. (When the heart rate is very rapid, however, the P waves may be hidden in the T waves of the preceding beats.)

4. The P waves and QRS complexes are related (the P-R intervals are constant).

5. The P waves are all alike, and the QRS complexes are similar. *The P waves are also similar to the dog's P waves when the heart rate is normal.*

Figure 4–11 demonstrates sinus tachycardia in a collie that had a temperature of 107.5° F. At first, when the rate was rapid, the P waves were lost in the T waves of the preceding beats (Fig. 4–11A). As the temperature came down, the rate slowed, and the P waves began to emerge (Fig. 4–11B). When the temperature and the heart rate fell to normal, the P waves could be easily seen (Fig. 4–11C). It can also be noted that the P waves seen during an episode of tachycardia are similar to those seen when the rate is normal (Fig. 4–11).

Part of the clinical significance of sinus tachycardia lies in its similarity to atrial tachycardia, which is usually a much more severe arrhythmia. The two can be virtually indistinguishable, both on physical examination and on the electrocardiogram. Their differentiation is discussed in detail on page 117 and in Table 4–4.

TREATMENT. Usually, no specific treatment is given for the sinus tachycardia. Treatment of the primary problem will resolve the sinus tachycardia, as in the case of the collie (Fig. 4–11).

Sinus Bradycardia

ASSOCIATIONS. Sinus bradycardia is an uncommon arrhythmia in the dog. It may occur secondary to moderate elevations of serum potassium level, or following the administration of drugs such as tranquilizers

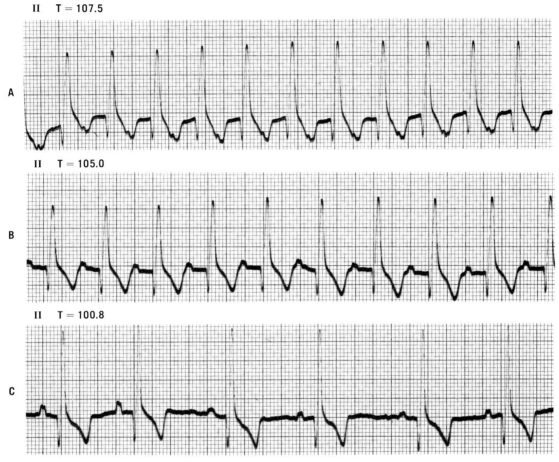

II   T = 107.5

A

II   T = 105.0

B

II   T = 100.8

C

Figure 4–11.   A. This lead II electrocardiogram was recorded from a collie that had a temperature of 107.5° F., and a sinus tachycardia. The heart rate is 250 beats per minute, and at this speed the P waves are buried in the T waves of the preceding beats. The P waves show up as a small notch at the bottom of each T wave. At this point the tracing is virtually indistinguishable from atrial tachycardia, but since the dog had such a high fever, it is safe to assume that this is probably a sinus tachycardia in response to the pyrexia.

B.   The dog was given a cold water bath, and when this strip was recorded his temperature was 105.0° F. The rate is now 200 beats per minute. The P waves are becoming visible as they begin to emerge from the T wave of each preceding beat. The morphology of the P waves can be seen.

C.   As a result of further cold water bathing the dog's temperature was only 100.8° F. when this tracing was recorded. Now the heart rate is normal, the P waves are easily seen, and a mild sinus arrhythmia is present. It can be seen that the P waves in this strip (when the rate was normal) look the same as the P waves in strip B (when tachycardia was present). This proves that this was a sinus tachycardia rather than an atrial tachycardia (see Figure 4–18). If this had been atrial tachycardia, the P waves would have been of a different configuration than the normal-rate P waves.

In this case, by knowing the dog and the circumstances, and by comparing normal heart rate P waves with the P waves during the tachycardia, a diagnosis of sinus tachycardia was made.

Paper speed = 50 mm./sec., 1 cm. = 1 mv.

TABLE 4–4. DIFFERENTIATION OF ATRIAL AND SINUS TACHYCARDIA

Atrial Tachycardia:	Sinus Tachycardia:
1. Tends to occur in older dogs with severe mitral insufficiency.	1. Can occur in any nervous or severely stressed animal.
2. Tends to occur in bursts or paroxysms.	2. Tends to be continuous.
3. Often terminates with ocular or carotid sinus pressure, and remains terminated until the next episode.	3. Usually does not terminate with ocular or carotid sinus pressure. If it does terminate, it resumes immediately when pressure is released.
4. On the electrocardiogram, the P waves during the tachycardia are positive, but different from the P waves when the heart rate is normal.	4. On the electrocardiogram, the tachycardia P waves are identical to the P waves when the heart rate is normal.
5. On the electrocardiogram, the R-R intervals tend to be exactly the same from beat to beat.	5. On the electrocardiogram, the R-R intervals tend to vary slightly because of sinus arrhythmia.

---

or sedatives. Often the bradycardia is mediated by the vagus nerve. Like sinus tachycardia, sinus bradycardia is usually a secondary complication of a pre-existing problem.

Clinical signs are absent unless the bradycardia is severe enough to cause a low cardiac output. Weakness, lethargy, or collapse could occur secondary to the slow heart rate.

PHYSICAL EXAMINATION. On auscultation, a heart rate of less than 70 beats per minute is the principal cardiac finding. There is neither a pulse deficit, nor is there a jugular pulse. When a slow heart rate is observed, the differential diagnosis must include sinus bradycardia, sinoatrial standstill (hyperkalemia), advanced heart block, ventricular or junctional escape rhythms, or occasionally sinus arrest (see Table 4–2). The electrocardiogram is essential for correct diagnosis.

ELECTROCARDIOGRAPHIC DIAGNOSIS

1. *The heart rate is less than 70 beats per minute.*

2. The rhythm may be regular or sinus arrhythmia may cause irregularity.

3. *There is a P wave for every QRS complex and a QRS complex for every P wave.*

4. The P waves and the QRS complexes are related (the P-R intervals may be prolonged as a result of the slow heart rate).

5. Wandering pacemaker may cause the P waves to vary in height, but the QRS complexes are all alike.

Figure 4–12 demonstrates a case of sinus bradycardia. This dog was given acepromazine without receiving atropine.

TREATMENT. Treatment is not necessary unless the sinus bradycardia is contributing to signs of weakness or collapse. Atropine usually will increase the heart rate, since sinus bradycardia is usually vagally induced. Isoproterenol may be used to increase the heart rate if atropine fails. Any primary abnormalities should be corrected.

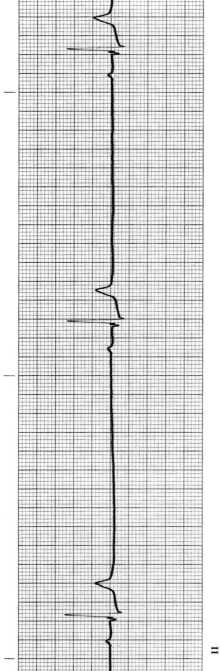

Figure 4–12. This lead II electrocardiogram demonstrates sinus bradycardia. The P waves and QRS complexes are related, and the heart rate is 37 to 42 beats per minute. Since most sinus bradycardias are vagally mediated, atropine might be used as a diagnostic aid to prove vagal involvement. Another thought would be to check the serum potassium levels to rule out hyperkalemia. If this were seen in an anesthetized dog, the anesthetic depth would be checked and lightened if necessary, or atropine would be given if the anesthetic depth were suitable. In this case, the dog had been given acepromazine without atropine.

Paper speed = 50 mm./sec., 1 cm. = 1 mv.

The Ectopic Arrhythmias

When an impulse originates from a site other than the sinoatrial node, it is ectopic. Ectopic impulses can arise from three areas: the atria (other than the sinoatrial node), the junctional tissues (tissues in the area of the atrioventricular node), or the ventricles (bundle of His or lower). If one of these areas becomes irritable and its rhythmicity is enhanced over that of the sinoatrial node, ectopic premature beats or ectopic tachycardia occurs. Tachycardias are more severe manifestations of the disease states that cause premature beats. Likewise, if something happens that depresses the sinoatrial node, such as increased vagal tone or hyperkalemia, the junctional (nodal) tissues or the ventricles can take over the rhythm at slower rates, and the escape rhythms are diagnosed.

Important in the study of the ectopic arrhythmias is proper application of the terms *supraventricular* and *ventricular*.

Atrial ectopic beats and junctional (nodal) ectopic beats are the two types of supraventricular ectopic arrhythmias (see Table 4–1). Supraventricular arrhythmias arise from the area of the atrioventricular node or higher (the atria). When these arrhythmias occur, *the P waves are altered* because the impulse arises from an unusual site, *but the QRS complexes remain normal,* since the impulse traverses the atrioventricular node and travels through the bundle of His, the Purkinje system, and the ventricular myocardium in a normal manner. Figure 4–13 shows an example of an atrial premature beat, and Figure 4–14 shows an example of a junctional (nodal) premature beat. These are discussed in detail later, but the important thing to remember now is that the P wave is abnormal and the QRS complex is normal. It is not very important to distinguish between atrial and junctional ectopic arrhythmias,

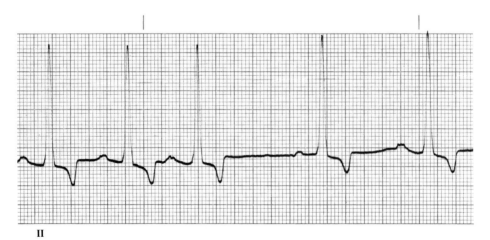

II

Figure 4–13. This lead II electrocardiogram demonstrates an atrial premature beat (third beat from left). It occurs early, is followed by a pause, the QRS complex remains normal, and the P wave is positive but different from the P waves of the normal beats. This tracing was recorded from an 11-year-old mixed breed dog that had signs of congestive heart failure due to severe mitral insufficiency. He eventually developed atrial fibrillation. He was successfully treated with digoxin, rest, and low sodium diet for almost 2 years.

Paper speed = 50 mm./sec., 1 cm. = 1 mv.

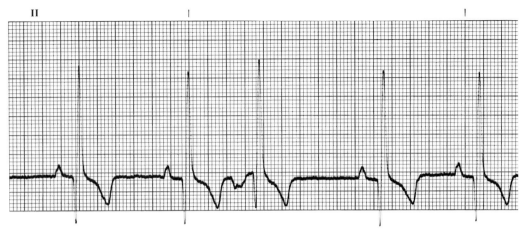

Figure 4–14. This lead II electrocardiogram demonstrates a junctional premature beat (third from left). It occurs early, is followed by a pause, the QRS complex remains normal, and the P wave is negative. This was recorded from a dog whose primary problem was posterior paresis. It was surmised that the dog had atrial myocarditis. The dog subsequently died.

Paper speed = 50 mm./sec., 1 cm. = 1 mv.

(Tracing courtesy of Dr. M. Lorenz, Athens, Ga.)

because their treatment is the same. It is more important to distinguish between the supraventricular and ventricular arrhythmias; their treatment is different.

When ectopic beats arise in the ventricles, the QRS complex is distorted. It is distorted because the normal sequence of ventricular depolarization is broken. Figure 4–24 shows a tracing taken from a dog that was intoxicated by digitalis and had both supraventricular and ventricular premature beats. It can be seen that the conformation of the QRS complex remains normal when the supraventricular premature beat occurs, but is grossly distorted and bizarre when the ventricular premature beats occur.

The other hallmark of ventricular premature beats is that they are not associated with P waves. This is because the ventricular focus becomes irritable and discharges prematurely without waiting for the atria to discharge first. As a result, either no P wave is seen, as in Figure 4–26, or the P waves that occur are obviously not related to the bizarre QRS complexes because the P-R interval is grossly different, as in Figure 4–25. This becomes important on occasion, because if a ventricular ectopic beat arises in or near the bundle of His, as in Figure 4–31, the ventricular complexes can look fairly normal, but still they are not associated with P waves.

The differentiation between supraventricular and ventricular arrhythmias is extremely important because the treatment for each is very different. The supraventricular arrhythmias in general are treated with digitalis, while the ventricular arrhythmias in general are treated with quinidine (antiarrhythmic agents). There are very few exceptions to this general rule, and mistakes may be fatal. Once again, remember that digitalis can cause every arrhythmia ever reported, and *any arrhythmia that develops after the institution of digitalis therapy should be considered a sign of digitalis intoxication until proved otherwise.*

The ectopic arrhythmias are first suspected during physical examination by auscultation of an irregular rhythm not associated with respiration, by auscultation of tachycardia or bradycardia, by detecting a pulse deficit, or by noting a jugular pulse (see pp. 90–92). The electrocardiogram then finally identifies the type of arrhythmia, allowing the clinician to begin the proper therapy.

Supraventricular Ectopic Arrhythmias

Atrial and Junctional Premature Beats. ASSOCIATIONS. Supraventricular premature beats most commonly occur in dogs that have severe atrioventricular valvular insufficiency, with resulting atrial enlargement (Patterson et al., 1961). The enlargement and stretching of the atrial fibers actually causes edema and foci of inflammation (Patterson et al., 1961); in turn, these very irritable atrial fibers tend to discharge prematurely. As the irritation becomes more severe, the supraventricular premature beats become more frequent, and eventually atrial tachycardia or, even worse, atrial fibrillation may occur. The classic case in which atrial and junctional (nodal) premature beats occur is the aged dog that has severe mitral valvular fibrosis and insufficiency.

Less commonly tumors, such as aortic body tumors or hemangiosarcomas, can infiltrate the atrial myocardium and cause atrial premature beats. Severe toxemias such as uremia can cause toxic myocarditis of the atria or the ventricles, and can give rise to atrial or junctional (nodal) premature beats. The vagus nerve depresses the sinoatrial and the atrioventricular nodes, but actually increases the excitability of the atrial fibers (Moe and Farah, 1970), and vagal hypertonia can cause supraventricular premature beats.

Digitalis intoxication frequently causes atrial and junctional (nodal) premature beats, so if either of these arrhythmias occurs while the dog is on digitalis it should be considered a sign of digitalis intoxication.

Clinical signs do not develop until the premature beats become frequent. When they are frequent, or when tachycardia begins to occur, the dog may show signs of weakness, lethargy, ataxia, collapse, or seizure. Signs of congestive heart failure may be present (since the dog usually has severe mitral insufficiency), but congestive heart failure is not always present. In an older dog that is known to have mitral insufficiency and is experiencing syncopal episodes, the supraventricular arrhythmias should be highly suspect.

If digitalis intoxication is the cause of the premature beats, the animal may also show physical signs of anorexia, vomiting, and diarrhea.

PHYSICAL EXAMINATION. On physical examination, premature beats that break the normal rhythm are heard, and are followed by a pause. It sounds like: lub dup, lub dup, lub dup dup—pause—lub dup, lub dup, lub dup, lub dup dup—pause. The murmur of mitral or tricuspid insufficiency, or perhaps both, may also be heard. If the atrial irritation is severe, paroxysms of tachycardia may also be heard. If the femoral pulse is compared with the heart beat, a pulse deficit may be felt when the premature beats occur. The supraventricular premature beats do not cause a jugular pulse.

ELECTROCARDIOGRAPHIC DIAGNOSIS

1. The heart rate is normal unless the premature beats are very frequent or unless the dog is in congestive heart failure.

2. *The rhythm is irregular, being broken by a premature PQRS complex or complexes followed by a pause.*

3. There is a P wave for every QRS complex and a QRS complex for every P wave (the P wave of the premature beat may be hidden in the T wave of the preceding beat).

4. The P waves are related to the QRS complexes (the P-R interval may be slightly shorter or longer).

5. *The P wave of the premature beat is altered.* In cases of atrial premature beat, the P wave is positive, but different from the normal P waves, while in cases of junctional (nodal) premature beat, the P wave is negative.

6. *The QRS complexes retain their normal configuration.*

Figure 4–13 demonstrates an atrial premature beat, while Figure 4–14 shows an example of a junctional (nodal) premature beat. In both, the PQRS complex occurs early and is followed by a pause, but the P wave of the atrial premature beat is positive and the P wave of the junctional premature beat is negative. In both instances it can be seen that the P wave of the premature beat is different in shape from the P waves of the normal beats.

In Figure 4–15, a premature beat is demonstrated, but a P wave cannot be identified because it is hidden in the T wave of the preceding beat. The beat can be recognized as supraventricular because the QRS complex is not altered, but it cannot be determined whether the P wave is positive or negative. In this instance all that can be said is that it is a supraventricular premature beat. This is sufficient, because supraventricular premature beats are treated the same, whether they are atrial or junctional. The important thing to recognize is that it is supraventricular.

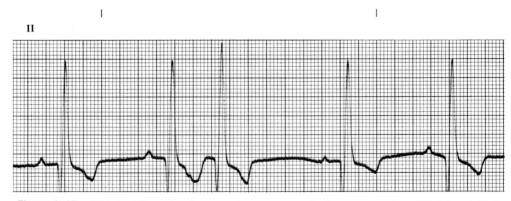

Figure 4–15. This lead II tracing demonstrates a supraventricular premature beat (third from left). It occurs early, is followed by a pause, and the QRS complex remains essentially normal. This time the P wave cannot be evaluated because it is hidden in the T wave of the preceding beat, so it is not possible to say whether this is an atrial or a junctional premature beat; however, the treatment of either condition is the same. This was recorded from the same dog as in Figure 4–14.

Paper speed = 50 mm./sec., 1 cm. = 1 mv.

(Tracing courtesy of Dr. M. Lorenz, Athens, Ga.)

The P-R interval may be slightly prolonged, because the premature beat may be so early that the atrioventricular node or the ventricles have not fully recovered from the last beat and thus may take slightly longer to conduct the impulse. Often for the same reason the QRS complex may be slightly shorter or taller than the normal ones, but the conformation is still the same. In the case of junctional premature beats, the P-R interval may be shorter because of the short distance to the atrioventricular node. Occasionally, if a junctional premature beat arises on the ventricular side of the atrioventricular node, the ventricles may depolarize before the impulse can go backward through the node and stimulate the atria. In these instances, a negative P wave may actually occur behind the QRS complex (usually between the QRS and the T wave).

When one premature beat occurs alone, it is called a single. When two in a row occur, it is called a pair. The occurrence of three such beats in a row is a run. Four or more premature beats in a row is called tachycardia. This applies to both supraventricular and ventricular ectopic beats. Figures 4-13, 4-14, and 4-15 demonstrate single supraventricular premature beats. Figure 4-16 demonstrates a pair of supraventricular premature beats.

When every other beat is a premature beat, this is called bigeminy. When every third beat is a premature beat, or when there are two premature beats to every normal beat, it is called trigeminy. Figure 4-17 demonstrates a supraventricular bigeminy.

TREATMENT. The treatment of choice for supraventricular premature beats is digitalis. Most dogs with these arrhythmias have severe mitral insufficiency and either are in congestive heart failure or are prone to it. Digitalis is the drug of choice for congestive heart failure; this drug also controls the heart rate by slowing conduction through the atrioventricular node, thus also preventing the development of tachycardia. If a dog with mitral insufficiency has even a few supraventricular premature

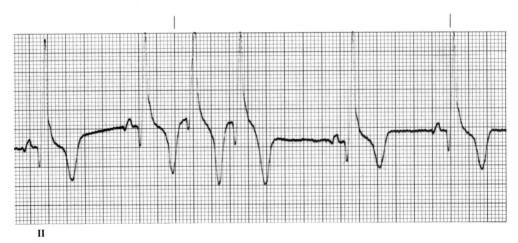

II

Figure 4-16. In this lead II tracing two supraventricular premature beats occur in a row. They are supraventricular because their QRS complexes are near-normal. It is not possible to determine whether they are atrial or junctional in origin, because their P waves are hidden in the T waves of the preceding beats. When two premature beats occur in succession they are called a pair.

Paper speed = 50 mm./sec., 1 cm. = 1 mv.

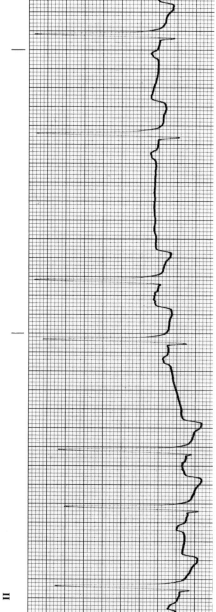

Figure 4–17. This lead II electrocardiogram demonstrates atrial bigeminy. The third and the fifth beats from the left are atrial premature beats. They occur early, are followed by a pause, their QRS complexes remain normal, and small positive P waves occur that are different from the P waves of the normal beats. When every other beat is a premature beat, it is called a bigeminy. This is an atrial bigeminy.

Paper speed = 50 mm./sec., 1 cm. = 1 mv.

beats, he should be digitalized whether he shows signs of cardiac decompensation or not.

Quinidine and procainamide should not be used for treatment of supraventricular arrhythmias. They would be very effective in controlling supraventricular premature beats, but they also depress the myocardium, which may be disastrous in a dog that is in congestive heart failure or is prone to it. These drugs can be used for supraventricular premature beats only if the premature beats are not caused by severe mitral or tricuspid insufficiency. Examples of their acceptable use are uncommon, but would include such conditions as uremic atrial myocarditis, neoplastic infiltration of the atria, traumatic atrial myocarditis, or bacterial endomyocarditis.

When the supraventricular premature beats arise after digitalis therapy is begun, they should be considered a sign of digitalis intoxication, and digitalis should be discontinued until the arrhythmias subside and the dog shows no physical signs of intoxication. The digitalis is then resumed at a slightly lower dosage. For instance, if the dog was receiving 0.25 mg. of digoxin b.i.d. when intoxication occurred, the dose would be reduced to 0.25 mg. in the morning, and 0.125 mg. in the evening. Treatment of digitalis intoxication is summarized by Ettinger and Suter (1970).

Atrial Tachycardia (Paroxysmal Atrial Tachycardia). ASSOCIATIONS. Atrial tachycardia is a more serious sign of the same disease states that cause atrial premature beats, and, as such, is seen as a more advanced stage of mitral insufficiency, when the atrial strain is more significant. It has also been reported in dogs with aortic body tumors infiltrating the atrial walls (Patterson et al., 1961; Roos, 1937).

Clinical signs include weakness, inability to exercise, lethargy, and ataxia, and a common presenting complaint is syncope. When many atrial premature beats or atrial tachycardia occurs, blood pressure decreases precipitously, causing syncope. This arrhythmia should be the prime suspect in any older dog that has severe mitral insufficiency and is experiencing syncopal episodes. Signs of congestive heart failure are usually, but not always, present. If the arrhythmia is due to digitalis intoxication, vomiting, anorexia, and diarrhea may occur.

PHYSICAL EXAMINATION. The usual finding is that of a burst of tachycardia, e.g., lub dup, lub dup, lub dup dup dup dup dup dup dup dup dup—pause—lub dup, lub dup, lub dup. Single premature beats may also be present, and mitral insufficiency is usually obvious. When tachycardia is continuous, it is virtually indistinguishable from sinus tachycardia on physical examination. If premature beats are present, a pulse deficit may be palpated, but there is no jugular pulse due to this arrhythmia.

When the bouts of tachycardia occur, the animal may become weak or may collapse. The syncopal episodes usually are of short duration (seconds), and may or may not be accompanied by seizures.

ELECTROCARDIOGRAPHIC DIAGNOSIS

1. *Intermittent (usually) or continuous (occasionally) tachycardia is present.*

2. *The tachycardia tends to be regular (R-R intervals are the same).*

3. There is a P wave for every QRS complex and a QRS complex for every P wave (the P waves may be hidden in the T wave of the preceding beat).

4. The P waves are related to the QRS complexes (P-R intervals are constant).

5. *The P waves during the tachycardia are positive, but different from the P waves when the heart rate is normal.* The QRS complexes are normal.

Figure 4–18 demonstrates atrial tachycardia in a dog. Atrial tachycardia and sinus tachycardia are difficult to distinguish both on physical examination and on electrocardiography (see page 106). There are several observations and procedures that can be used to make the differentiation.

First, and most valuable, is the patient and his clinical signs. Atrial tachycardia most often occurs in the older dog that has severe mitral insufficiency and is in congestive heart failure or is experiencing syncopal episodes. Sinus tachycardia can occur in any dog that is severely ill, and a common cause of physiological sinus tachycardia is nervousness or excitement. It can also occur secondary to congestive heart failure, however.

Secondly, atrial tachycardia tends to occur in bursts or paroxysms (paroxysmal atrial tachycardia), and atrial premature beats may occur between paroxysms. Sinus tachycardia tends to be continuous. Atrial tachycardia may be continuous, however.

Thirdly, a clinical test can be done. Digital pressure on the eyeballs or in the area of the bifurcation of the carotid artery will reflexly increase vagal tone. Such ocular or carotid sinus pressure often will terminate a bout of atrial tachycardia, and, after the pressure is released, the rhythm will remain normal until the next episode. Sinus tachycardia, on the other hand, usually cannot be terminated by this procedure, and even when it does terminate, the tachycardia will resume immediately after the pressure is released.

Fourthly, the P waves of atrial tachycardia are positive, but different from the P waves when the heart rate is normal (Fig. 4–18). With sinus tachycardia, the P waves during the tachycardia are the same as the P waves when the heart rate is normal (Fig. 4–11).

Lastly, the R-R intervals of atrial tachycardia tend to be exactly the same, while the R-R intervals of sinus tachycardia may vary slightly because of the influence of sinus arrhythmia. This is not a good criterion, however, since sinus tachycardia can be regular, and atrial tachycardia may be slightly irregular.

Although none of the foregoing criteria are perfect, collectively they make it possible to decide in most instances whether one is dealing with sinus tachycardia or atrial tachycardia. Table 4–4 summarizes the methods used to differentiate atrial and sinus tachycardia.

If the P waves during the tachycardia are hidden in the T waves of the preceding beats, as in Figure 4–19, it can still be said that the tachycardia is supraventricular in origin, because during the burst of tachycardia the QRS complexes retain a relatively normal conformation. Again, the important thing is to recognize it as a supraventricular arrhythmia, for treatment purposes.

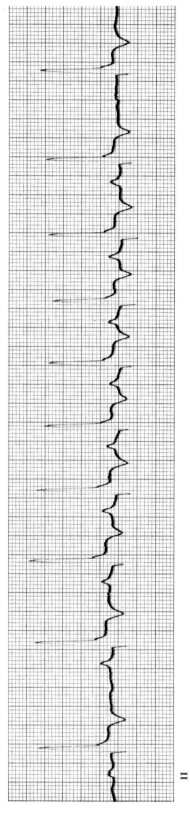

Figure 4–18. In the middle of this tracing, a burst of atrial tachycardia occurs. This is paroxysmal atrial tachycardia (PAT), because it occurs in paroxysms, the QRS complexes remain normal, and the P waves during the tachycardia are positive, but different from the P waves when the rate is normal. This differentiates it from sinus tachycardia, in which the P waves during the tachycardia are the same as the P waves when the rate is normal (see Figure 4–11). The normal heart rate in this tracing is about 100 beats per minute, while the tachycardia occurs at about 180 beats per minute.
Paper speed = 50 mm./sec., 1 cm. = 1 mv.

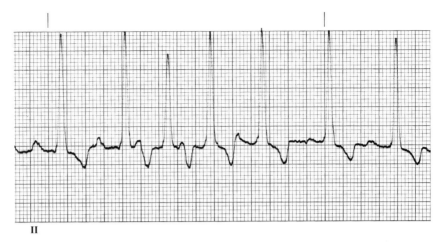

II

Figure 4–19. In the middle of this lead II tracing a burst of three supraventricular premature beats occurs. Since the P waves are hidden in the T waves of the preceding beats, it cannot be determined whether these are atrial or junctional in origin. It would appear that they are atrial premature beats because the P waves do show a little between the QRS complex and the T wave in each of the preceding beats, and they appear to be positive and slightly different than the normal P waves. Although the QRS complex of the first premature beat is slightly shorter than the others, it still has a similar morphology. Technically this is an atrial run, since there are three premature beats in a row. Four or more in a row is an atrial tachycardia. This was recorded from the 11-year-old mixed breed dog in Figure 4–13 that had severe mitral insufficiency. These atrial arrhythmias became worse, and the dog eventually developed atrial fibrillation.
    Paper speed = 50 mm./sec., 1 cm. = 1 mv.

TREATMENT.   The treatment of choice for atrial tachycardia is digitalis. Digitalis controls the tachycardia by slowing conduction through the atrioventricular node. It also increases myocardial contractility and controls symptoms of congestive heart failure.

Again, although quinidine or procainamide would effectively control this arrhythmia, these drugs are depressing to the myocardium and would be likely to precipitate or aggravate congestive heart failure. If atrial tachycardia were due to an extracardiac lesion, such as a heart base tumor, quinidine could be used, but in most instances of atrial tachycardia quinidine is contraindicated.

Ocular or carotid sinus pressure can be used as a temporary measure to break the episodes of atrial tachycardia. Another method that has been used to increase vagal tone and break the arrhythmia is the intravenous injection of vasopressors such as phenylephrine or methoxamine. This increases blood pressure, reflexly stimulates the vagus nerve, and breaks the arrhythmia (Ettinger and Suter, 1970). One should think twice about the use of these drugs in a dog with severe mitral insufficiency. Cholinergic drugs such as neostigmine or edrophonium have been used in man to increase vagal effect (Bellet, 1973), but these could also be stressing to a dog that is predisposed to congestive heart failure.

If the arrhythmia occurs as a result of digitalis intoxication, digitalis is stopped until the arrhythmia and all physical signs of digitalis overdose disappear. The digitalis is then resumed at a slightly lower dosage.

Atrial Fibrillation. ASSOCIATIONS. Atrial fibrillation is another supraventricular tachycardia. It is a more severe consequence of the same abnormalities that cause atrial premature beats and atrial tachycardia. When atrial fibrillation occurs it is a grave sign because it indicates that the atrioventricular valvular insufficiency is severe and atrial enlargement and stretching are severe. In man, atrial fibrillation can occur in the absence of primary heart disease (Friedberg, 1966), but in the dog it indicates severe atrial disease.

There are several types of dogs in which this arrhythmia tends to occur. The old dog with severe mitral insufficiency may develop atrial fibrillation when left atrial enlargement becomes severe. Dogs with idiopathic cardiomyopathy consistently develop atrial fibrillation secondary to the severe atrioventricular valvular insufficiencies that develop (Ettinger and Suter, 1970). A few of the congenital heart defects, such as patent ductus arteriosus, ventricular septal defect, congenital mitral insufficiency (Dear, 1971; Ettinger and Suter, 1970; Weirich, 1974), tricuspid valvular hypoplasia, pulmonic stenosis (Detweiler, 1957), and aortic stenosis (Flickenger and Patterson, 1967), can cause atrial fibrillation. In these defects, severe atrioventricular valvular insufficiency develops secondary to ventricular dilatation.

By the time atrial fibrillation is diagnosed, signs of biventricular congestive heart failure are usually present. A prominent presenting complaint by the owner is the pot-bellied appearance of the dog, which is caused by the accumulation of ascitic fluid. On closer examination shortness of breath, exercise intolerance, coughing, and dyspnea are usually present, although the signs of right heart failure predominate. Clinical signs may develop rapidly. Dogs with idiopathic cardiomyopathy often present with a two-week history of weight loss, ascites, and dyspnea. Hydrothorax may develop, and the respiratory signs may be severe. Sometimes fainting occurs.

Occasionally, a larger breed of dog may have atrial fibrillation but have no symptoms (Buchanan, 1961). The author has seen two Irish wolfhounds that were in atrial fibrillation but were asymptomatic. They can apparently defy the rules, although they may have primary atrial disease.

PHYSICAL EXAMINATION. The physical examination of the dog in atrial fibrillation is classic. The heart rate is rapid and irregular, there is a pulse deficit, and a jugular pulse is present. To confuse the picture further, a gallop rhythm (third heart sound) is usually present. Murmurs may or may not be heard. Sometimes the valvular insufficiency is so great that blood just sludges from atrium to ventricle and back again without any turbulence, and no murmur is produced. The rapid, irregular rate and the abnormal heart sounds present a picture of utter chaos in the chest when the heart is heard on auscultation. There is simply no rhyme or reason to the heart beat.

In both of the asymptomatic Irish wolfhounds the heart rate was normal despite atrial fibrillation. The heart beat was still grossly irregular, and a pulse deficit was present. No murmurs were heard.

ELECTROCARDIOGRAPHIC DIAGNOSIS

1. *The heart rate exceeds 160 beats per minute, and often exceeds 220 beats per minute.*

2. *The rhythm is irregular*, although at very rapid heart rates it may not appear spectacularly so.

3. *There are no P waves or P-R intervals*.

4. The P waves are replaced by fine baseline undulations called "f" waves, which represent the chaotic electrical activity of the fibrillating atria.

5. The QRS complexes are fairly normal, and no P waves are present.

Figure 4–20 is an electrocardiogram recorded from a Doberman pinscher that was in atrial fibrillation as a result of idiopathic cardiomyopathy. The top tracing was taken before digitalis was given. The bottom tracing was taken after administration of the digitalis. It can be seen that the heart beat is rapid, it is irregular, and no P waves can be found, not even when pauses occur. Instead, small "f" waves are seen as the atria

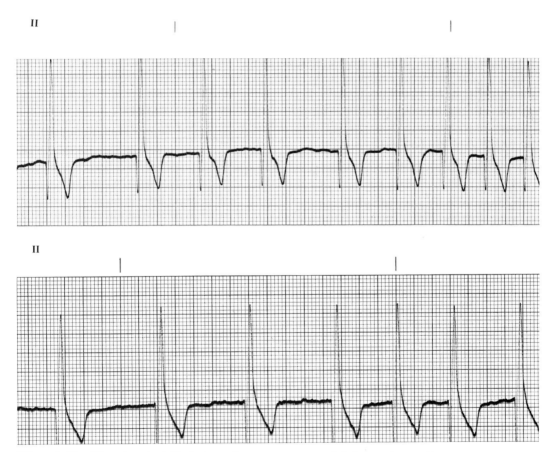

Figure 4–20. These two lead II electrocardiograms were recorded from a 4-year-old Doberman pinscher that was in atrial fibrillation because of idiopathic cardiomyopathy. The top tracing was taken prior to digitalization. The QRS complexes look like relatively normal lead II complexes, which indicates that this is a supraventricular tachycardia. The heart rate is rapid and irregular and no P waves can be found, not even when pauses in the rhythm occur. An irregular supraventricular tachycardia with no P waves is diagnostic of atrial fibrillation. The minute fasciculations of the baseline are "f waves," and represent chaotic atrial activity. In the bottom tracing, taken at a later date, the heart rate has been controlled with digoxin. The rhythm is still irregular, the "f waves" can be seen, and the lack of P waves is readily apparent. The dog lived for 2 years on treatment, even though his atrial fibrillation was permanent.

Paper speed = 50 mm./sec., 1 cm. = 1 mv.

fibrillate. There is no coordinated atrial beat, and the atrioventricular node is bombarded by millions of impulses. Many go through the atrioventricular node and stimulate a ventricular contraction, but they do so irregularly. Some cancel each other out, while others go through in a random and irregular manner. The QRS complexes often vary slightly in height, as in Figure 4–20, because the ventricles are depolarized so quickly that parts of the ventricle are not yet completely repolarized when the next beat occurs, and, as a result, conduction is slightly aberrant, and the complex is slightly different.

Cases of paroxysmal atrial fibrillation, in which the arrhythmias have come and gone spontaneously, have been reported (Bolton and Ettinger, 1971).

TREATMENT.   The treatment of choice for atrial fibrillation, as with all the supraventricular arrhythmias, is digitalis. Digitalis improves the congestive heart failure and controls the heart rate by delaying conduction through the atrioventricular node. Digitalis actually increases the fibrillatory pattern of the atria (Moe and Farah, 1970). This increases the number of impulses that cancel each other out, which also decreases the heart rate. The aim of digitalis therapy is to reduce the heart rate to less than 160 beats per minute. Diuretics or aminophylline may be needed when ascites is present, and a low sodium diet and enforced rest are also indicated.

Once the heart rate and the congestive heart failure are under control with digitalis, quinidine can be added to the treatment regime in an attempt to restore the chaotic atrial rhythm to a sinus rhythm. Digitalis therapy is continued while quinidine is being given. Quinidine therapy is usually unsuccessful, but occasionally the rhythm may convert to normal. When it does convert, it is usually only temporary, because the severe atrial disorder is still present. In the author's opinion, attempts at quinidine conversion are unwarranted except in special cases such as the Newfoundland described below. As long as the heart rate can be controlled with digitalis, quinidine therapy does not seem either to alter the course of the disease or to increase the longevity of the patient.

Recently a young Newfoundland was presented to our clinic. She had been hit by a car one day previously. She had an acetabular fracture, and atrial fibrillation was diagnosed (Fig. 4–21). Traumatic myocarditis was diagnosed when no atrial enlargement could be seen in radiographs of the chest. She was first treated with digitalis, and, once the heart rate was controlled, quinidine was given, and on the second day of quinidine therapy she converted to a sinus rhythm (Fig. 4–21). In this instance, quinidine was used because it was hoped that the atrial bruising would heal itself, and that sinus rhythm could be maintained. After 6 weeks on quinidine (digitalis therapy was discontinued), sinus rhythm was present, and she was well. One week after withdrawal of the quinidine, atrial fibrillation reoccurred. This time quinidine therapy failed to convert the rhythm, and D.C. cardioversion was successfully employed to reconvert her to sinus rhythm. The dog is now doing well and is being maintained indefinitely on quinidine.

D.C. cardioversion is a reliable method of converting atrial fibrillation if the proper equipment is available (Ettinger, 1968; Ettinger and Suter, 1970). A shock is applied over the heart precisely 2.5 milliseconds after the R wave of the electrocardiogram. This method of cardio-

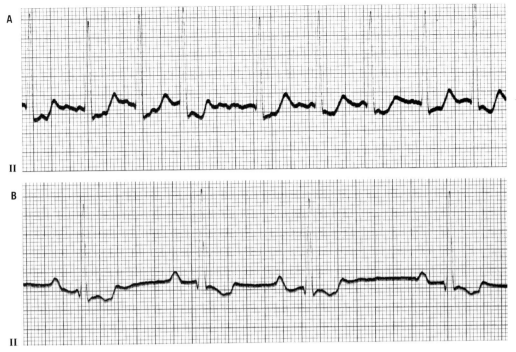

Figure 4–21. A. This lead II electrocardiogram was recorded from a 5-year-old New-foundland dog that had been hit by a car and had traumatic myocarditis and atrial fibrillation. The heart rate averages about 220 per minute and is irregular. The QRS complexes look fairly normal for lead II, as one would expect with a supraventricular tachycardia. When the pauses occur, no specific P waves can be seen. An irregular supraventricular tachycardia with no P waves is diagnostic of atrial fibrillation.

B. The dog was treated with digoxin until the heart rate was under control, and then quinidine was added to the treatment regime. On the second day of quinidine therapy she converted to sinus rhythm, and this lead II tracing was recorded after she converted. The heart rate is normal, P waves are present now, and the QRS complexes are the same as they were during the tachycardia. A mild sinus arrhythmia is also present.

Paper speed = 50 mm./sec., 1 cm. = 1 mv.

version requires anesthesia. It has been used with success, but, in most instances, as with quinidine therapy, the rhythm soon reverts to atrial fibrillation because of the severe atrial disease.

The prognosis when atrial fibrillation occurs is guarded. Most dogs are well during treatment for approximately 4 to 6 months, although some have lived for 2 years.

Atrial Flutter. ASSOCIATIONS. This is an uncommon arrhythmia in the dog (Clark et al., 1966), but it carries the same significance as the other supraventricular tachycardias and indicates severe atrial disease. It has been reported (Detweiler, 1957; Gratzl, 1960; Pedini, 1954; and Robertson, 1970), and in Detweiler's report, two cases occurred while atrial fibrillation was being treated with quinidine. We have seen atrial flutter in a 17-year-old German shepherd that was suspected of having ruptured chordae tendineae (Fig. 5–105).

ELECTROCARDIOGRAPHIC DIAGNOSIS

1. The heart rate may be normal or rapid.
2. The rhythm is usually regular, but may be irregular.

3. *There are no P-R intervals, but the ventricles may respond in a periodic manner, usually in a 2:1, 3:1, or 4:1 manner.*

4. *The QRS complexes are normal, P waves are absent and replaced by baseline "f" waves, and there are several "f" waves for every QRS complex.*

Figure 4–22 demonstrates atrial flutter. Atrial flutter may be easily misdiagnosed when trembling artifacts occur on the electrocardiogram (Fig. 3–43).

TREATMENT. Atrial flutter is a supraventricular tachycardia, and the treatment of choice is digitalis, which controls the heart rate. Once the dog is stabilized on digitalis therapy, quinidine can be added to the treatment regime in an attempt to convert the arrhythmia to a sinus rhythm. Robertson (1970) reports the successful conversion of atrial flutter using digitalis and quinidine in combination.

Junctional (Nodal) Tachycardia. ASSOCIATIONS. Junctional tachycardia is most often due to digitalis intoxication, although it may occur secondary to severe atrioventricular valvular insufficiency or vagal hypertonia, or in response to inflammatory changes in the atria (atrial myocarditis).

Clinical signs may be those of digitalis intoxication, namely, vomiting and anorexia. Signs of weakness, lethargy, or syncope may also occur during the bouts of tachycardia.

PHYSICAL EXAMINATION. The physical examination may not be remarkable, because there may be a normal heart rate in junctional tachycardia. The spontaneous rhythm of the junctional tissues is 40 to 60 beats per minute, as indicated in Chapter 1. Therefore tachycardia of the junctional tissues often occurs within the normal limits of heart rate for the dog. Tachycardia may be heard to occur in paroxysms. There may be a pulse deficit if premature beats are also present. Usually no jugular pulse is detected.

ELECTROCARDIOGRAPHIC DIAGNOSIS

1. *Heart rate may be normal or tachycardia may be present.*

2. The rhythm is usually regular; tachycardia may occur in bursts.

3. There is a P wave for every QRS complex, and a QRS complex for every P wave (the P waves may be hidden in the T waves of the preceding beats).

4. The P waves and the QRS complexes are related.

5. *The P waves are negative while the QRS complexes are normal.*

Figure 4–23 demonstrates junctional tachycardia. The word "tachycardia" can be misleading in this instance. Since the spontaneous rate of the junctional tissues is 40 to 60 beats per minute, any heart rate above 60 beats per minute constitutes tachycardia of the junctional tissues. The heart rate in Figure 4–23 is about 150 beats per minute, so this is junctional tachycardia. The negative P waves indicate that the beats originate near the junctional tissues in the area of the atrioventricular node and travel backward through the atria toward the sinoatrial node.

TREATMENT. Since this arrhythmia is usually due to digitalis intoxication, withdrawal of the drug is necessary until the arrhythmia abates and there is no vomiting or anorexia. Digitalis is then resumed at a slightly lower dosage. If the dog is not on digitalis and junctional

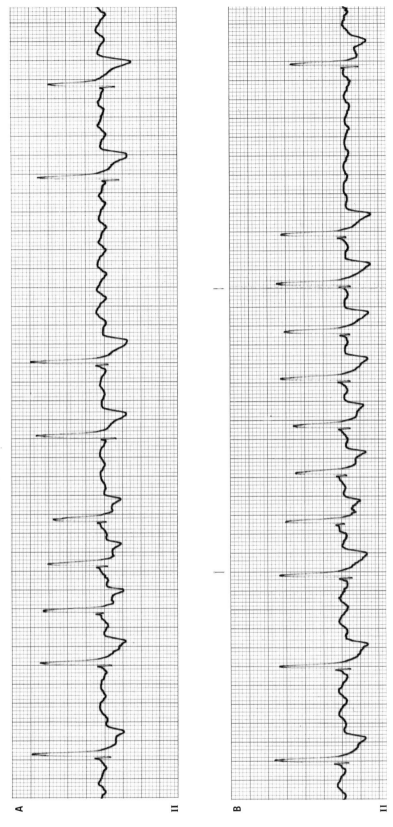

Figure 4-22. These continuous lead II electrocardiograms were recorded from a 10-year-old male border collie with chronic mitral valvular fibrosis and congestive heart failure, being treated with digitalis. Atrial flutter is demonstrated by the regular baseline fasciculations, called "f waves". The ventricular responses in these tracings are irregular; however, the ventricles may respond in a regular manner. As the bursts of tachycardia occur, the QRS complexes become slightly altered because the ventricles begin to depolarize so quickly that some parts of the ventricles are still refractory when the next impulse originates, and conduction must proceed via a slightly aberrant pathway. The basic conformation of the QRS complexes remains the same, but they become shorter. Slurring of the S-T segment is also present, which indicates left ventricluar hypertrophy.

Paper speed = 50 mm./sec., 1 cm. = 1 mv.

(Tracing courtesy of Dr. W. Thomas, Philadelphia, Pa.)

II

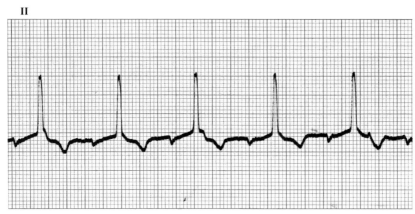

Figure 4–23. This junctional tachycardia was recorded from a miniature poodle with digitalis intoxication. The P waves and QRS complexes are consistently related, and the P waves are negative, which indicates that their origin is in the junctional tissues. The spontaneous rate of the junctional tissues is 40 to 60 per minute, so in this case a rate of 150 per minute is a tachycardia for the junctional tissues.
Paper speed = 50 mm./sec., 1 cm. = 1 mv.

tachycardia occurs, digitalization is the treatment of choice, since it is a supraventricular arrhythmia.

Ventricular Arrhythmias

Ventricular Premature Beats and Ventricular Tachycardia. ASSOCIA-TIONS. Ventricular premature beats and ventricular tachycardia are caused by irritation or inflammation of the ventricular myocardium. Thus, they indicate ventricular myocarditis. Primary disease of the myocardium occurs infrequently in dogs; whenever myocarditis does occur, it is usually secondary to another disease state, such as viral, bacterial, mycotic, or protozoal infection, hyperthyroidism, hypothyroidism, anemia, malnutrition, electrolyte imbalance, parasitic infections, uremia, pyometra, pancreatitis, endotoxemia, neoplasia, trauma, diabetes mellitus, endocarditis, pericarditis, and pleural effusion, to mention a few (Bolton, 1973; Ettinger and Suter, 1970).

Ventricular premature beats may occur secondary to drugs such as digitalis, phenothiazine derivative tranquilizers, and anesthetics (see Chapter 3). Stress and anxiety can cause them to occur (Ettinger and Suter, 1970). Some cardiac diseases—for example, mitral insufficiency, aortic stenosis, and idiopathic cardiomyopathy—are frequently associated with ventricular premature beats. Also, older dogs commonly have multiple microscopic intramural myocardial infarcts in the left ventricle (Jonsson, 1972; Patterson, 1961). Although they are clinically insignificant, these minute areas of ischemia result in irritation and stimulate an occasional ventricular premature beat. So if occasional ventricular premature beats occur in an older dog, they are due probably to one of these minute ischemic areas, and carry little clinical significance unless they occur frequently.

Hypoxia and acidosis can cause the ventricular myocardium to become irritable and stimulate ventricular arrhythmias. A dog that is poorly ventilated and oxygenated during anesthesia and surgery may develop ventricular premature beats and ventricular tachycardia. Severe congestive heart failure may cause hypoxic myocarditis after pulmonary edema develops and makes adequate oxygen intake impossible.

Since there are so many equally likely causes of ventricular arrhythmia, a thorough and careful search for the cause of any such arrhythmia must be made. Any critically ill patient should have his cardiac status carefully evaluated to ascertain whether the myocardium is secondarily affected.

Regardless of the cause, ventricular premature beats and ventricular tachycardia are dangerous arrhythmias. Ventricular tachycardia is critical, and is the more serious consequence of ventricular myocarditis. The myocarditis-induced arrhythmia can be quickly fatal, and it may be necessary first to control the arrhythmia, to keep the dog alive long enough to treat the primary disease.

In a disturbing number of cases, no cause can be found for the ventricular arrhythmias. When a complete search for a cause reveals nothing, the myocarditis is said to be primary, or idiopathic. The author has treated patients that died from uncontrollable ventricular arrhythmias in which even postmortem examination did not reveal the cause of these arrhythmias. Arteriosclerosis of the smaller coronary arteries, as well as myocardial necrosis and fibrosis, has been reported in four dogs that had bouts of paroxysmal ventricular tachycardia (Patterson et al., 1961).

Clinical signs do not occur until the ventricular premature beats become frequent or until ventricular tachycardia occurs. When they do become significant, signs of weakness, exercise intolerance, lethargy, collapse, seizure, coma, and sudden death may occur. The dog may periodically collapse and recover, or he may suddenly collapse and die. Seizures may or may not occur when the dog collapses. Death from myocarditis is usually sudden and dramatic; it is this unpredictability that makes these arrhythmias worrisome.

PHYSICAL EXAMINATION. Signs of the primary disease condition may predominate. For example, if a seven year old female dog that was in heat four weeks previously presents with anorexia, polydipsia, emesis, and a mucopurulent vaginal discharge, her cardiac status should be evaluated before attempting surgery for the pyometra, because ventricular arrhythmias may occur with pyometra.

On auscultation the only finding may be an arrhythmia not associated with respiration. The premature beats may be heard as lub dup, lub dup, lub dup, lub dup dup — pause — lub dup, lub dup dup — pause, or bursts of ventricular tachycardia may be heard as lub dup, lub dup, lub dup dup dup dup dup dup dup dup dup — pause — lub dup, lub dup. When a burst of ventricular tachycardia occurs the dog may become weak, or collapse, or suffer a seizure.

If the femoral pulse is compared with the heart beat, a pulse deficit will be detected when the premature beats or tachycardia occurs. A jugular pulse may also be present if the right atrium contracts against a right

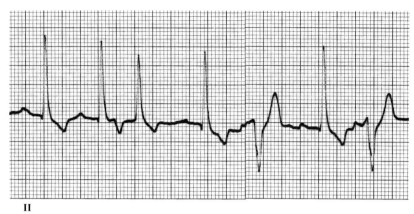

II

Figure 4-24. This tracing demonstrates the difference between supraventricular and ventricular premature beats. The third beat from the left is a supraventricular premature beat. It occurs early, is followed by a pause, and the QRS complex is slightly shorter but still of near-normal conformation. When the two bizarre ventricular premature beats occur toward the end of the tracing, they occur early, are followed by a pause, and the distortion of the QRS complex is obvious. They are not associated with P waves. A P wave occurs just before the last ventricular premature beat, but the P-R interval is obviously much shorter than those of the normal beats, which proves that the P wave is unrelated to the abnormal ventricular beat. Digitalis intoxication was present at the time of this recording.

Paper speed = 50 mm./sec., 1 cm. = 1 mv.

atrioventricular valve that has been closed prematurely by a ventricular premature beat.

It is not possible to tell with certainty what type of premature beat or tachycardia is present during the physical examination; thus, the electrocardiogram is essential when working with these arrhythmias.

ELECTROCARDIOGRAPHIC DIAGNOSIS

1. The heart rate is usually normal.

II

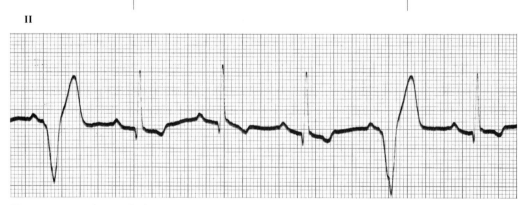

Figure 4-25. Two ventricular premature beats occur on this lead II tracing. They obviously distort the QRS complex. Although it may appear that they are stimulated by a P wave, they are not, as evidenced by the fact that the P-R intervals are much shorter than those of the normal beats. When they occur one at a time like this, they are called *singles*. The also arise from a unifocal source, as can be determined by their similarity.

Paper speed = 50 mm./sec., 1 cm. = 1 mv.

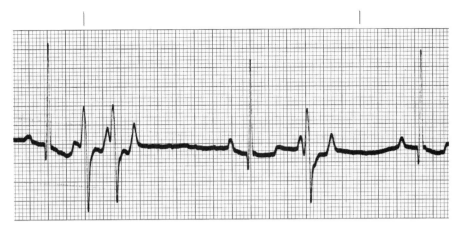

Figure 4–26. In this lead II electrocardiogram, two ventricular premature beats occur in succession, then a normal beat occurs, and a single ventricular premature beat occurs. Ventricular premature beats obviously distort the QRS complex, and are not associated with P waves. When two premature beats occur in a row, it is called a pair. Since all three of the ventricular premature beats in this tracing look similar, they all arose from the same source (they are unifocal).
Paper speed = 50 mm./sec., 1 cm. = 1 mv.

2. *The normal rhythm is broken by premature beats that are usually followed by a pause. When ventricular tachycardia occurs, the rhythm is broken by a string of premature beats*.

3. *There are no P waves associated with the premature beats*.

4. The normal QRS complexes are related to P waves, but *the abnormal beats have no consistent P-R interval*.

5. The P waves that can be seen are normal, but *the premature beats have bizarre QRS complexes*.

Figure 4–24 demonstrates a tracing from a dog that was intoxicated

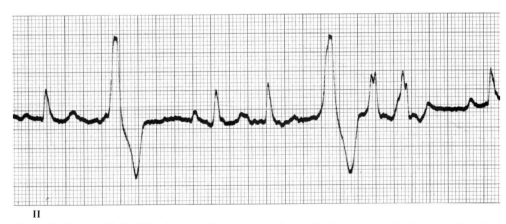

II

Figure 4–27. In this lead II electrocardiogram, a single ventricular premature beat occurs, then two normal beats, and finally three ventricular premature beats in a row are discharged. When three premature beats occur in succession, it is called a run. This is a more worrisome situation; because now the ventricular premature beats are of multifocal origin in that they have different conformations. In the run, they are all different. This should be considered a dangerous prefibrillatory rhythm.
Paper speed = 50 mm./sec., 1 cm. = 1 mv.

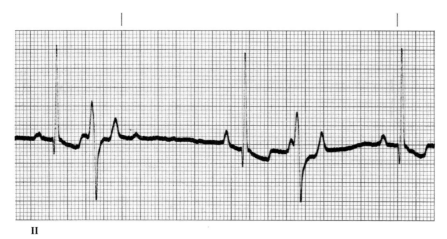

II

Figure 4–28. This lead II tracing demonstrates a ventricular bigeminy. Every other beat is a ventricular premature beat. These are bizarre and not associated with P waves, and are of unifocal origin.
    Paper speed = 50 mm./sec., 1 cm. = 1 mv.

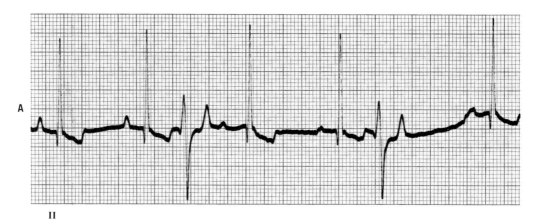

A

II

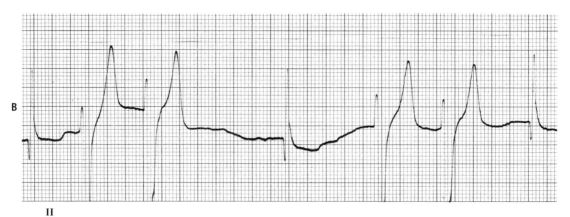

B

II

Figure 4–29.   A. When every third beat is a ventricular premature beat, as in this tracing, it is called a ventricular trigeminy. These ventricular premature beats are unifocal in origin.
    B. This tracing also demonstrates a trigeminy when there are two ventricular premature beats to one normal beat. This rhythm goes normal, veep veep, normal, veep veep, normal.
    Paper speed = 50 mm./sec., 1 cm. = 1 mv.

by digitalis and had both supraventricular and ventricular premature beats. The QRS complex is quite normal when the supraventricular premature beat occurs, but the two ventricular premature beats that occur at the end of the tracing are obviously bizarre, and not associated with P waves.

As mentioned previously, if one ventricular premature beat occurs at a time, it is called a single (Fig. 4–25). When two ventricular premature beats occur in succession, they are called a pair (Fig. 4–26). Three ventricular premature beats in a row are called a run (Fig. 4–27). Four or more ventricular premature beats in a row constitute a ventricular tachycardia (Fig. 4–33). If every other beat is a ventricular premature beat, it is called ventricular bigeminy (Fig. 4–28). When every third beat is a ventricular premature beat, or when there are two ventricular premature beats for every normal beat, it is termed ventricular trigeminy (Fig. 4–29).

If all of the ventricular premature beats are from a single source, they are said to be of unifocal origin, and they look identical (Figs. 4–25, 4–26, 4–28, 4–29, and 4–33). If they arise from several different areas of the ventricular myocardium, they are said to be of multifocal origin, and they vary in conformation (Figs. 4–27, 4–30, and 4–36). Multifocal types of ventricular premature beats and of ventricular tachycardia are more dangerous than the unifocal types because several areas of the myocardium are irritable.

When a ventricular premature beat arises near the bundle of His, as in Figure 4–31, its QRS complex may not be very bizarre in conformation, but is still not associated with a P wave. Occasionally, ventricular premature beats may occur without being followed by a pause. In these instances they do not break the normal rhythm, but instead occur be-

II

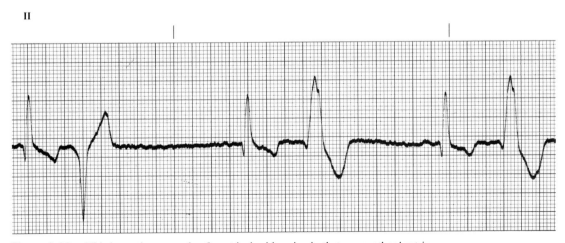

Figure 4–30. This is another example of ventricular bigeminy in that every other beat is a ventricular premature beat, but this time they are of multifocal origin. The first ventricular premature beat is different in conformation from the two that occur toward the end of the tracing. This is more worrisome than if they were all from the same source.
    Paper speed = 50 mm./sec., 1 cm. = 1 mv.

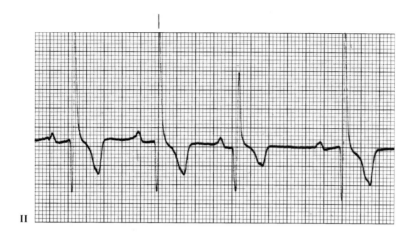

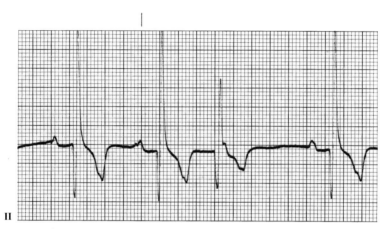

Figure 4–31. The top and bottom lead II strips represent continuous recordings from an Irish Setter that had myocarditis of undetermined origin. The third beat from the left in each strip is a ventricular premature beat. Although there appears to be a P wave associated with the premature beat in the top strip, its P-R interval is different than the P-R interval of the normal beats, so it really is not associated with that premature beat. The premature beat in the bottom tracing obviously has no P wave. The QRS conformation of the ventricular premature beats is not markedly different from the normal QRS complexes, because their origin is near the bundle of His and thus depolarization travels a nearly normal pathway. The important observation here is that they are not associated with P waves.

Paper speed = 50 mm./sec., 1 cm. = 1 mv.

tween two normal beats (Fig. 4–32). When this occurs, it is termed an interpolated ventricular premature beat. Interpolation is of no particular clinical significance.

Ventricular tachycardia is diagnosed when four or more bizarre ventricular beats occur in a row (Fig. 4–33). In the bottom tracing of this electrocardiogram it can be seen that two normal complexes break the string of bizarre ventricular premature beats. These normal beats are called capture beats, because the P wave managed to slip through the atrioventricular node at just the right time and "captured" the ventricles for one beat. The normal beats, then, are capture beats. Figure 4–34 demonstrates another hallmark of ventricular tachycardia. Two capture

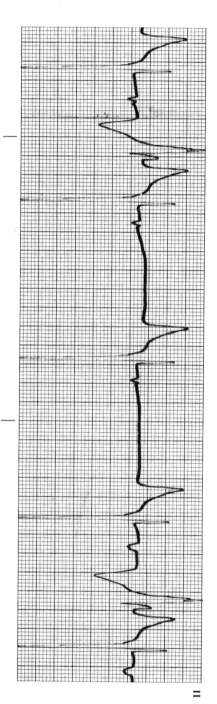

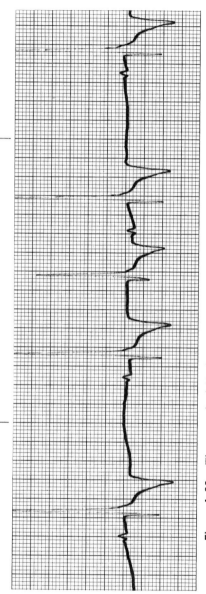

Figure 4–32. These two lead II electrocardiograms demonstrate an unusual form of ventricular premature beat. These are interpolated ventricular premature beats. They are interpolated because they do not break the normal rhythm, but simply slip in between two normal beats. This is an interesting variation, but is of no particular significance. In the bottom strip, the ventricular premature beat arises near the bundle of His; note that the QRS complex is nearly normal but is not associated with a P wave. Since the beat is of a different configuration than the ventricular premature beats in the top tracing, this dog has multifocal ventricular premature beats. These recordings are from the same Irish Setter as in Figure 4–31.

Paper speed = 50 mm./sec., 1 cm. = 1 mv.

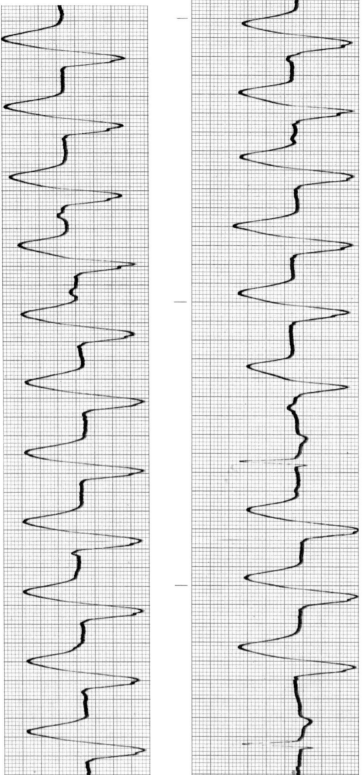

II

II

Figure 4-33. These continuous lead II recordings demonstrate ventricular tachycardia. In the top strip, all of the beats are ventricular premature beats. Toward the end of the strip, two P waves can be seen. They are not associated with those two ventricular complexes because their P-R intervals vary. P waves are also occurring at their own rate during the rest of the tracing but are hidden in the QRS complexes. In the bottom strip two normal PQRST complexes can be seen to break the string of bizarre ventricular beats; one at the beginning, and one 4 beats later. These are "capture beats" in which those P waves happened to occur at just the right time to "capture" the ventricles for one beat and produce a normal complex. Capture beats are diagnostic of ventricular tachycardia. These tracings were recorded from a Great Dane that had autoimmune hemolytic anemia and thrombocytopenia.

Paper speed = 50 mm./sec., 1 cm. = 1 mv.

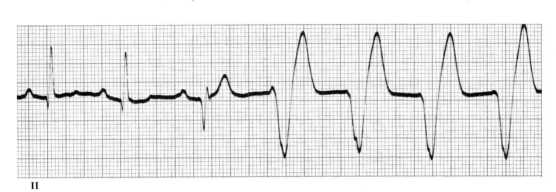

II

Figure 4–34. This electrocardiogram is also of the same Great Dane as in Figure 4–33, and demonstrates, from the left, two capture beats, a fusion beat, and then ventricular tachycardia. The two capture beats are the dog's normal beats. The fusion beat occurs when the P wave fires, then a normal P-R interval occurs, and, as the P wave comes out of the atrioventricular node and begins to depolarize the ventricles, the ectopic ventricular focus also discharges. The result is a complex that has a normal P-R interval and is midway in form between the normal beats and the ventricular premature beats. Capture and fusion beats are both diagnostic of ventricular tachycardia.
 Paper speed = 50 mm./sec., 1 cm. = 1 mv.

beats occur, an abnormal beat occurs, and then a paroxysm of ventricular tachycardia is present. The beat that occurs between the normal capture beats and the string of ventricular premature beats is called a fusion beat. This beat has a normal P-R interval. The P wave occurred, traversed the atrioventricular node normally, and began to depolarize the ventricles. Just as the P wave began to depolarize the ventricles, the irritable focus in the ventricle also discharged and tried to depolarize the ventricles at the same time. This resulted in a beat that has a P wave and a normal P-R interval, but is different from either the normal beats or the ventricular premature beats. Capture and fusion beats are diagnostic of ventricular tachycardia. Figure 4–35 demonstrates a ventricular tachycardia that is broken by a capture beat, which is then followed by a fusion beat, which is, in turn, followed by resumption of the ventricular tachycardia. Ventricular tachycardia of multifocal origin is dangerous and should be considered a prefibrillatory rhythm (Fig. 4–36).

 Atrioventricular dissociation is a confusing term. It refers to a form of ventricular tachycardia in which the rate of the P waves is almost equal to that of the ventricles. *Of importance is the fact that the P waves and the QRS complexes are not associated with one another.* There are two types of atrioventricular dissociation: synchrony and accrochage.

 Synchrony is diagnosed when the P wave rate and the ventricular rate are exactly equal and occur almost simultaneously, but are not associated (Fig. 4–37). Accrochage is a form of atrioventricular dissociation in which the P waves move into and out of the QRS complexes, demonstrating the lack of relationship between the P waves and the QRS complexes (Fig. 4–38). Atrioventricular dissociation is almost always due to digitalis intoxication, although it has been reported in a dog with ruptured chordae tendineae (Ettinger and Buergelt, 1968).

Text continued on page 139.

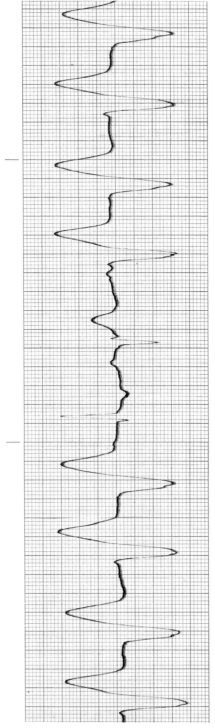

Figure 4–35. This recording also demonstrates a ventricular tachycardia in the same Great Dane. The string of four ventricular premature beats is interrupted by a capture beat, followed by a fusion beat, and then the ventricular tachycardia resumes.

Paper speed = 50 mm./sec., 1 cm. = 1 mv.

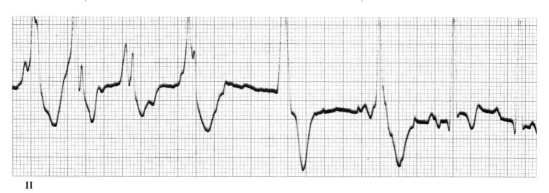

II

Figure 4–36. This rhythm indicates a dangerous situation! The first six beats in this tracing are ventricular premature beats of multifocal origin. Two capture beats occur at the end of the tracing. This multifocal ventricular tachycardia is a prefibrillatory rhythm.

Paper speed = 50 mm./sec., 1 cm. = 1 mv.

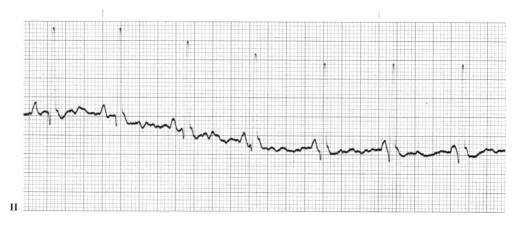

II

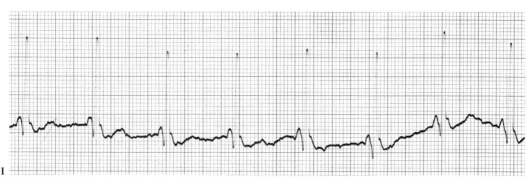

II

Figure 4–37. These continuous lead II electrocardiograms demonstrate a form of ventricular tachycardia called atrioventricular dissociation. In this rhythm there is no correlation between the P waves and the QRS complexes, but the rates of the P waves, and of the QRS complexes is exactly equal, and the P waves fall almost on top of the QRS complexes. At the beginning, the P waves can be seen to move toward the QRS complexes with each beat, which shows the lack of relationship between the P waves and QRS complexes. In the bottom tracing, as the rhythm continues, the rate of the P waves and QRS complexes is almost exactly the same. When the P waves and QRS complexes are unrelated, but occur at the same rate, it is called synchrony, and is diagnostic of atrioventricular dissociation. It is a form of ventricular tachycardia that is most often caused by digitalis toxicity, as in this case.

Paper speed = 50 mm./sec., 1 cm. = 1 mv.

(Tracings courtesy of Dr. L. Tilley, New York, N.Y.)

137

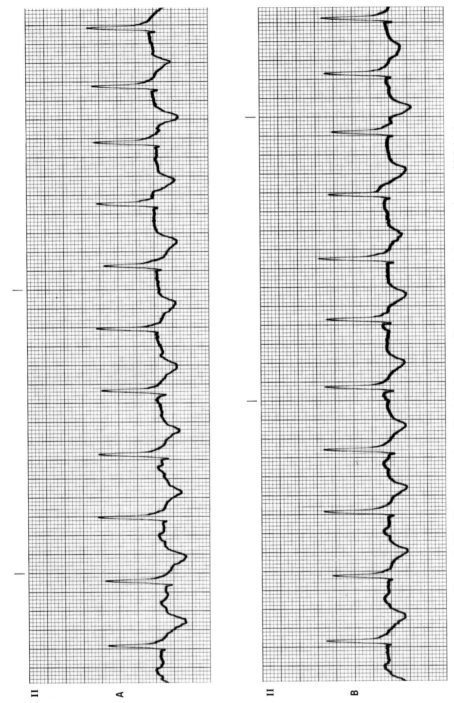

Figure 4–38. These two strips of lead II electrocardiogram demonstrate accrochage, which is also diagnostic of atrioventricular dissociation. The bottom strip is a continuation of the top strip. Accrochage is diagnosed when the P wave moves in and out of the QRS complexes, as it does in these tracings. It signifies that the P waves are not related to the QRS complexes. In the third and fourth beats from the right side of strip A, the P waves can actually be seen to occur as small bumps just behind the QRS complexes of those beats. This dog was also experiencing digitalis intoxication. Paper speed = 50 mm./sec., 1 cm. = 1 mv.

TREATMENT. Antiarrhythmic agents such as quinidine and procainamide are the treatment of choice for the ventricular arrhythmias. The only time when they should not be used is when the ventricular premature beats or tachycardias are caused by congestive heart failure. In these cases, quinidine would depress the myocardium and only further aggravate the congestive heart failure. When the ventricular arrhythmias are due to congestive heart failure, the failure is usually very severe, and pulmonary edema is present. In these instances, cage rest, digitalis, diuretics, morphine, and oxygen are used, because the ventricular premature beats are due to myocardial hypoxia. If myocardial oxygenation can be improved, the arrhythmia will be resolved. In all other instances, digitalis is contraindicated for the treatment of ventricular arrhythmias because it will enhance the excitability of the ventricular myocardium and aggravate the arrhythmia.

Antiarrhythmic agents act by depressing the irritable foci. Results of quinidine therapy can be spectacular (Fig. 4–39).

The choice of which antiarrhythmic agent to use depends on the urgency of the situation. If the dog has collapsed or is comatose, 2 per cent lidocaine without epinephrine should be used intravenously, and will act in seconds (Fig. 4–40). If the situation is not as critical, oral therapy is adequate. Of the oral quinidine preparations, quinidine sulfate acts most rapidly and reaches high blood concentrations within one hour. The longer-acting preparations have the advantage of being given only two or three times daily, while quinidine sulfate must be given every 4 to 6 hours. If the ventricular arrhythmias are frequent, quinidine sulfate should be used at first to achieve rapid blood levels, and after the arrhythmias are alleviated, the dog may be switched to the longer-acting forms.

Quinidine or lidocaine therapy is usually highly effective, but the results may vary from dog to dog. Most of the time the patient responds quickly and completely to the medication. A few patients will respond only partially, while occasionally control will be poor. If a primary disease can be identified and successfully treated, quinidine therapy eventually can be discontinued. Of those dogs in which the cause cannot be established, some will be on quinidine indefinitely while others can eventually be withdrawn from the drug.

If one antiarrhythmic agent is not working effectively, another regime should be tried. Dilantin may control an arrhythmia when quinidine and procainamide have failed. The dog in Figures 4–26, 4–28, and 4–29A was incompletely controlled on high doses of quinidine, but his arrhythmia is now successfully controlled with diphenylhydantoin. Quinidine and procainamide can be used in combination at lower doses of each with synergistic effects (Ettinger and Suter, 1970). In this way greater effects can be obtained without added toxicity. Some other combinations of antiarrhythmic agents that have been tried in man are quinidine and propranolol, procainamide and diphenylhydantoin, and quinidine and diphenylhydantoin (Mason et al., 1973). These combinations might be tried if the arrhythmia is proving difficult to control.

One new antiarrhythmic agent that shows promise is bretylium tosylate, which may exert its effect because of its antiadrenergic proper-

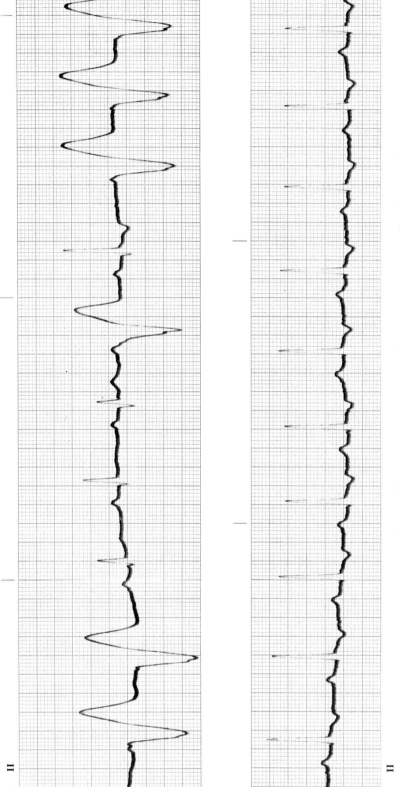

Figure 4-39. Therapy with quinidine can be rewarding. In tracing A. there are many unifocal ventricular premature beats. Strip B was recorded just one hour after the administration of 5 mg/lb. of quinidine sulfate. The arrhythmia is completely controlled.

Paper speed = 50 mm./sec.. 1 cm. = 1 mv.

140

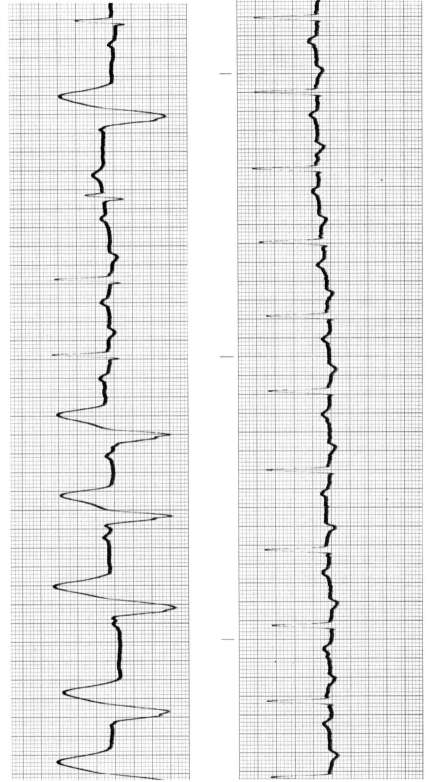

Figure 4–40. These two continuous lead II recordings were taken during the treatment of ventricular tachycardia with lidocaine. The string of ventricular premature beats is broken on top by two capture beats, then a fusion beat, then one more ventricular ectopic beat occurs, and then the normal rhythm takes over in the bottom tracing. The response is dramatic; this all happened within seconds.
Paper speed = 50 mm./sec., 1 cm. = 1 mv.

ties. In man it has been used alone and in combination with other agents with some success (Mason et al., 1973).

When myocarditis is idiopathic, the dog should be given a 2- to 3-week course of broad-spectrum antibiotics on general principle because of the known association of endocarditis with myocarditis.

There are other methods of therapy for the ventricular ectopic arrhythmias. D.C. cardioversion can be used to convert ventricular tachycardia to normal sinus rhythm, but requires special equipment. Atropine may be given on a short-term basis. The principle behind this is that atropine will increase the rate of discharge of the sinoatrial node so that it will override that of the irritable focus in the ventricular myocardium, thus controlling the rhythm.

Occasionally a situation occurs that forces a difficult decision, such as the following. Severe congestive heart failure can cause myocardial hypoxia and ventricular tachycardia, and in these situations digitalis, along with other methods of therapy, should be used to improve the congestive heart failure and thus eliminate the arrhythmia. On the other hand, if ventricular tachycardia occurs and persists, congestive heart failure may result secondary to the arrhythmia. In these situations lidocaine will break the ventricular tachycardia and improve the congestive heart failure. But, if a dog is presented in severe congestive heart failure with pulmonary edema, extreme dyspnea, and ventricular tachycardia, which came first? Is the ventricular tachycardia secondary to the congestive heart failure, or is the congestive heart failure secondary to the ventricular tachycardia? Fortunately, this does not occur often, but what should be done when it does occur?

The chances are overwhelming that congestive heart failure occurred first; therefore, the dog should be given intramuscular or intravenous injections of aminophylline and Lasix. Morphine is given subcutaneously, and ouabain is given intravenously. Oxygen therapy should be administered and the dog monitored closely. Ouabain peaks within 30 minutes and is practically gone in an hour. Meanwhile, a syringe with lidocaine can be kept ready in case this was the wrong approach and the arrhythmia becomes worse. If the condition improves or at least stabilizes, then the therapy was correct. If the arrhythmia becomes more severe, lidocaine is used to control the rhythm until the ouabain is gone, and a longer-acting antiarrhythmic agent can be begun. The total dose of ouabain is 0.02 mg./lb., and one-fourth to one-half of the total dose is given intravenously. This is one of the rare times that the author recommends the use of ouabain.

Quinidine should be continued for six to eight weeks. At the end of the first six to eight weeks, if the arrhythmia is no longer present, quinidine may be gradually withdrawn over one to two weeks with electrocardiographic monitoring, preferably every second or third day. If the ventricular arrhythmias reoccur, therapy is reinstituted for another six to eight weeks. As long as the rhythm is under complete control, the dog can do well on quinidine indefinitely. If a primary disease such as pyometra is diagnosed and successfully corrected, the quinidine can be withdrawn as soon as the dog has recovered.

When the arrhythmia is difficult to control, the owner should be warned that the situation is an unpredictable one. Dogs may do well on medication for a long time, but as long as the arrhythmias persist, there is danger of sudden death. To illustrate the point, ventricular tachycardia was diagnosed in a 6-year-old Welsh terrier. Amazingly, the dog was virtually asymptomatic, but the arrhythmia was discovered on a routine physical examination, and an electrocardiogram revealed ventricular tachycardia. A complete medical work-up failed to disclose any cause. The owner was warned of the seriousness of the situation, and quinidine was given. At first control was good, but the ventricular tachycardia reoccurred during quinidine therapy. Over a period of time quinidine, procainamide, quinidine and procainamide in combination, and diphenylhydantoin were all used with only partial success. On each visit the owner was warned of the possibility of sudden death. The dog was asymptomatic at all times. One night, while going out for her nightly walk, she walked happily down the first porch step, and was dead when she reached the second. This dramatic way of dying is the way that dogs with myocarditis usually end their lives.

Ventricular Fibrillation. ASSOCIATIONS. When ventricular fibrillation is diagnosed, the dog is often beyond resuscitation. This is the most serious consequence of ventricular myocardial irritability. In the surgical suite, premonitory signs of hypoxia and acidosis usually occur and are diagnosed on the electrocardiogram before the ventricles fibrillate. By the time fibrillation occurs, the changes due to hypoxia and acidosis are already advanced, and the chances of saving the dog are slim.

Ventricular fibrillation may be the terminal event of a severe illness or, as in the case of the Welsh terrier (mentioned earlier), may result from uncontrollable myocarditis. Sudden death, presumably also due to ventricular fibrillation, is common among dogs with aortic stenosis.

Clinical signs are acute collapse, with or without seizures, followed by death throes and agonal gasps.

PHYSICAL EXAMINATION. The outstanding features on physical examination are a prostrate dog with no heart beat or femoral pulse, and bilaterally dilated pupils.

ELECTROCARDIOGRAPHIC DIAGNOSIS
1. No coordinated heart beat can be detected.
2. *Specific P waves and QRS complexes are absent.*
3. *A series of baseline undulations is seen.*

When cardiac arrest occurs, it may be due either to ventricular fibrillation or to cardiac standstill (Bolton, 1973). An electrocardiogram differentiates these two. Cardiac standstill produces a straight, steady baseline, opposed to the baseline undulations of ventricular fibrillation. Figures 4–41 and 4–42 illustrate two prefibrillatory rhythms. Coarse or fine fibrillations may occur (Fig. 4–43). Cases of ventricular fibrillation in which the coarse type are seen are more prone to successful defibrillation.

TREATMENT. An emergency tray should be available for just such an event. A list of drugs for the emergency tray, their indications, and their dosages is given in Table 4–5.

External or internal cardiac massage is begun immediately. A rapid intravenous drip containing sodium bicarbonate should be secured if

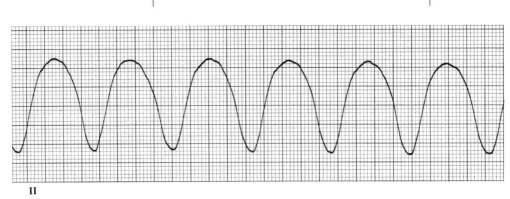

II

Figure 4–41. This lead II tracing was recorded from a dog that was dying of myocarditis. There is no co-ordinated beat, merely a series of bizarre rhythmic baseline undulations (called ventricular flutter). This proceeded to ventricular fibrillation in a matter of seconds.
    Paper speed = 50 mm./sec., 1 cm. = 1 mv.

possible and oxygen should be given with assisted ventilation. Anesthesia should be terminated. The heart is monitored, and one or two sharp blows are delivered over the cardiac area. If the heart fails to restart, D.C. defibrillation is attempted. If electrical defibrillation fails, massage is continued, and sodium bicarbonate and epinephrine are given intracardially. Epinephrine hopefully converts fine fibrillation to coarse fibrillation, which is more suitable for defibrillation. Bicarbonate alleviates the severe acidosis that develops, reducing myocardial irritability.

After massaging the heart and administering epinephrine and bicarbonate, defibrillation should again be attempted. If this fails, epinephrine and bicarbonate are repeated, and calcium is given to improve myocardial tone. Again defibrillation is attempted. If it still fails, the outlook is

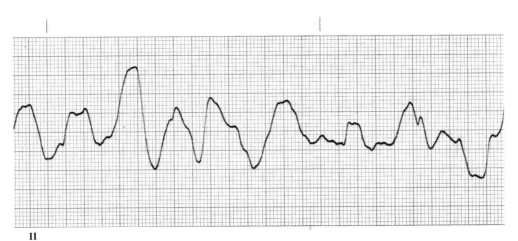

II

Figure 4–42. This tracing demonstrates a more chaotic prefibrillatory rhythm that developed into ventricular fibrillation.
    Paper speed = 50 mm./sec., 1 cm. = 1 mv.

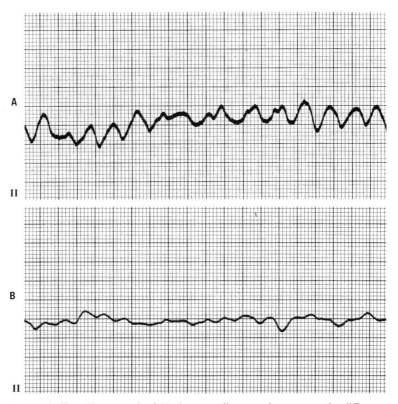

Figure 4–43. These two lead II electrocardiograms demonstrate the difference between coarse fibrillation and fine fibrillation.

A. This tracing represents coarse ventricular fibrillation. The baseline undulations are much more exaggerated than those in tracing B. Defibrillation is more likely to be successful in this tracing than in tracing B.

B. The fibrillations in this tracing are much finer than the ones in tracing A. If defibrillation were unsuccessful epinephrine might be given, since epinephrine could produce a more coarse pattern.

Paper speed = 50 mm./sec., 1 cm. = mv.

poor. If the heart fails to restart after 10 minutes and the pupils are fixed and dilated, resuscitation attempts are discontinued. A step-by-step approach to the treatment of cardiac arrest, including ventricular fibrillation and cardiac standstill, is given in the veterinary literature (Bolton, 1973).

Bretylium tosylate is a new drug that has antiarrhythmic properties that may be helpful in the treatment of ventricular fibrillation (Bacaner, 1968; Mason, 1973.) Bretylium's antiarrhythmic properties may be due to its antiadrenergic properties, but its actions are not yet completely understood (Mason, 1973).

Escape Rhythms

The escape rhythms occur when the rate of spontaneous discharge of the sinoatrial node becomes depressed. The lower pacemaker centers in either the junctional tissues near the atrioventricular node or the ventricles eventually beat on their own, because they fail to receive stimulation from the sinoatrial node. The two types of escape beats are the

TABLE 4–5. DRUGS FOR THE EMERGENCY TRAY; DOSAGES AND RATIONALE FOR USE*

1. **Levarterenol bitartrate (norepinephrine)** – (Levophed)
   Winthrop Labs – 2 mg./ml. in ampules. Given in an intravenous drip to effect. Dilute 1 to 2 ml. in 250 ml. of drip. Used as a potent vasopressor to increase blood pressure. Does have some chronotropic and inotropic effects on the heart.
2. **Epinephrine HCl** – 1:10,000
   Give 1 to 5 ml. intracardially. Used primarily in an attempt to convert cardiac standstill to either ventricular fibrillation or a normal heart beat. Epinephrine causes coarse ventricular fibrillation which can be more successfully converted to sinus rhythm by direct current electric shock. Fine fibrillations may be converted to coarse fibrillations by the intracardiac administration of epinephrine.
3. **Isoproterenol** – (Isuprel)
   Winthrop Labs – 1 or 5 ml. ampules, .2 mg./ml. Given intravenously in a drip. Dilute 1 mg. in 250 ml. of solution, and give as needed to maintain heart rate between 80 and 140 beats per minute. Isuprel is used for its positive inotropic and chronotropic effects. It also causes peripheral vasodilatation.
4. **Phenylephrine HCl** – (NeoSynephrine)
   Winthrop Labs – 1 ml. ampules, 2 mg./ml. Give .8 mg. intravenously. Phenylephrine is used to raise blood pressure because of its potent vasopressive action. It has no direct effect on the heart.
5. **Doxapram HCl** – (Dopram)
   Robins Co. – 20 mg./ml. Give .5 mg./lb. intravenously as a potent analeptic to reverse respiratory depression. May need to be repeated frequently.
6. **Atropine sulfate** – .5 mg./cc.
   Give 1 ml. per 20 lbs. of body weight intravenously to block vagal reflexes and prevent severe bradycardias.
7. a. **Calcium gluconate** – 10 per cent solution
      Give 5 to 10 ml. intravenously or intracardially.
   b. **Calcium chloride** – 10 per cent solution
      Give 1 to 2 ml. intravenously or intracardially.
   Calcium solutions strengthen myocardial contraction. They also increase myocardial excitability, which may be helpful during cardiac arrest.
8. **Lidocaine HCl** – (Xylocaine) – WITHOUT EPINEPHRINE!
   Astra Pharmaceutical – 20 mg./ml. Give 2 to 4 mg./lb. by slow intravenous bolus and follow with a 2 mg./ml. intravenous drip if needed. Xylocaine is used as an antiarrhythmic drug to control ventricular arrhythmias. It may be used if ventricular fibrillation tends to recur.
9. **Ouabain** – .25 mg./ml.
   Eli Lilly – Initial dose is one-quarter of calculated total dose, given intravenously. Total dose is .02 mg./lb. Repeat In 30 minutes if necessary. Digitalis strengthens myocardial contraction, increases cardiac output, and thus controls congestive heart failure. It controls supraventricular tachycardias by delaying conduction through the atrioventricular node and by vagal effects on the sinoatrial node.
10. **Sodium bicarbonate**
    Abbott Labs – 44.6 mEq./50 ml. Given in an intravenous drip. Dilute 25 to 50 ml. in 250 ml. of drip. May give 10 to 20 mEq. intracardially. The administration of sodium bicarbonate helps alleviate acidosis during cardiac arrest.
11. **Aminophylline**
    Searle – 250 mg./ml., ampules of 2 ml. Give 2 to 4 mg./lb. intravenously. Aminophylline causes bronchodilation for effective exchange of gases, and has a myocardial stimulatory effect.

---

*Reproduced from Bolton, G. R.: Prevention and Treatment of Cardiovascular Emergencies During Anesthesia and Surgery. Vet. Clin. N. Am. 2(2) (1972):411.

junctional type and the ventricular type. If only one escape beat occurs it is called an escape beat. If the escape beats dominate the rhythm, the heart beats at a slow rate, and the rhythm is termed an escape rhythm. There are junctional and ventricular escape beats as well as junctional and ventricular escape rhythms.

Junctional (Nodal) Escape Rhythm. ASSOCIATIONS. Junctional escape patterns in the dog are often caused by digitalis intoxication. Occasionally, if the vagus nerve depresses the sinoatrial node, junctional escape rhythms may occur, and occasionally the pause that follows a premature beat may be so long that a junctional beat discharges before the sinoatrial node does (Fig. 5–20). Hamlin et al. (1972) reported junctional escape beats during sinoatrial syncope episodes in miniature schnauzers.

Clinical signs of digitalis intoxication may be present. When the arrhythmia is induced by vagal tone, the dog is asymptomatic unless the heart rate becomes slow enough to cause signs of weakness, fatigue, or syncope upon exercise.

PHYSICAL EXAMINATION. On physical examination long pauses, as well as bradycardia, are noted. No pulse deficit is present. The electrocardiogram is the only way to specifically identify these escape rhythms.

ELECTROCARDIOGRAPHIC DIAGNOSIS

1. The heart rate is normal or slow.

2. *The rhythm is irregular, with long pauses when isolated escape beats occur, but is regular when junctional rhythm persists.*

3. There is a P wave for every QRS complex, and a QRS complex for every P wave.

4. The P waves may occur before, during, or just after the QRS complex. When a P-R interval is present, it may be slightly shorter than the normals.

5. The QRS complexes are normal, *but the P waves are negative*.

Isolated junctional escape beats may occur (Figs. 4–44 and 4–45), or a junctional escape rhythm may predominate (Fig. 4–46). Sinus arrhythmia or sinus arrest may also be present on the tracing. Premature ectopic beats may also be occurring. *The distinguishing characteristics of the junctional escape beats is that they occur late, after a long pause, and their P waves are negative.*

The position of the P wave in relation to the QRS complex depends on the site of origin of the impulse. If the impulse arises on the atrial side of the atrioventricular node, the P wave precedes the QRS complex, and the P-R interval may be slightly shorter than normal because the beat arose so near the node. When the junctional beat arises on the ventricular side of the atrioventricular node, the ventricles are stimulated almost immediately, but atrial depolarization is delayed while the impulse is conducted backward through the node and into the atrial tissues. As a result, the QRS complex can actually precede its accompanying P wave. The negative P wave usually appears between the QRS complex and the T wave (Fig. 4–45).

TREATMENT. If digitalis is being given in overdose, it is stopped until the physical signs improve and the arrhythmias are resolved. It is then resumed at a slightly lower dosage. Atropine will improve the

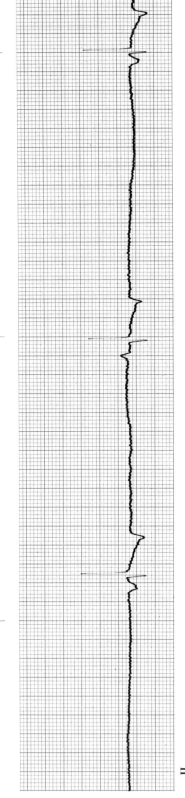

II

Figure 4–44. Two junctional escape beats occur in this lead II electrocardiogram. It can be seen that they occur after long pauses in the rhythm. The junctional tissues wait and wait for an impulse to come from the sinoatrial node, but none comes, and they finally initiate an impulse. The negative P waves indicate the junctional origin of the impulse. This dog was suffering from digitalis intoxication.

Paper speed = 50 mm./sec., 1 cm. = 1 mv.
(Tracing courtesy of Dr. L. Tilley, New York, N.Y.)

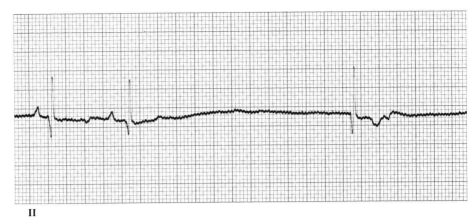

II

Figure 4–45. This lead II tracing is from the same dog as in Figure 4–44. The last beat on the strip is a junctional escape beat in which the negative P wave can actually be seen to occur behind the QRS complex, between the QRS and the T wave.
Paper speed = 50 mm./sec., 1 cm. = 1 mv.
(Tracing courtesy of Dr. L. Tilley, New York, N.Y.)

vagally induced form of this arrhythmia. If the dog has only a few vagally induced junctional escape beats and is asymptomatic, no treatment is required.

Ventricular Escape Beats and Rhythms. ASSOCIATIONS. Ventricular escape beats may occur singly, after long pauses in the rhythm. If they do not occur very often, they carry no more significance than do occasional junctional escape beats. They may also occur after long pauses in the rhythm, as a result of exaggerated vagal tone. Digitalis intoxication can cause both ventricular escape beats and ventricular escape rhythms.

When ventricular escape beats control the rhythm, the heart beats

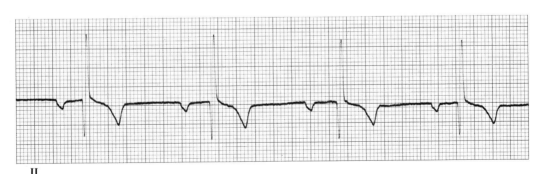

II

Figure 4–46. When all of the beats are junctional escape beats and the junctional tissues control the rhythm, as in this tracing, it is a junctional escape rhythm. Actually, to be a junctional escape rhythm, the heart rate should be 60 beats per minute or lower, which is the natural spontaneous rate of the junctional tissues. Here, the heart rate is 85 beats per minute, so by strict definition, this is really a junctional tachycardia. This dog was experiencing digitalis intoxication when this tracing was recorded.
Paper speed = 50 mm./sec., 1 cm. = 1 mv.
(Tracing courtesy of Dr. L. Tilley, New York, N.Y.)

at a very slow rate, and this is termed an idioventricular rhythm. Idioventricular rhythms should be thought of as pre-death rhythms. They represent a final attempt by the ventricles to maintain life. This situation may occur before, during, or after cardiac arrest during anesthesia and surgery; as the terminal rhythm of a dying dog; or secondary to hyperkalemia with resultant atrial standstill. In complete heart block situations the ventricles also have to beat on their own, because no stimuli emerge from the atrioventricular node.

No clinical signs occur when occasional ventricular escape beats occur. If the heart rate becomes sufficiently slow, signs of weakness, lethargy, exercise intolerance, fatigue, and collapse may occur. When an idioventricular rhythm is present, the heart rate is usually so slow that the dog shows profound weakness and may collapse, and coma and death may occur.

PHYSICAL EXAMINATION. On physical examination, long pauses in the rhythm, bradycardia or both may be noted. No pulse deficit is present. If the dog is in the terminal stages, the ventricular beats may be ineffectual, producing no pulse even though they can be heard on auscultation.

ELECTROCARDIOGRAPHIC DIAGNOSIS

1. The heart rate is normal or slow.
2. *The rhythm is irregular if isolated ventricular escape beats occur, but is regular if an idioventricular rhythm occurs.*
3. P waves may or may not occur on the tracing.
4. *The ventricular escape beats are not associated with P waves.*
5. *The P waves are normal when they occur, but the QRS complexes may be bizarre.*

Figure 4–47 demonstrates a single ventricular escape beat. *The distinguishing characteristics are that it occurs late, after a long pause, is bizarre, and is not associated with a P wave.* The dog in Figure 4–48 was dying. His ventricles were beating on their own as a final attempt to maintain life. At this stage, the dog was essentially dead. These beats were not producing a femoral pulse and the pupils were fixed and dilated. The electrocardiogram was recorded after a cardiac arrest episode in surgery. Idioventricular rhythms also occur secondary to hyper-

II

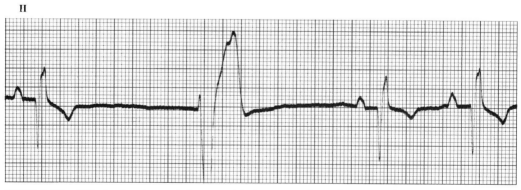

Figure 4–47. This tracing demonstrates a ventricular escape beat. It occurs after a pause, is bizarre, and has no P wave preceding it. This occurred in a Doberman pinscher after the administration of acepromazine without the simultaneous use of atropine.
    Paper speed = 50 mm./sec., 1 cm. = 1 mv.

II

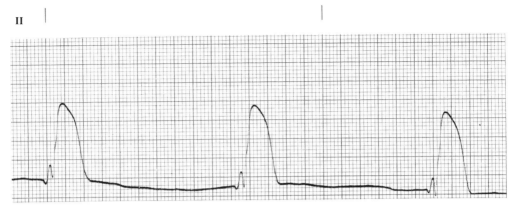

Figure 4–48. This electrocardiogram was recorded just after this dog had undergone cardiac arrest. All of the beats are ventricular escape beats, and this is called an idioventricular rhythm. Since no P waves are present, atrial standstill is also occurring. This represents a last-ditch effort by the ventricles to maintain life. No femoral pulse was produced when these beats occurred. Isoproterenol would be given now to increase the rate and force of contraction, and atropine would be given, should the atrial standstill be due to exaggerated vagal tone. Whatever the treatment, the prognosis is poor.
 Paper speed = 50 mm./sec., 1 cm. = 1 mv.

kalemia and atrial standstill (Fig. 3–32C), or when complete heart block occurs (Fig. 4–53). In both of these situations no impulses emerge from the atrioventricular node to stimulate the ventricles and they eventually beat at their own slow rate.

TREATMENT. The treatment depends on the cause. If hyperkalemia is the cause of the atrial standstill or complete heart block, correction of the hyperkalemia and the disease that caused it will improve the rhythm (Fig. 3–32D). If the complete heart block is idiopathic in nature, atropine, isoproterenol, or an artificial pacemaker may be used to increase the ventricular rate (see page 156). If the dog is in the terminal stage with a slow idioventricular rhythm, fluids, sodium bicarbonate, and isoproterenol are given to support the rate and strength of myocardial contraction. In cases of digitalis intoxication, the digitalis is stopped until the rhythm improves. Vagally induced ventricular escape beats will respond to atropine therapy, but treatment is not necessary if the dog is asymptomatic.

The Conduction Disturbances

The conduction disturbances arise when transmission of the cardiac impulse is either delayed or blocked completely. All of the conduction disturbances may be differentiated electrocardiographically.

Atrioventricular Heart Block. ASSOCIATIONS. Atrioventricular heart block is caused by a delay in transmission of the impulse through the atrioventricular node. The atrial impulse may be delayed only slightly or may be completely blocked. Three classifications useful in describing the degree or the severity of the interference with transmission of the cardiac impulses from the atria to the ventricles are first degree heart block, second degree heart block, and third degree heart block.

First degree heart block is the least severe of the three types of heart block, and is seen as a delay in the speed of impulse transmission through the atrioventricular node. All of the atrial impulses are successfully conducted to the ventricles but are delayed.

Second degree heart block is characterized by a higher degree of impulse interference. One or several of the atrial impulses are completely prevented from reaching the ventricles, while other atrial impulses are able to traverse the atrioventricular node and successfully stimulate ventricular depolarization. First degree heart block and second degree heart block may occur together on the same electrocardiogram.

Third degree heart block is the highest degree of impulse interference. All of the atrial impulses are completely blocked by the atrioventricular node, none of them reaching the ventricles. Also termed complete heart block, this arrhythmia carries grave implications.

Digitalis intoxication is probably the most important cause of serious atrioventricular heart block in the dog (Ettinger and Suter, 1970).

First degree heart block is most often due to digitalis intoxication. It may occur in apparently normal dogs (Ettinger and Suter, 1970; Patterson et al., 1961), and is significant only if a clinical abnormality or drug intoxication is present. Exaggerated vagal tone may delay impulse transmission through the atrioventricular node and cause first degree heart block (Ettinger and Suter, 1970). Reflex vagal stimulation can result from thoracic or cervical masses, or hypoxia, or may occur in brachycephalic dogs whose stertorous respirations aggravate the vagal reflex. Antiarrhythmic drugs such as quinidine, procainamide, and propranolol delay atrioventricular conduction and can produce first degree heart block. Tranquilizers and sedatives may cause first degree heart block when they cause bradycardia. Potassium also delays atrioventricular impulse transmission and hyperkalemia can produce all degrees of heart block. Of twelve dogs with first degree heart block reported by Patterson et al. (1961), seven had other evidence of cardiac disease, four had no evidence of cardiac disease, and one had widespread myocardial degeneration occurring in association with a severe anemia.

Second degree heart block also is frequently a result of digitalis intoxication. Like first degree heart block, it may also occur secondary to reflex vagal stimulation. Of twelve dogs that were reported by Patterson, et al. (1961) to have this arrhythmia, eight had other signs of heart disease. One had a parasitic granuloma in the region of the atrioventricular node, and another had no detectable pathologic changes in the heart at necropsy. It has been reported to occur secondary to toxins from infectious processes (Robertson and Ramy, 1968), and in dogs with pericardial effusion and heartworms (Buchanan, 1965).

Complete heart block (third degree heart block) can also result from digitalis intoxication and has been reported to occur secondary to hyperkalemia and to aortic body tumor (Patterson et al., 1961). In the same study it was diagnosed in a dog with severe chronic valvular disease, but necropsy was not done. Ettinger (1969) also reported complete heart block and chronic heart disease, as has Buchanan et al. (1968). It has been seen with vegetative endocarditis (Robertson, 1972), and with infarction of the atrioventricular node (Hamlin, 1966). It was diagnosed in another dog with myocardial infarction (Jaffe and Bolton, 1974), although in this report the complete heart block was not proved to be due to the infarction. Third degree heart block has been associated with congenital heart defects (Hamlin, 1966), and a possible case of congenital third degree heart block is reported (Dear, 1970b). Most dogs that develop this arrhythmia are over 5 years of age, but occasionally younger dogs have been reported to have it (Dear, 1970a and 1970b). In the majority of the cases the cause of complete heart block cannot be determined ante mortem and sometimes not even at necropsy. When complete heart block occurs it is usually a permanent abnormality, but reversion to sinus rhythm has been reported occasionally (Dear, 1970a; Ettinger, 1969; Patterson et al., 1961).

Although clinical signs may be absent when first or second degree heart block occurs, third degree heart block almost always causes signs of exercise limitation, weakness, fatigue, lethargy, or syncope. Exertion exacerbates these signs. Clinical signs due to first or second degree heart block do not occur unless they are accompanied by significant bradycardia. They are little cause for concern if the dog is clinically normal. When they do occur with significant bradycardia, signs similar to those described for complete heart block occur. Signs referable to drug intoxication may also be present. First and second degree heart block are signs of mild digitalis intoxication, while complete heart block indicates a much more serious degree of intoxication.

PHYSICAL EXAMINATION. First degree heart block is not detectable on physical examination. Second degree heart block is characterized by pauses caused by dropped beats, and can be difficult to distinguish from sinus arrhythmia and sinus arrest. When complete heart block occurs, marked bradycardia is noted. On auscultation, the loud booming ventricular beats are heard, with the soft atrial beats occurring in between. It is impressive, and sounds like: boom! pit pit pit pit boom! pit pit pit pit boom! Jugular pulses (cannon "a" waves) occur with complete heart block when atrial contraction occurs after the atrioventricular valves have been previously closed by one of the ventricular beats. There is no pulse deficit.

ELECTROCARDIOGRAPHIC DIAGNOSIS

A. First degree heart block

1. The heart rate is usually normal.
2. The rhythm is regular, but other arrhythmias, such as second degree heart block or premature beats, may also be present.
3. There is a P wave for every QRS complex and a QRS complex for every P wave (sinus rhythm).
4. The P-R intervals are consistent and prolonged beyond 0.13 second.
5. The P waves and the QRS complexes are normal.

B. Second degree heart block

1. The heart rate is usually normal, but may be slow.

2. The rhythm is broken by the omission of one or several QRS complexes.

3. There is a P wave for every QRS complex, but *some P waves occur without a QRS complex*.

4. *The P-R intervals of the normal complexes are consistent*.

5. The P waves and QRS complexes are normal.

C. Complete heart block (third degree heart block)

1. *Bradycardia below 60 beats per minute is present*.

2. The rhythm is usually regular.

3. *There are more P waves than QRS complexes*.

4. *The P-R intervals vary, and no consistent relationship can be shown to occur between the atrial and the ventricular beats*.

5. The P waves are normal, but while the QRS complexes are usually near-normal, they may be bizarre.

First degree heart block is diagnosed whenever the P-R interval is prolonged beyond 0.13 second (Fig. 4–49). Second degree heart block usually appears as an occasional P wave that occurs without a QRS complex (Fig. 4–50), but can be much more advanced (Fig. 4–51). When third degree heart block occurs, the atria and ventricles beat independently of one another (Fig. 4–53), and no relationship can be seen between the P waves and the QRS complexes. The ventricular rate is much less than the atrial rate, and, since the ventricles beat at their own rate, complete heart block is a form of idioventricular rhythm.

The literature classifies second degree heart block in humans into two categories: Mobitz type I (Wenkebach phenomenon), and Mobitz type II (Friedberg, 1966). In Mobitz type I second degree heart block the P-R intervals become prolonged just prior to the omission of a QRS complex (Fig. 4–52). The P-R interval is not prolonged before the dropped QRS complex in Mobitz type II second degree heart block (Fig. 4–50). Differentiation is of little clinical significance, although there is a greater association of the Wenkebach phenomenon with digitalis intoxication.

II

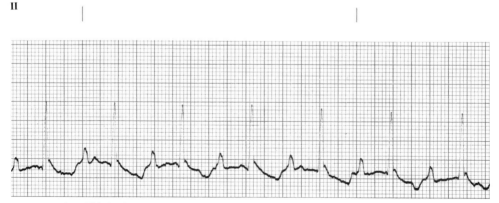

Figure 4–49. This lead II electrocardiogram was recorded from a dog that was digitalis toxic, and first degree heart block is present. The P-R interval is 0.16 second. First degree heart block is present whenever the P-R interval exceeds 0.13 second.

Paper speed = 50 mm./sec., 1 cm. = 1 mv.

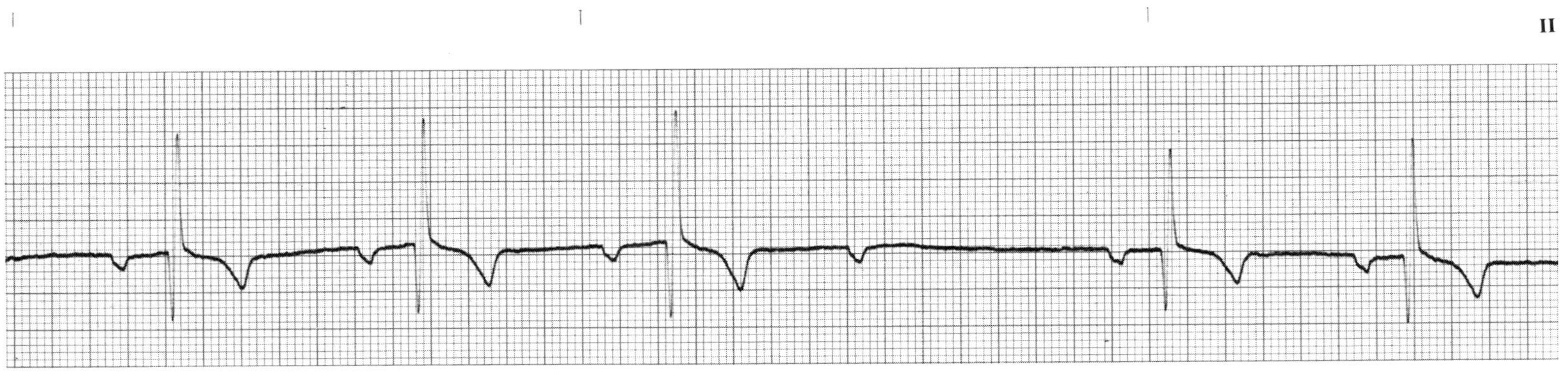

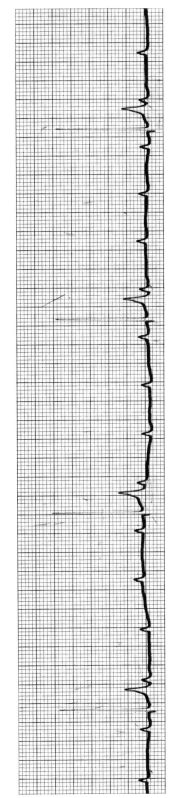

Figure 4–50. This lead II electrocardiogram demonstrates two arrhythmias. Since the P waves are negative, the dominant rhythm arises in the junctional tissues. The heart rate is 90 per minute, so this is a junctional tachycardia. In the middle of the tracing a P wave occurs without a QRS complex, which indicates second degree heart block. Since the P-R intervals of the preceding beats remain constant, this is a so-called Mobitz type II second degree heart block. This dog was suffering from digitalis intoxication.

Paper speed = 50 mm./sec., 1 cm. = 1 mv.

(Tracing courtesy of Dr. L. Tilley, New York, N.Y.)

Figure 4–51. This is an example of 4:1 second degree heart block. There are four P waves for every QRS complex. The P waves that do occur with QRS complexes all have the same P-R interval. This was recorded from a normal dog that had been given xylazine (Rompun).

Paper speed = 50 mm./sec., 1 cm. = 1 mv.

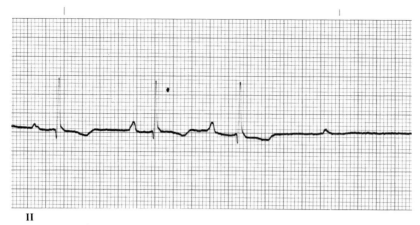

II

Figure 4–52. At the end of this tracing a P wave occurs without a QRS complex, which indicates second degree heart block. In this case, the P-R interval of the beat preceding the dropped QRS complex is prolonged over that of the other normal beats. This is the Wenkebach, or so-called Mobitz type I second degree heart block. There is no particular clinical significance to this other than that most Wenkebach second degree blocks are due to digitalis toxicity. This was recorded from an older dog with severe mitral and tricuspid insufficiency and a right atrial tear.

Paper speed = 50 mm./sec., 1 cm. = 1 mv.

(Tracing courtesy of Dr. L. Tilley, New York, N.Y.)

TREATMENT. First or second degree heart block does not require treatment if the dog is clinically normal. Whenever any of the heart blocks develop after the institution of digitalis therapy, digitalis intoxication is indicated, and the drug should be temporarily withdrawn until the arrhythmias are corrected.

Whenever these arrhythmias occur without apparent cause, exaggerated vagal reflex may be suspected. Abolition of the arrhythmia with atropine is proof of vagal causation. It is rarely necessary to treat the vagally induced heart blocks.

Diphenylhydantoin is an antiarrhythmic drug with special properties that may make it useful for treating incomplete atrioventricular heart block. It has the unique effect of enhancing and accelerating conduction through the atrioventricular node (Helfant et al., 1967; Damato, 1966; Mason et al., 1973). It is not useful for complete heart block because its effect on atrioventricular conduction time lags behind its effect of depressing the ventricular myocardium (Damato, 1966).

Complete heart block responds poorly to medical therapy. If digitalis intoxication or hyperkalemia is the case, correction of the condition will convert the complete heart block to sinus rhythm. In the other instances, atropine and isoproterenol are used. Atropine therapy is usually unsuccessful, and is pursued no further than to give one subcutaneous injection of atropine and record an electrocardiogram 30 minutes to 1 hour later. Isoproterenol is the drug of choice for complete heart block. The dog is given 0.1 to 0.2 mg. intramuscularly or subcutaneously every 4 hours, or is given 15 to 30 mg. orally four to six times a day. Isoproterenol does not relieve the atrioventricular block, but is used to increase the ventricular rate to 80 to 120 beats per minute so that the dog can undergo at least minimal activity without developing clinical

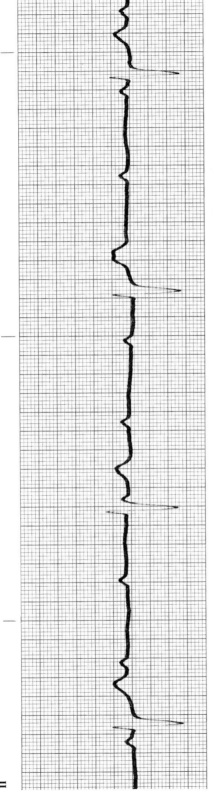

Figure 4–53. Complete heart block (third degree) occurs in this lead II electrocardiogram. The main indication is that there are more P waves than QRS complexes, and the varying P-R intervals indicate that there is no relationship between the P waves and the QRS complexes. The atria are beating at their own rate (140 beats per minute), and the ventricles are beating at their own rate (60 beats per minute). Some of the P waves are lost in the QRS complexes. The etiology of this case was never determined, not even on post-mortem examination.

Paper speed = 50 mm./sec., 1 cm. = 1 mv.

signs. The elixir and sublingual forms of isoproterenol are not recommended for use with this arrhythmia (Ettinger and Suter, 1970).

Empirically, the dog is also given broad spectrum antibiotics and corticosteroids, on the chance that the cause is bacterial endomyocarditis with edema or inflammation in the region of the atrioventricular node or bundle of His. One case has responded in this manner (Fig. 5–43), but results are generally poor (Hamlin, 1966).

Some medications are contraindicated in heart block situations. These include digitalis, quinidine (and other antiarrhythmic agents), and potassium. All of these medications delay conduction through the atrioventricular node and would aggravate the heart block, with the exception of diphenylhydantoin and lidocaine, which may accelerate atrioventricular conduction (Mason et al., 1973). In no case should any antiarrhythmic drug (not even diphenylhydantoin or lidocaine) be used when complete heart block is present (page 156).

Surgical implantation of an artificial pacemaker is the ideal treatment for permanent third degree heart block, but economic considerations usually preclude this procedure, and anesthesia is difficult in these patients. This form of therapy has been successfully performed (Buchanan et al., 1968). In that report, the types of pacemakers are discussed, and the installment procedure is described.

The prognosis is always guarded when complete heart block occurs. Even though the dog may do well for weeks or even months, death may occur at any time.

Sinoatrial Standstill. ASSOCIATIONS. Hyperkalemia is the most common cause of atrial standstill. It can occur any time the serum K$^+$ rises above 7 meq./l. Adrenal insufficiency and terminal renal insufficiency are the two most frequent causes of hyperkalemia and atrial standstill. Occasionally, dogs with cardiac arrest have shown this rhythm (Fig. 4–48). Sinoatrial standstill may be thought of as a pre-death rhythm. Since the ventricles do not receive stimulation from the higher pacemaker centers, they beat very slowly, at their own spontaneous rate. The idioventricular rhythm is a final attempt by the ventricles to maintain life.

Profound weakness, collapse, syncope, and coma occur as a result of asystole and poor cardiac output, and hypotension is severe (Ettinger and Suter, 1970). Gastrointestinal upsets may be reported in the past history, and episodes of exercise intolerance, weakness, or lethargy may also have occurred previously.

PHYSICAL EXAMINATION. On physical examination bradycardia is the outstanding finding, and the heart rate is usually 60 beats per minute or less. Sinoatrial standstill should be on the list of possible diagnoses whenever a profoundly weak or comatose dog is presented with bradycardia. Unlike complete heart block, there is total silence between ventricular beats, and no jugular pulse is present.

ELECTROCARDIOGRAPHIC DIAGNOSIS

1. Bradycardia is present, the heart rate usually being 60 beats per minute or less.

2. The rhythm may be regular or irregular.

3. There are no P waves. The QRS complexes occur alone, with a straight, steady baseline between them.

4. There are no P-R intervals.

5. The QRS complexes are nearly normal if they arise near the bundle of His or are bizarre if they originate in the ventricular muscle mass.

Sinoatrial standstill is demonstrated in a dog with hyperkalemia due to terminal renal insufficiency in Fig. 3–32C. Figure 4–48 demonstrates atrial standstill with an idioventricular rhythm that occurred following a cardiac arrest episode. *The chief characteristics of the diagnosis are the absence of P waves and the slow idioventricular heart rate with smooth, steady baseline between ventricular complexes.*

TREATMENT. The treatment for hyperkalemia includes intravenous dextrose and saline, intravenous and intramuscular hydrocortisone, intramuscular desoxycorticosterone acetate (DOCA), sodium bicarbonate intravenously, and regular insulin intravenously or subcutaneously. The dosages are outlined in the veterinary literature (Bolton, 1974; Lorenz, 1972). Proper therapy can result in dramatic improvement (Fig. 3–32D).

Treatment for the dog in Figure 4–48 should include an intravenous fluid drip to maintain blood volume, and intravenous fluids containing 1 mg. of isoproterenol per 250–500 cc. of fluid and up to 9 meq./kg. of body weight of sodium bicarbonate could be given intravenously to reverse the acidosis caused by cardiac arrest. The isoproterenol drip is run as needed to improve the heart rate and strength of myocardial contraction. Atropine should be given intravenously, should the atrial standstill be due to reflex vagal stimulation.

Atrial standstill carries a grave prognosis, and treatment must be given immediately because the dog could undergo cardiac arrest at any moment.

Bundle Branch Block

Bundle branch block refers to disruption of impulse transmission through the right or left branches of the bundle of His. When bundle branch block occurs, ventricular depolarization occurs in an abnormal sequence, and the QRS complexes become distorted. The ventricle on the affected side is delayed in its depolarization. Rather than receiving stimulation via the Purkinje system, it must wait and receive stimulation from the muscle cells of the normal ventricle. This muscle cell transmission is much slower than the normal conduction velocity, so the complexes become wide. Since the ventricles do not discharge simultaneously, the normal canceling of forces no longer occurs and the complexes usually become large.

Right Bundle Branch Block (RBBB). ASSOCIATIONS. Right bundle branch block most often is an incidental electrocardiographic finding (Bolton and Ettinger, 1972), but has been associated with congenital heart disease (Clark et al., 1970; Hill et al., 1968) and chronic valvular fibrosis (Bolton and Ettinger, 1972; Patterson et al., 1961), and has been seen in normal, healthy dogs wihout apparent disease (Bolton and Ettinger, 1972; Detweiler et al., 1960; Ettinger and Suter, 1970; Patterson et al., 1961). The author has reported right bundle branch block occurring after a cardiac arrest episode (Bolton and Ettinger, 1972), and an example of transient right bundle branch block is shown that occurred during experimental hypothermia for cardiac surgery (Fig. 5–32). It was also reported to occur after the surgical correction of a ventricular septal defect (Breznock et al., 1970). Right bundle branch block occurs most often in older dogs, but may also be seen in young dogs.

Right bundle branch block does not appear to cause any cardiac dysfunction; its clinical significance lies in the fact that electrocardiographically it can mimic severe right ventricular hypertrophy and ventricular tachycardia of left ventricular origin (Fig. 4–55).

No clinical signs are attributable to right bundle branch block, but it has been seen in association with right ventricular dilatation (Patterson et al., 1961).

PHYSICAL EXAMINATION. A helpful clue in diagnosis is the presence of a split second heart sound. The delayed right ventricular depolarization causes the pulmonic valve to close slightly later than the aortic valve. This splitting of the second heart sound is not present in all cases, however.

ELECTROCARDIOGRAPHIC DIAGNOSIS
1. The heart rate is usually normal.
2. The rhythm is regular unless sinus arrhythmia is present.
3. There is a P wave for every QRS complex and a QRS complex for every P wave (i.e., sinus rhythm is present).
4. The P waves and QRS complexes have constant P-R intervals.
5. The P waves are normal, but *the QRS complexes have large wide S waves in leads I, II, III, and aVF. An S wave is usually present in lead V_{10}.*

An electrocardiogram recorded from a 10-year-old beagle dog revealed complete right bundle branch block (Fig. 4–54). The rhythm is sinus in origin, and large wide S waves are seen in leads I, II, III, and aVF. An S wave is present in lead V_{10}, although this is not present in all cases of right bundle branch block. On autopsy, no gross or microscopic lesions could be found to explain the cause of right bundle branch block in this dog. This tracing could be confused with severe right ventricular hypertrophy because of the S_1, S_2, S_3 pattern, and because the mean electrical axis is about −130 degrees. Right ventricular hypertrophy, however, seldom causes the S waves to be so wide (Fig. 4–55). Another way to confirm that this is right bundle branch block is to examine thoracic radiographs. The electrocardiogram indicates that, if right ventricular hypertrophy were present, it would have to be very severe. If the thoracic radiographs do not show this severe right ventricular enlargement, right bundle branch block is diagnosed. Ventricular premature beats and tachycardia of left ventricular origin can also resemble right bundle branch block complexes, but this would not be a sinus rhythm (Fig. 4–55).

Right bundle branch block may occur intermittently, as in Figure 4–56, and may be transient, as in Figure 5–32, but most often it is a permanent conduction abnormality.

If one of the smaller ramifications of the right bundle branch is blocked, incomplete right bundle branch block can occur. This is characterized on the electrocardiogram by the presence of S waves in leads I,

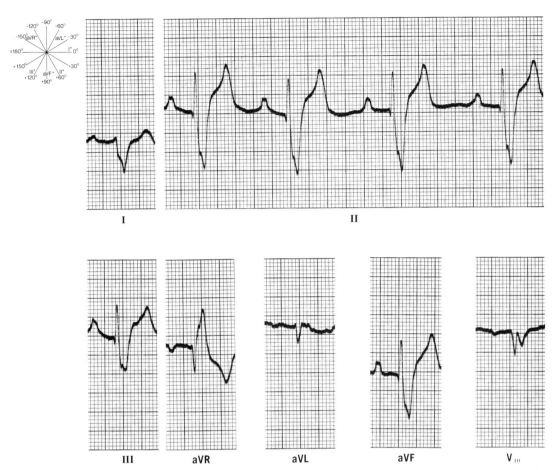

Figure 4–54. Right bundle branch block is present on this tracing recorded from a 10-year-old beagle. Right bundle branch block is characterized by the large, wide S waves in leads I, II, III, and aVF. Right ventricular hypertrophy does not tend to cause the terminal forces to be this wide. There is also an S wave present in lead V_{10}, which is frequently present with right bundle branch block, although it is not present in all cases. The dog had a Grade 3 of 6 left atrioventricular valvular insufficiency, but showed no clinical signs. Only mild right ventricular enlargement was seen on thoracic radiographs, which confirms the diagnosis of right bundle branch block, because right ventricular hypertrophy would have to be very severe to produce an electrocardiogram such as this one.

Paper speed = 50 mm./sec., 1 cm. = 1 mv.

II, III, and aVF, but their size and width are smaller, and the complexes are of normal duration (Bolton and Ettinger, 1972; Hill, 1968). Figure 4–57 was recorded from a Doberman pinscher female with posterior weakness and ataxia. In addition to incomplete right bundle branch block, as characterized by the S waves in leads I, II, III, and aVF that are delayed terminally, she had multifocal ventricular premature beats in other parts of the tracing. It was suspected that myocarditis was causing both the premature beats and the conduction disturbance. Treatment with antibiotics and corticosteroids failed to reverse the right bundle branch block. Thoracic radiographs were normal, as were spinal radiographs and myelography.

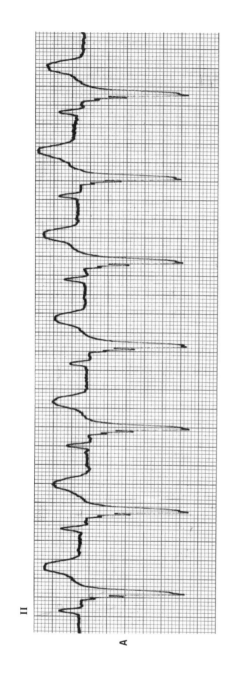

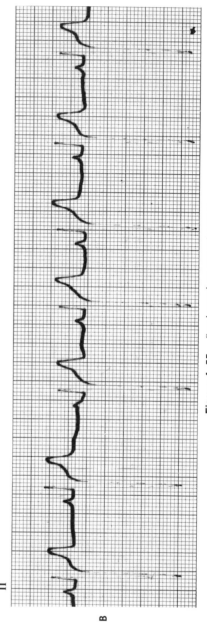

II

A

II

B

Figure 4–55. *See legend on opposite page.*

(Illustration continued on opposite page.)

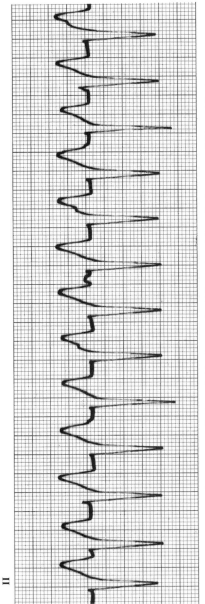

II

C

Figure 4–55. Right bundle branch block must be differentiated from both severe right ventricular hypertrophy and from ventricular tachycardia that originates in the left ventricle.

A. This lead II electrocardiogram was recorded from a 14-year-old Chihuahua with complete right bundle branch block. Note the similarity of this to the lead II recording below it. The important points to note in the tracing are that the rhythm is of sinus origin as opposed to the ventricular tachycardia in strip C where the P waves and QRS complexes are not related, and that the large negative terminal forces are much wider than those in strip B, which were recorded from a dog that had severe right ventricular hypertrophy due to a tetralogy of Fallot.

B. This lead II tracing was recorded from a wirehaired fox terrier with severe right ventricular hypertrophy due to tetralogy of Fallot. Sinus rhythm is present, but note that the large S wave in this tracing is not as wide as the one produced by the complete right bundle branch block in tracing A.

C. This episode of ventricular tachycardia occurred in a boxer dog. The small positive R wave followed by a large negative S wave indicates that the tachycardia arose in the left ventricular mass. This is differentiated from the complete right bundle branch block in tracing A by the fact that the P waves and the QRS complexes are not associated with each other in this tracing, which indicates that this is not a sinus rhythm. One P wave can be seen at about the middle of the tracing, and the other P waves are lost in the larger QRS complexes.

Paper speed (A, B, and C) = 50 mm./sec., 1 cm. = 1 mv.

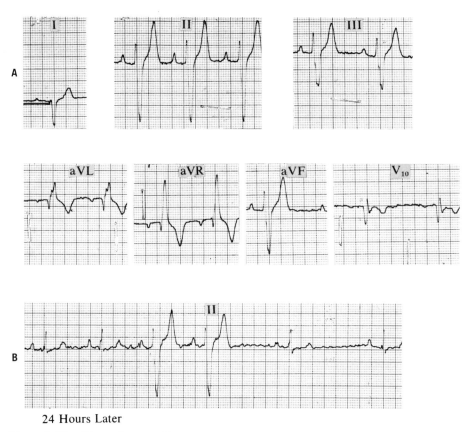

24 Hours Later

Figure 4-56. These electrocardiograms were recorded from a 10-year-old miniature poodle that had intermittent right bundle branch block.

A. This initial tracing indicates complete right bundle branch block by the large, negative, wide terminal forces in leads I, II, III, and aVF, and by the presence of an S wave in lead V_{10}.

B. This lead II tracing was recorded 24 hours later, and shows the right bundle branch block to be only intermittently present. Note that the P-R interval of a right bundle branch block complex is the same as that of a normal complex, which indicates that it is a sinoatrial impulse.

Paper speed = 50 mm./sec., 1 cm. = 1 mv.

(From Ettinger, S. J., and Suter, P. F.: *Canine Cardiology.* W. B. Saunders Co., Philadelphia, 1970.)

TREATMENT. No specific treatment is required for right bundle branch block. Therapy is directed at any other problems that the dog might have, but the right bundle branch block itself is usually an incidental finding.

Left Bundle Branch Block (LBBB). ASSOCIATIONS. Unlike right bundle branch block, left bundle branch block is usually associated with heart disease (Buchanan, 1965; Detweiler et al., 1960; Ettinger and Suter, 1970; Patterson et al., 1961; Romagnoli, 1953). It is commonly associated with severe left ventricular hypertrophy.

Clinical signs do not occur from the arrhythmia per se, but signs of cardiac decompensation may occur in dogs that have myocardial disease or severe left ventricular hypertrophy.

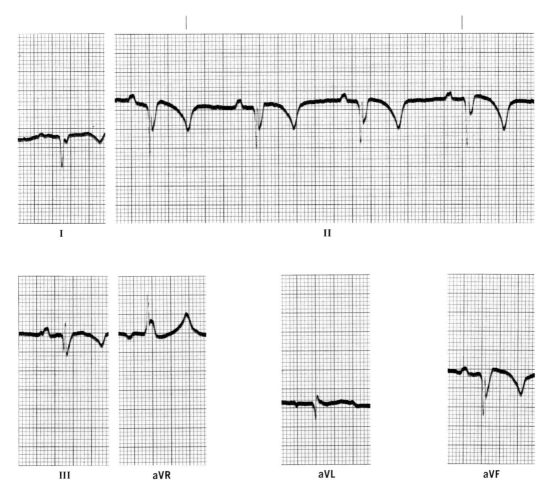

I   II   III   aVR   aVL   aVF

Figure 4–57. This electrocardiogram was recorded from a Doberman pinscher that was presented for posterior weakness and ataxia. The electrocardiogram was taken when premature beats were auscultated on cardiac examination. Incomplete right bundle branch block is indicated here by the presence of S waves in leads I, II, III, and aVF. The delay in the terminal forces is easily seen. The width of the QRS complexes remains normal with incomplete right bundle branch block. In other parts of the lead II rhythm strip ventricular premature beats were present, and it was hypothesized that the dog had myocarditis that was causing the premature beats and that this might also be the etiology of the conduction disturbance that was involving a branch of the right bundle. Thoracic radiographs were normal. No cause was found for the neurologic problem, and the dog was sent home on broad spectrum antibiotics and diphenylhydantoin. Neither quinidine nor diphenylhydantoin have completely controlled the ventricular premature beats.

Paper speed = 50 mm./sec., 1 cm. = 1 mv.

PHYSICAL EXAMINATION. A splitting of the second heart sound may also occur with left bundle branch block when the aortic valve closes late as a result of the delay in left ventricular depolarization.

ELECTROCARDIOGRAPHIC DIAGNOSIS

1. The heart rate is usually normal.

2. The rhythm is regular or sinus arrhythmia is present.

3. There is a P wave for every QRS complex and a QRS complex for every P wave (i.e., sinus rhythm is present).

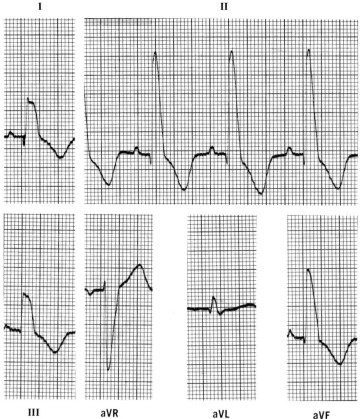

Figure 4–58. This electrocardiogram was recorded from an older dog that was diagnosed as having endocarditis. Thoracic radiographs were not taken, but the electrocardiogram demonstrates a complete left bundle branch block pattern. The QRS complexes are large, wide, and positive in leads I, II, III, and aVF. Whenever the QRS complexes are wider than 0.07 second (3½ boxes), left bundle branch block is diagnosed. These QRS complexes are 0.08 to 0.09 second wide (4 to 4½ boxes). Complete left bundle branch block does not tend to deviate the mean electrical axis, as does complete right bundle branch block. The mean electrical axis is +70° in this tracing.

Paper speed = 50 mm./sec., 1 cm. = 1 mv.

(Tracing courtesy of Dr. J. Kazmierczak, Plainfield, N.J.)

4. The P-R intervals are similar (P waves and QRS complexes are related).

5. The P waves are normal. *The QRS complexes are positive and wider than 0.07 second in leads I, II, III, and aVF.*

Left bundle branch block and severe left ventricular hypertrophy can occur together and are indistinguishable. *When the QRS complexes are wider than 0.07 second, left bundle branch block is diagnosed* (Figs. 3–28 and 4–58). The electrocardiographic findings are compared with thoracic radiographs to determine whether left ventricular enlargement is present along with left bundle branch block.

TREATMENT. No specific therapy is given for the conduction disturbance, but if myocardial disease is suspected, broad spectrum antibiotics and corticosteroids might be given, should there be an inflammatory lesion causing the left bundle branch block. Signs of cardiac decompensation should be treated accordingly.

Wolff-Parkinson-White Syndrome (W-P-W). ASSOCIATIONS. This is a rare conduction abnormality in dogs. Its significance is unknown, but it has been described in the veterinary literature (Patterson et al., 1961). In man it is considered to be a congenital abnormality in which an accessory pathway bypasses the atrioventricular node and conducts atrial impulses directly to the ventricles (Bellet, 1972). Another theory holds that conduction is somehow accelerated through the normal conduction system, but at this time evidence favors the theory of one or more accessory pathways, possibly the bundle of Kent, the James fibers, or the Mahaim fibers (Bellet, 1972).

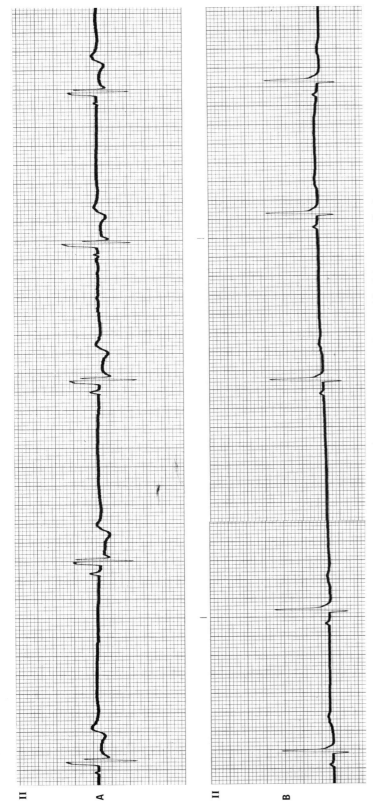

Figure 4–59. These two lead II tracings were recorded from an 8-year-old miniature poodle that presented because of tenesmus and coughing. A Grade 1 to 2 of 6 left atrioventricular valvular insufficiency and a bradycardia were auscultated.

A. This tracing was recorded on the day of admittance. Wolff-Parkinson-White (W-P-W) syndrome was diagnosed because the P-R intervals are short and vary from 0.05 to 0.06 second. there is a mild slurring of the upstroke of the R wave (delta wave), and the QRS complexes are too wide for this breed (0.06 second). The QRS complexes are also aberrant in form, which indicates that they enter the ventricular conduction system at an aberrant site. Sinus arrhythmia and wandering pacemaker are also present. Generalized cardiomegaly was seen on thoracic radiography, but the lung fields were clear.

B. Quinidine therapy alleviated the conduction disturbance and this electrocardiogram was recorded about one month later. The P-R interval is now 0.06 to 0.07 second, and the QRS complexes look more normal. Sinus arrhythmia is still present.

Paper speed = 50 mm./sec., $^1/_2$ cm. = 1 mv.

(Tracings courtesy of Dr. L. Tilley. New York. N.Y.)

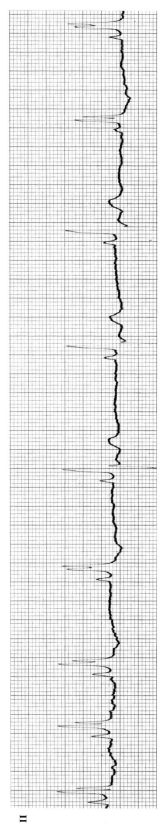

Figure 4–60. This lead II electrocardiogram was recorded on a different day from the same dog as in Figure 4–59. In this tracing, the "delta waves" are much better demonstrated. Also, the three ventricular beats in the middle are different in form than the other QRS complexes, which indicates that they were conducted via a different pathway than the others. These three complexes are similar to the complexes in Figure 4–59 (these are recorded at full sensitivity, while Figure 4–59 was recorded at one-half sensitivity). The alternation between types of QRS complexes may indicate that there is more than one accessory conduction pathway that can bypass the normal atrioventricular conduction system in this dog.

Paper speed = 50 mm./sec., 1 cm. = 1 mv.
(Tracing courtesy of Dr. L. Tilley, New York, N.Y.)

II

Clinical signs have not been reported in the dog. The one case reported was a wirehaired fox terrier that was healthy except for demodectic mange. In man, episodes of supraventricular tachycardia which are distressing to the patient are associated with this syndrome (Friedberg, 1966). No specific physical findings are associated with this arrhythmia.

ELECTROCARDIOGRAPHIC DIAGNOSIS

1. The heart rate is normal.

2. The rhythm is regular or sinus arrhythmia is present.

3. There is a P wave for every QRS complex and a QRS complex for every P wave (i.e., it is a sinus rhythm).

4. *The P-R intervals are constant and shorter than 0.06 second.*

5. The P waves are normal, but *the QRS complexes are prolonged and may be aberrant, and there is slurring of the upstroke of the R wave (delta wave).*

Wolff-Parkinson-White syndrome was diagnosed in an 8-year-old male miniature poodle seen by Dr. L. Tilley at the Animal Medical Center, New York, New York. The dog was presented because of a perineal hernia with tenesmus, and a persistent cough. A Grade 1 to 2 of 6 mitral insufficiency was detected on auscultation, and the heart rate was 80 beats per minute. An electrocardiogram recorded at this time revealed the presence of this syndrome (Fig. 4–59A). The QRS complexes were aberrant in configuration, and the P-R intervals were 0.05 to 0.06 second long. The delta waves were not well visualized. Generalized cardiomegaly, especially of the right side, was seen on thoracic radiographs, but the lung fields were normal. At times, the QRS complexes varied in configuration (Fig. 4–60). Also in Figure 4–60 the delta waves are more prominent.

TREATMENT. No treatment is required if the dog is free of clinical signs. In man, bouts of supraventricular tachycardia are controlled with antiarrhythmic agents such as propranolol and quinidine (Phibbs, 1973). Quinidine and procainamide have been used in man to abolish the Wolff-Parkinson-White syndrome by increasing the refractory period of the fibers in the accessory pathway, permitting conduction to occur over the normal pathway via the atrioventricular junction (Bellet, 1972).

Surgical treatments have been used with limited success in man. An attempt is made, by using endocardial and epicardial mapping, to locate the accessory pathways and interrupt them surgically (Bellet, 1972).

Quinidine was successfully used to treat the Wolff-Parkinson-White syndrome in the miniature poodle (Fig. 4–59B).

REFERENCES

Bacaner, B.: Treatment of Ventricular Fibrillation and Other Acute Arrhythmias with Bretylium Tosylate. Amer. J. Cardiol., 21 (1968):530.

Bellet, S.: Essentials of Cardiac Arrhythmias, Diagnosis and Mangement. W. B. Saunders Co., Philadelphia, 1972.

Bellet, S.: Treatment of Atrial Arrhythmias. In *Cardiac Arrhythmias.* Edited by L. S. Dreifus. Grune & Stratton, New York. (1973), p. 171.

Bolton, G. R., and Ettinger, S. J.: Paroxysmal Atrial Fibrillation in the dog. J.A.V.M.A., 158 (1971):64.

Bolton, G. R.: Prevention and Treatment of Cardiovascular Emergencies During Anesthesia and Surgery. In Vet. Clin. N. Am., 2 (1972a):411.

Bolton, G. R.: Cardiomyopathy. In *A Manual of Clinical Cardiology*. American Animal Hospital Association, Elkhart, Indiana. (1972b), p. 47.

Bolton, G. R., and Ettinger, S. J.: Right Bundle Branch Block in the Dog. J.A.V.M.A., 160 (1972c):1104.

Bolton, G. R.: Tachyarrhythmias. In *Current Veterinary Therapy V*, edited by R. W. Kirk. W. B. Saunders Co., Philadelphia. 1974, p. 312.

Breznock, E. M., Hilwig, R. W., Vasko, J. S., and Hamlin, R. L.: Surgical Correction of an Interventricular Septal Defect in the Dog. J.A.V.M.A., 157 (1970):1343.

Buchanan, J. W.: Spontaneous Arrhythmias and Conduction Disturbances in Domestic Animals. Ann. N.Y. Acad. Sci., 127 (1965):224.

Buchanan, J. W., Dear, M. G., Pyle, R. L., and Berg, P.: Medical and Pacemaker Therapy of Complete Heart Block and Congestive Heart Failure in a Dog. J.A.V.M.A., 152 (1968):1099.

Clark, D. R., Szabuniewicz, M., and McCrady, J. D.: Clinical Use of the Electrocardiogram in Animals. Vet. Med., 61 (1966):751, 86, 1973.

Clark, D. R., Anderson, J. G., and Paterson, C.: Imperforate Cardiac Septal Defect in a Dog. J.A.V.M.A., 156 (1970):1020.

Damato, A. N.: Diphenylhydantoin: Pharmacological and Clinical Use. Progr. Cardiovasc. Dis., 8 (1966):364.

Dear, M. G.: Spontaneous Reversion of Complete A-V Block to Sinus Rhythm in the Dog. J. Small Anim. Pract., 11 (1970a):17.

Dear, M. G.: Complete atrio-ventricular block in the dog: a possible congenital case. J. Small Anim. Pract., 11 (1970b):301.

Dear, M. G.: Mitral Incompetence in Dogs. J. Small Anim. Pract., 12 (1971):1.

Detweiler, D. K.: Electrocardiographic and Clinical Features of Spontaneous Auricular Fibrillation and Flutter (Tachycardia) in Dogs. Zbl. Veterinaermed., 4 (1957):509.

Detweiler, D. K., Hubben, K., and Patterson, D. F.: Survey of Cardiovascular Disease in Dogs: Preliminary Report on the First 1,000 Dogs Screened. Am. J. Vet. Res., 21 (1960):329.

Ettinger, S. J.: Conversion of Spontaneous Atrial Fibrillation in Dogs, Using Direct Current Synchronized Shock. J.A.V.M.A., 152 (1968a):41.

Ettinger, S. J., and Buergelt, C. D.: Atrioventricular Dissociation (Incomplete) with Accrochage in a Dog with Ruptured Chordae Tendineae. Amer. J. Vet. Res., 29 (1968b):1499.

Ettinger, S. J.: Isoproterenol Treatment of Atrioventricular Block in the Dog. J.A.V.M.A., 154 (1969):398.

Ettinger, S. J., and Suter, P. F.: Canine Cardiology. W. B. Saunders Co., Philadelphia, 1970.

Fisher, E. W.: Fainting in Boxers—the Possibility of Vasovagal Syncope (Adam-Stokes attacks). J. Small Anim. Pract., 12 (1971):347.

Flickenger, G. L., and Patterson, D. F.: Coronary Lesions Associated with Congenital Subaortic Stenosis in the Dog. J. Path. Bact., 93 (1967):133.

Friedberg, C. K.: Diseases of the Heart. 3rd edition. W. B. Saunders Co., Philadelphia, 1966.

Gratzl, F.: Tachykardien beim Hund, eine klinische und elektrokardiographische Studie. Wien. Tieraerztl. Mschr., 47 (1960):281.

Hamlin, R. L.: Heart Block. In *Current Veterinary Therapy, 1966–1967*. Edited by R. W. Kirk. W. B. Saunders Co., Philadelphia, 1966, p. 79.

Hamlin, R. L., Smetzer, D. L., and Breznock, E. M.: Sinoatrial Syncope in Miniature Schnauzers, J.A.V.M.A., 161 (1972):1023.

Helfant, R. H., Law, S. H., Cohen, S. I., and Damato, A. N.: Effects of Diphenylhydantoin on Atrioventricular Conduction in Man. Circulation, XXXVI (1967):686.

Hill, J. D., Moore, E. N., and Patterson, D. F.: Ventricular Epicardial Activation Studies in Experimental and Spontaneous Right Bundle Branch Block in the Dog. Am. J. Cardiol., 21 (1968):232.

Jaffe, K. R., and Bolton, G. R.: Myocardial Infarction in a Dog with Complete Heart Block. Vet. Med. Small Anim. Clin., 69 (1974):197.

Jonsson, L.: Coronary Arterial Lesions and Myocardial Infarcts in the Dog. A Pathologic and Microangiographic Study. Acta Scand., Suppl. 38, 1972.

Mason, D. T., Amsterdam, E. A., Massumi, R. A., Mansour, E. J., Hughes, J. L., and Zelis, R.: Combined Actions of Antiarrhythmic Drugs: Electrophysiologic and Therapeutic Considerations. In Cardiac Arrhythmias, edited by L. S. Dreifus. Grune & Stratton, New York, 1973, p. 531.

Moe, G. K., and Farah, A. E.: Digitalis and Allied Cardiac Glycosides. In *The Phar-*

macological Basis of Therapeutics. 4th edition. Edited by L. S. Goodman and A. Gilman. The Macmillan Company, London, 1970, p. 677.

Patterson, D. F., Detweiler, D. K., Hubben, K., and Botts, R. P.: Spontaneous Abnormal Cardiac Arrhythmias and Conduction Disturbances in the Dog. (A Clinical and Pathologic Study of 3000 Dogs.) Amer. J. Vet. Res., 22 (1961):355.

Pedersoli, W. M., and Brown, M. K.: A New Approach to the Etiology of Arrhythmogenic Effects of Thiamylal Sodium in Dogs. Vet. Med. Small Anim. Clin., 68 (1973):1286.

Pedini, B.: Flutuazione Atriale Pura e Bigeminismo Extrasistolico in un Cane. Vet. Italiana, 5 (1954):1003.

Phibbs, B.: The Cardiac Arrhythmias. C. V. Mosby Co., St. Louis, 1973.

Robertson, B. T., and Ramy, C. T.: Reversible Heart Block in a Dog. J.A.V.M.A., 152 (1968):1110.

Robertson, B. T.: Correction of Atrial Flutter with Quinidine and Digitalis. J. Small Anim. Pract., 11 (1970):251.

Robertson, B. T., and Giles, H. D.: Complete Heart Block Associated with Vegetative Endocarditis in a Dog. J.A.V.M.A., 161 (1972):180.

Roos, J.: Atrioventrikularer Herzrhythmus beim Hund. (Paroxysmalie Tachycardie mit periodischem Herzstillstand.) Tijdschr. Diergeneesk, 64 (1937):969. (Abstract in Wien. Tieraerztl. Mschr., 24 (1938):151.)

Weirich, W. E., Blevins, W. E., Conrad, C. R., Ruth, G. R., and Gallina, A. N.: Congenital Tricuspid Insufficiency in a Dog. J.A.V.M.A., 164 (1974):1025.

Chapter 5 is a series of case studies, and is designed to be used as a self-study aid. In each instance, a short description of the dog or the circumstances is given, and questions are asked concerning the electrocardiogram that accompanies that case. Please study each case, answer the questions, and then compare your answers to those that are provided. As a study aid each answer has been referenced to direct the reader to the appropriate area of the book if further clarification is needed.

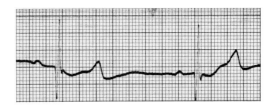

Chapter 5

SELF-ASSESSMENT

1. These continuous lead II electrocardiograms were recorded from a 16-year-old, small mixed breed dog. The dog had no clinical signs, but an arrhythmia was detected during routine physical examination.

Paper speed = 50 mm./sec., 1 cm. = 1 mv.
(Tracings courtesy of Dr. W. Thomas, Philadelphia, Pa.)

Questions:

a. Which arrhythmias are present?

b. What is a likely cause?

c. What treatment should be given?

Answers:

a. The basic rhythm is sinus in origin, and the long pauses are greater than twice the normal R-R interval, indicating that sinus arrest is present (refer to Figures 4–9 or 4–10). At the end of the pauses, escape beats occur. In the top electrocardiogram, the first pause is terminated by a ventricular escape beat. The P-R interval of the beat following the ventricular escape beat is prolonged, because the ventricles were refractory to the sinus impulse for a short time following the previous beat. The second sinus arrest pause in the top tracing is terminated by a junctional escape beat. The negative P wave can be seen to occur behind the QRS deflection and in front of the T wave (refer to Figures 4–44, 4–45, and 4–47. In the bottom tracing, the first escape beat is either a junctional escape beat, in which the P wave is lost in the QRS complex, or a ventricular escape beat arising in the bundle of His. Since the QRS complex has a slightly different configuration from the other complexes, this is probably a ventricular escape beat. After the second pause in the lower electrocardiogram, another junctional escape beat occurs, with a negative P wave following it. This electrocardiogram resembles the sick sinus syndrome described in miniature schnauzers by Hamlin et al. (1972). The sinus arrest episodes in this dog are not as long as those in the schnauzers, and the dog was asymptomatic. The schnauzers experienced episodic syncope.

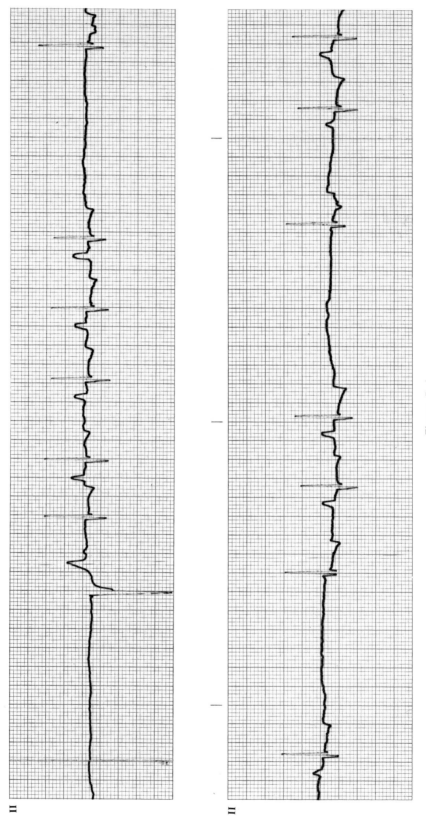

Figure 5-1.

b. The periods of sinus arrest may be caused by an exaggerated vagal reflex.

c. Since the dog shows no clinical signs, treatment is unnecessary. Atropine may be given to prove whether hypertonic vagal reflex is the cause. If the dog showed signs of weakness or syncope, isoproterenol could also be used to increase the ventricular rate. Isoproterenol was not effective in treating the schnauzers (Hamlin et al., 1972).

2. These lead II electrocardiograms were recorded from a 10-year-old male border collie with chronic mitral valvular fibrosis and congestive heart failure. He was being treated with digitalis.

    A. Paper speed = 50 mm./sec., 1 cm. = 1 mv.
    B. Paper speed = 25 mm./sec., 1 cm. = 1 mv.
(Tracings courtesy of Dr. W. Thomas, Philadelphia, Pa.)

Questions:

    a. What is the arrhythmia?

    b. What is its cause?

    c. What is the treatment?

Answers:

a. Atrial flutter. The rhythmic undulations of the baseline between the QRS complexes are "f" waves, indicating atrial flutter. The ventricular response is uneven, and when a burst of tachycardia occurs in the lower tracing, the QRS complexes discharge so quickly that depolarization is initiated while some parts of the ventricles are still refractory from the previous beat, and conduction is slightly aberrant. This is the same dog as in Figure 4–22.

b. Since this arrhythmia was not present when digitalis therapy was instituted, digitalis intoxication should be suspected until proved otherwise.

A second possible cause is that left atrial enlargement and stretching secondary to the mitral valvular insufficiency is becoming severe enough to cause the arrhythmia.

c. Digitalis therapy should be discontinued to see if the arrhythmia improves. When the arrhythmia is abolished, digitalis would then be given in slightly smaller amounts.

If discontinuation of digitalis did not improve the arrhythmia (improvement usually occurs in 24 hours but may take up to 7 days), and progression of the disease is thought to cause the atrial flutter, digitalis would be given to control the congestive heart failure, and then quinidine would be added to the therapeutic regime. Conversion of atrial flutter to sinus rhythm by using digitalis and quinidine in combination has been reported (Robertson, 1970).

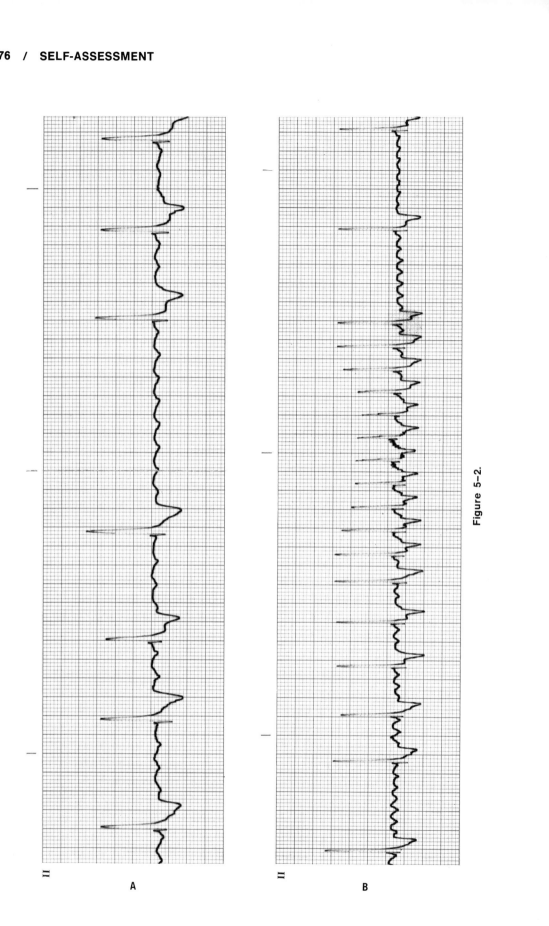

II

A

II

B

Figure 5–2.

3. For these lead II recordings, a normal Husky dog was given xylazine (Rompun). Tracing A was recorded after giving 0.5 mg./lb. intramuscularly. Tracing B was recorded 52 seconds after the dog was given 0.8 mg. (0.02 mg./lb.) of atropine intravenously. Tracing C was recorded 10 seconds after tracing B.

Paper speed = 50 mm./sec., 1 cm. = 1mv.

Questions:

a. What arrhythmia is present in tracing A?

b. What arrhythmia is present in tracing B?

c. What is occurring in tracing C?

Answers:

a. Sinus bradycardia has occurred. The heart rate is 32 to 40 beats per minute. Sinus arrhythmia is also present; note that the R-R intervals vary (refer to Figures 4–4, 4–5, and 4–12).

b. Second degree heart block. The occurrence of two P waves with no QRS complexes, followed by two PQRS complexes, and then followed by two more P waves with no QRS complexes indicates second degree atrioventricular block (refer to Figures 4–50, 4–51, and 4–52). In the normal complexes, the P waves are associated with the QRS complexes, so this is not complete heart block. Atropine, when given intravenously, exerts an initial vagal effect before it blocks vagal activity, and this initial vagal stimulation was apparently strong enough to block a few of the P waves from entering the ventricular conduction system.

c. In this tracing, one more episode of second degree block occurs (third P wave from left), and then the vagal blocking action of atropine became dominant and increased the heart rate. The initial vagal effect of the atropine lasted about 10 seconds. The P-R interval in this tracing averages 0.14 second, so first degree heart block is still present despite atropine therapy.

4. This lead II tracing was recorded after administering xylazine and atropine to a dog for examination purposes.

Paper speed = 50 mm./sec., 1 cm. = 1 mv.

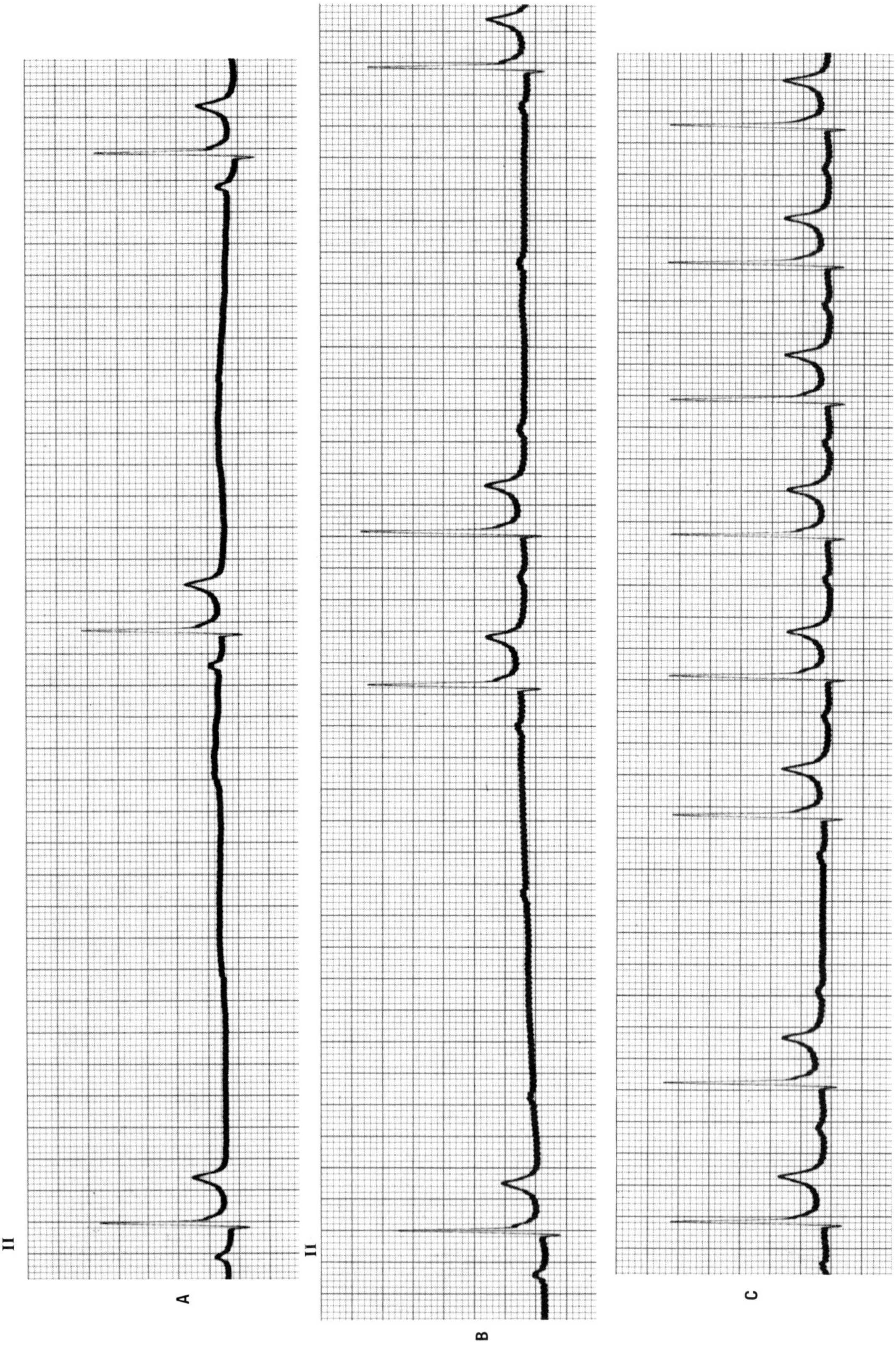

Figure 5–3.

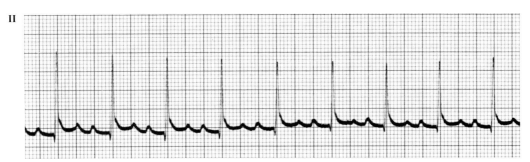

Figure 5–4.

Questions:

    a. What is the arrhythmia?

    b. Why is this not atrial tachycardia?

    c. What is the treatment?

Answers:

    a. Sinus tachycardia. The heart rate is 200 beats per minute, and it is a sinus rhythm.

    b. In this case, knowing the situation is enough to diagnose this as sinus tachycardia. The dog is normal and has a normal heart rate, but, after atropine is given the heart rate accelerates, as expected. Atrial tachycardia usually occurs in an older dog that has severe mitral valvular incompetence (see Table 4–4 for the differentiation of atrial tachycardia and sinus tachycardia). Another way to confirm the diagnosis of sinus tachycardia would be to record a tracing when the dog's heart rate had returned to normal. The P waves of the normal heart rate should be identical to the P waves during the tachycardia if this is sinus tachycardia (refer to Figure 4–11).

    c. No treatment is necessary. The heart rate will return to normal when the atropine is eliminated from the system.

5. This electrocardiogram was recorded from a 4-year-old mixed breed female dog weighing 6.8 kg. On physical examination, the dog had a continuous murmur of patent ductus arteriosus. The heart rate was rapid and irregular, and there was a pulse deficit. The dog was presented in biventricular congestive heart failure.

    Paper speed = 50 mm./sec., 1 cm. = 1 mv.

Questions:

    a. Interpret the electrocardiogram.

    b. What is the treatment?

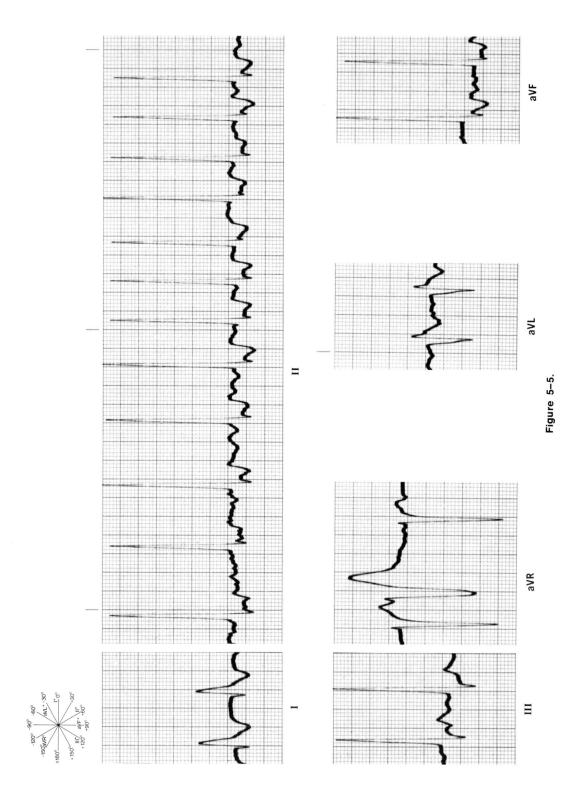

Figure 5–5.

Answers:

   a. Heart rate = 220 to 240 beats per minute

     Heart rhythm = atrial fibrillation. One ventricular premature beat is present in lead aVR (the middle beat)

     Mean electrical axis = +75°

     Measuring and multiplying:

       1. P waves: none present

       2. P-R interval: none present

       3. QRS width = 0.05 second (2½ boxes)

       4. R wave height = 3.4 mv. (average = 34 boxes)

       5. S-T segment and T wave: S-T segment depression of 0.3 mv. (3 boxes) in leads II, III, and aVF

       6. Q-T interval = 0.16 second (8 boxes)

     Miscellaneous criteria: none

Electrocardiographic diagnosis: atrial fibrillation, ventricular premature beat, left ventricular hypertrophy (probably biventricular, because the axis remained normal).

The atrial fibrillation was suspected on physical examination because of the rapid, irregular heart beat and the pulse deficit. On the electrocardiogram irregular tachycardia with fairly normal-looking lead II complexes, indicating supraventricular beats, is seen. When the pauses occur there are no P waves; only baseline undulations called "f" waves (refer to Figures 4–20 and 4–21). Severe mitral insufficiency can occur secondary to left ventricular dilatation in patent ductus arteriosus, and the resultant left atrial enlargement and stretching caused atrial fibrillation. The ventricular premature beat could be caused by the congestive heart failure and myocardial hypoxia.

Left ventricular hypertrophy was diagnosed because of the tall R waves and the S-T segment depression (refer to Figures 3–20 and 3–22). Since the axis did not shift leftward, it may be suspected that right ventricular hypertrophy has also occurred, although no specific indications for this were found. On thoracic radiographs, both ventricles, as well as the left atrium, were markedly enlarged.

The depression of the S-T segment might also be caused by myocardial hypoxia, resulting from the severe congestive heart failure.

Leads I and aVL are about equally close to being isoelectric, although neither is perfect. If lead I is used, aVF is perpendicular and aVF is positive. The positive pole of aVF is +90°. If lead aVL is used as isoelectric, lead II is perpendicular and positive. The positive pole of lead II is +60°. The average of +60° and +90° is taken, and the axis is about +75° (refer to Figure 3–12).

   b. The treatment of choice is digitalization. Once the heart rate is controlled below 160 beats per minute and the congestive heart failure is alleviated, quinidine could be added and used in conjunction with digitalis to try to convert the atrial fibrillation to sinus rhythm.

This dog was treated with digitalis, which controlled the condition. Surgery for the patent ductus arteriosus was successful. For one year the dog has had to remain on digitalis therapy postoperatively, and three different attempts at cardioversion with quinidine have failed. The changes on thoracic radiographs have not reversed themselves.

6. These two lead II electrocardiograms were recorded from the same Irish Terrier just 15 minutes apart.

Paper speed = 50 mm./sec., 1 cm. = 1 mv.

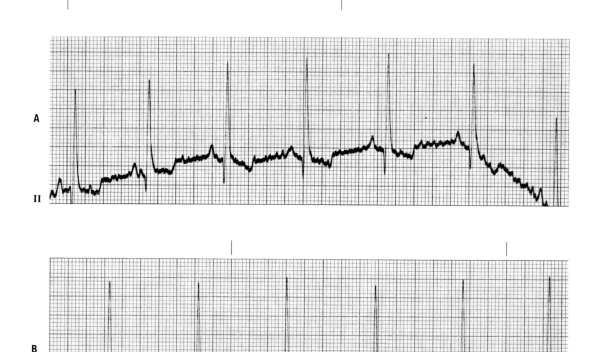

Figure 5-6.

Questions:

a. What does strip A indicate?

b. What was done to correct it in strip B?

Answers:

a. This is a sinus rhythm that is slightly irregular because the R-R intervals vary slightly. The baseline shifts up and down, and there is a trembling artifact present.

b. This recording was made after tranquilizing the dog with acepromazine and atropine. The R-R intervals are still not exactly regular, so some sinus arrhythmia is present (refer to Figure 4–3). The trembling and respiratory fluctuations are gone now that the dog is tranquil.

7. This electrocardiogram was taken as a part of the case evaluation of a 10-year-old miniature poodle with a Grade 4 of 6 systolic murmur of chronic mitral valvular insufficiency. The dog had a BB-shot pulse, the heart rate was normal, and no significant arrhythmias were found. The dog showed no clinical signs. Thoracic radiographs revealed mild right ventricular enlargement and slight left atrial enlargement.

Paper speed = 50 mm./sec., 1 cm. = 1 mv.

Questions:

a. Read the electrocardiogram.

b. What should the owner be told?

Answers:

a. Heart rate = 81 to 120 beats per minute
Heart rhythm: sinus arrhythmia, wandering pacemaker
Mean electrical axis = +70°
Measuring and multiplying:
  a. P waves = 0.03 second (1½ boxes) by 0.3 mv. (3 boxes on the average). P waves vary in height
  b. P-R interval = 0.08 second (4 boxes)
  c. QRS width = 0.05 second (2½ boxes)
  d. R wave height = 1.5 mv. (15 boxes average)
  e. S-T segment and T wave = normal
  f. Q-T interval = 0.185 second (9½ boxes)
Miscellaneous criteria: positive T wave in lead V_{10}

Electrocardiographic diagnosis: sinus arrhythmia, wandering pacemaker, and right ventricular hypertrophy.

The sinus arrhythmia and wandering pacemaker are normal variations of the canine rhythm (refer to Figure 4–6). The positive T wave in lead V_{10} indicates right ventricular hypertrophy (refer to Figure 3–27). Since the axis is +70° (normal), there may be some left ventricular hypertrophy also. It is worth a good look at the thoracic radiographs.

Lead aVL was used as the closest to isoelectric. Lead II was perpendicular and positive, so the axis is about +60°. Since lead aVL was not perfectly isoelectric and it was more negative than positive, the axis was shifted from +60° a little toward aVL's negative pole and was interpolated to about +70°.

b. Since the dog is showing no clinical signs and the electrocardiographic and radiographic signs are mild, the owner is given a diagnosis of compensated mitral insufficiency and is told to recheck the dog

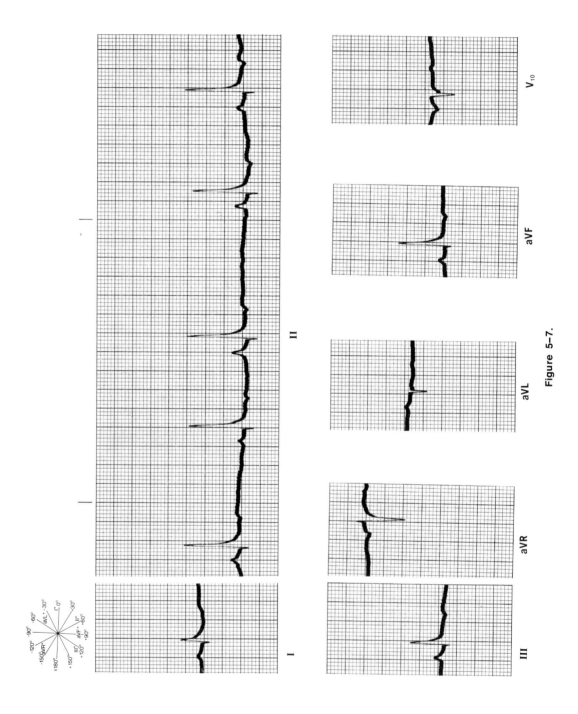

Figure 5–7.

every 3 to 6 months. No treatment is necessary, but the owner is given a list of signs to be aware of if the disease should progress.

8. This lead II electrocardiogram was recorded from a 5-year-old stand-ard poodle that was being rechecked while being treated for Addison's disease. He was doing well and this was a routine check.

Paper speed = 50 mm./sec., 1 cm. = 1 mv.

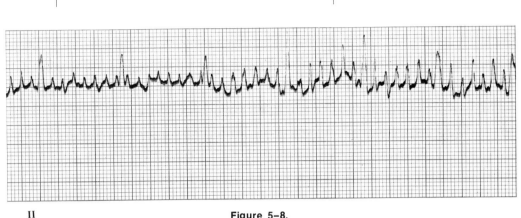

II   Figure 5–8.

Questions:

a. What arrhythmia is present?

b. What treatment is necessary?

Answers:

a. No arrhythmia is present. The dog is trembling and shaking, which makes the baseline jump wildly. The clue is the irregularity of the trembling artifact. It is so large in the end of the tracing that the R waves of the QRS complexes cannot even be seen (refer to Figure 3–43). This could falsely resemble atrial flutter.

b. The dog could be tranquilized if the electrocardiogram were vital to the recheck visit. Since the dog was well, attempts to record an elec-trocardiogram were discontinued.

9. Paper speed = 50 mm./sec., 1 cm. = 1 mv.

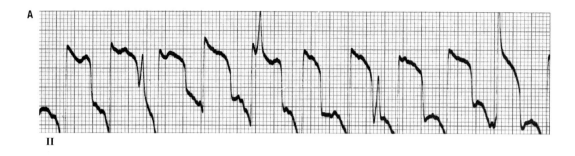

A

II

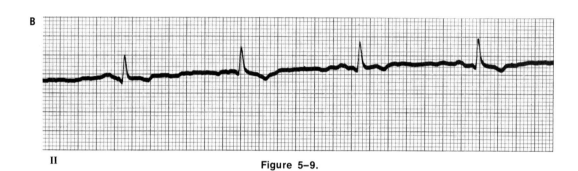

B

II

Figure 5–9.

Questions:

    a. What is the diagnosis in tracing A?

    b. What treatment was given to produce tracing B?

Answers:

    a. This is panting artifact. This is lead I, and as the front legs bounced up and down when he panted, the tracing bounced up and down. This could resemble the bizarre QRS complexes of ventricular tachycardia and lead to misdiagnosis (refer to Fig. 3–46).

    b. A rolled-up wad of paper towels was wedged between the dog's front legs to steady them.

10. Paper speed = 50 mm./sec., 1 cm. = 1 mv.

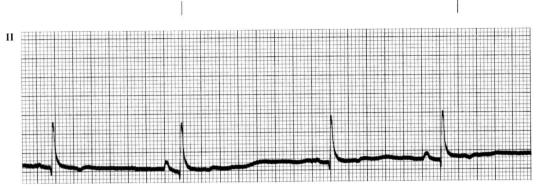

Figure 5–10.

Questions:

    a. What is the rhythm?

    b. What causes this rhythm?

Answers:

    a. Sinus arrhythmia and wandering pacemaker. The rhythm is sinus in origin (the P waves and QRS complexes are related), and the R-R intervals vary, which indicates an irregular sinus rhythm. Wandering pacemaker is evidenced by the variation in the height of the P waves (refer to Figures 4–6 and 4–7).

    b. Sinus arrhythmia is caused by variations in vagal tone secondary to respiration. On inspiration the vagal reflex diminishes and the heart rate increases. On expiration the vagal tone increases and the heart rate decreases. The pacemaker site varies (wanders) slightly. As the vagal tone increases it depresses the sinoatrial node, and the pacemaker site may shift within the node or even the atria.

11. This lead II electrocardiogram was recorded from a 14-year-old mixed breed female dog with mitral insufficiency. At the time of this recording she was suffering from digitalis intoxication. She was anorexic and vomiting. She had been given 0.375 mg. digoxin once daily for 5 days when she became ill.

    Paper speed = 50 mm./sec., 1 cm. = 1 mv.

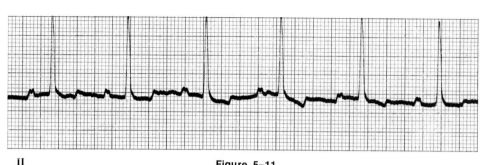

II   Figure 5–11.

Questions:

a. Is there any evidence of digitalis intoxication here?

b. Are there any criteria present for enlargement of any of the cardiac chambers?

Answers:

a. No. The P-R interval is within normal limits, (0.12 second or 6 boxes). There are no arrhythmias. Since we do not know what her P-R interval was at the start of digitalization, we do not know how much it is prolonged. If it were 0.08 second in the beginning, then 0.12 second is excessive prolongation for her. Also, although electrocardiographic changes usually occur before the physical signs of digitalis intoxication, they do not always precede the physical signs.

b. There is no evidence of any sign of cardiac enlargement. The P waves are notched, but they are only 0.04 second (2 boxes) wide. They must be wider than 0.04 second to indicate left atrial hypertrophy. There was mild left atrial enlargement and mild right ventricular enlargement on the thoracic radiographs.

12. This electrocardiogram was recorded from a 9-year-old female miniature poodle. She had asymptomatic mitral insufficiency and severe emesis from a gastric carcinoma. This tracing was recorded while she was under anesthesia for an abdominal exploratory operation.

Paper speed = 50 mm./sec., 1 cm. = 1 mv.

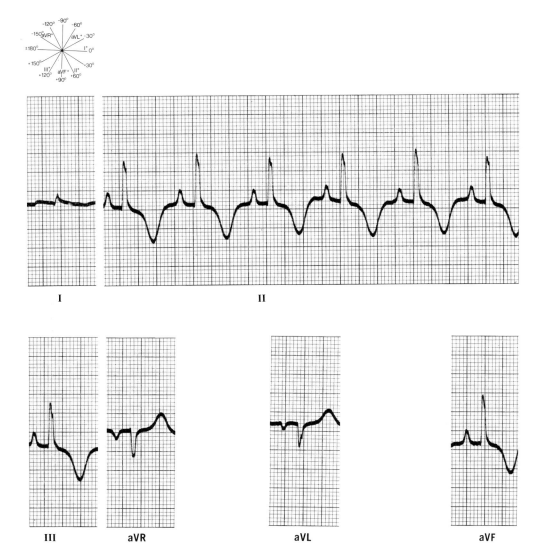

Figure 5–12.

Question:

Please interpret her electrocardiogram.

Answer:

Heart rate = 150 beats per minute
Heart rhythm = normal sinus rhythm (NSR)
Mean electrical axis = +85° to +90°
Measuring and multiplying:
  P wave = 0.4 mv. (4 boxes) by 0.04 second (2 boxes)
  P-R interval = 0.10 second (5 boxes)
  QRS width = 0.05 second (2½ boxes)

R wave height = 1.3 mv. (13 boxes average)
S-T segment and T wave: S-T segment normal, but T wave large
Q-T interval = 0.24 to 0.26 second (12 to 13 boxes)
Miscellaneous criteria: none

Electrocardiographic diagnosis: The prolonged Q-T interval may be suggestive of imbalances in serum K^+ or Ca^{++} (refer to Figures 3–32, 3–34, 3–35 and 3–36). It would be worth checking. The large T waves might indicate hyperkalemia, or she may be hypoxic under the anesthesia (refer to Figures 3–32 and 3–38). Serum Ca^{++} was normal in this dog, and serum K^+ was 3.2 meq./lb. (slightly low for our laboratory). There is no evidence of cardiac hypertrophy.

13. This electrocardiogram was recorded from an 11-year-old male cocker spaniel that was being treated with digoxin. He was depressed and lethargic, and was losing weight. On physical examination paroxysms of tachycardia were detected, and mitral insufficiency was present.

Paper speed = 25 mm./sec., 1 cm. = 1 mv.
(Tracing courtesy of Dr. E. Grano, Briarcliff Manor, N. Y.)

Questions:

a. What two arrhythmias are present?

b. What is the significance?

Answers:

a. Paroxysmal atrial tachycardia (PAT) and second degree heart block. This is called paroxysmal atrial tachycardia with block. In the beginning of the tracing two P waves occur without QRS complexes. When the burst of tachycardia occurs, the QRS complexes remain normal, indicating that it is a supraventricular tachycardia (refer to Figures 4–18 and 4–19). Also, P waves can be seen between the QRS complexes and the T waves of some of the preceding beats in the tachycardia, and those P waves are positive but slightly different (shorter) than normal ones.

b. Paroxysmal atrial tachycardia with block is most commonly associated with digitalis intoxication. Serum potassium level should also be checked, since it might be either low or high (Bellet, 1972). If the dog were not already on digitalis, the paroxysmal atrial tachycardia would be treated with digitalis; however, there were already signs of digitalis intoxication when this recording was taken.

14. This is the electrocardiogram of an English Bulldog male being treated for urethral prolapse.

Paper speed = 50 mm./sec., 1 cm. = 1 mv.

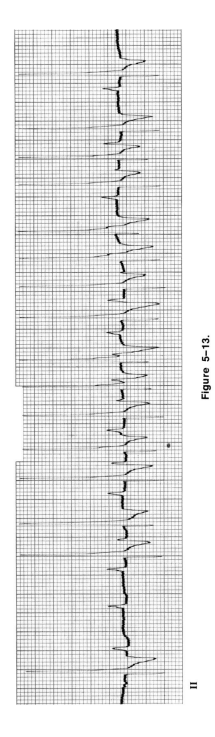

Figure 5–13.

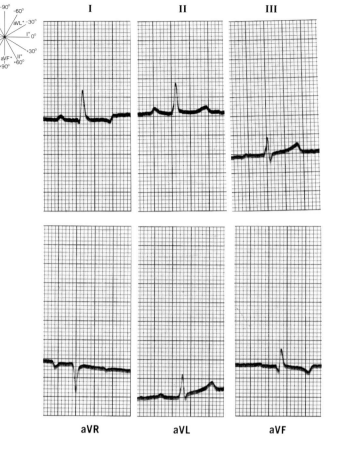

Figure 5-14.

Questions:

  a. What is the mean electrical axis?

  b. Are there any other criteria for cardiac hypertrophy present?

Answers:

  a. The mean electrical axis is +15°. Leads III and aVF are equally close to being isoelectric. If lead III is used, the perpendicular is lead aVR, which is negative. Lead aVR's negative pole is +30°. If lead aVF is used as isoelectric, the perpendicular lead is I, which is positive. Lead I's positive pole is 0°. If we average 0° and +30°, the result is +15°. This is a left axis deviation and indicates left ventricular hypertrophy.

  b. No other criteria are present.

15. This is a lead II tracing.

  Paper speed = 50 mm./sec., 1 cm. = 1 mv.

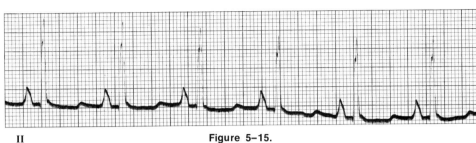

II   Figure 5–15.

Question:

Are there any abnormalities?

Answer:

Yes. The P waves are 0.5 mv. (5 boxes) tall, and 0.05 second (2½ boxes) wide. The tall P waves indicate "P pulmonale," or right atrial hypertrophy. The wide P waves indicate "P mitrale," or left atrial hypertrophy. The notching in the QRS complex is not significant unless the QRS complex is prolonged. The electrocardiographic diagnosis is biatrial hypertrophy (refer to Figures 3–15, 3–16, and 3–18).

16. This lead II electrocardiogram was recorded from a standard poodle being rechecked while on treatment for adrenal insufficiency.

Paper speed = 50 mm./sec., 1 cm. = 1 mv.

Question:

What is happening?

Answer:

The dog began to struggle and made the baseline jump. This could resemble bizarre ventricular beats and could lead to erroneous diagnosis (refer to Figure 3–45).

17. Paper speed = 50 mm./sec., 1 cm. = 1 mv.

Question:

Please interpret this electrocardiogram and render an electrocardiographic diagnosis.

Answer:

Heart rate = 70 to 100 beats per minute (approximately)
Heart rhythm: sinus arrhythmia, wandering pacemaker

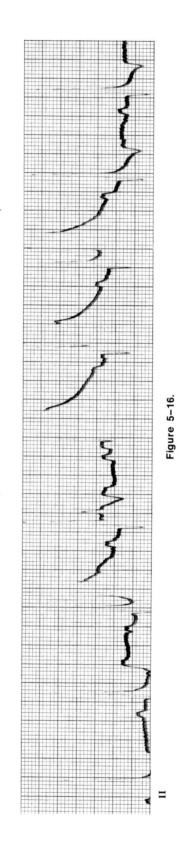

Figure 5–16.

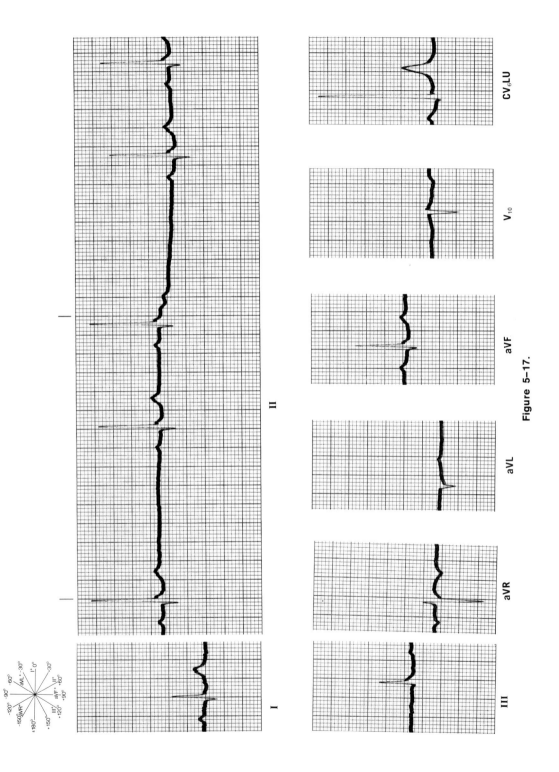

Figure 5–17.

Mean electrical axis = +65° to +70°
Measuring and multiplying:
  P wave = 0.2 mv. (2 boxes) by 0.03 second (1½ boxes)
  P-R interval = 0.11 second (5½ boxes)
  QRS width = .05 to .06 second (2½ to 3 boxes)
  R wave height = 1.8 mv. (18 boxes average)
  S-T segment and T wave: normal
  Q-T interval = 0.18 second (9 boxes average)
Miscellaneous criteria: none
Electrocardiographic diagnosis: normal

The rhythm is irregular and the pauses are shorter than twice the normal R-R interval, which makes this sinus arrhythmia rather than sinus arrest (refer to Figures 4–4, 4–5, and 4–9). Wandering pacemaker is seen; the P waves in this electrocardiogram vary slightly in height (refer to Figures 4–6 and 4–7).

18. This lead II electrocardiogram was recorded from a 3-year-old Doberman pinscher male with idiopathic cardiomyopathy. He was in biventricular congestive heart failure and had a rapid, irregular heart rate and a pulse deficit.

Paper speed = 50 mm./sec., 1 cm. = 1 mv.

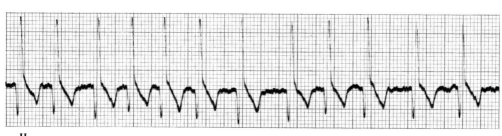

II

Figure 5–18.

Questions:

  a. What arrhythmia is present?

  b. What is the treatment?

Answers:

  a. Atrial fibrillation. This is a supraventricular tachycardia; note that the QRS complexes are fairly normal. It is rapid (heart rate = 260 beats per minute) and irregular. When pauses occur, no P waves are present. The P waves are replaced by minute baseline undulations ("f" waves). A rapid, irregular, supraventricular tachycardia with no P waves is diagnostic of atrial fibrillation (refer to Figures 4–20 and 4–21).

b. Digitalization is the treatment of choice. Diuretics, a low sodium diet, and rest may also be required. Once the heart failure is alleviated, quinidine could be added to the treatment in an attempt to convert the arrhythmia to a sinus rhythm.

19. Tracings A and B were recorded from an 11-year-old miniature schnauzer. The dog was experiencing syncopal attacks. On physical examination, premature beats and bursts of tachycardia were occurring, and a prominent murmur of mitral insufficiency was detected. A pulse deficit was occasionally present. He showed no signs of congestive heart failure.

    Paper speed = 50 mm./sec., 1 cm. = 1 mv.
(Tracings courtesy of Dr. L. Tilley, New York, N.Y.)

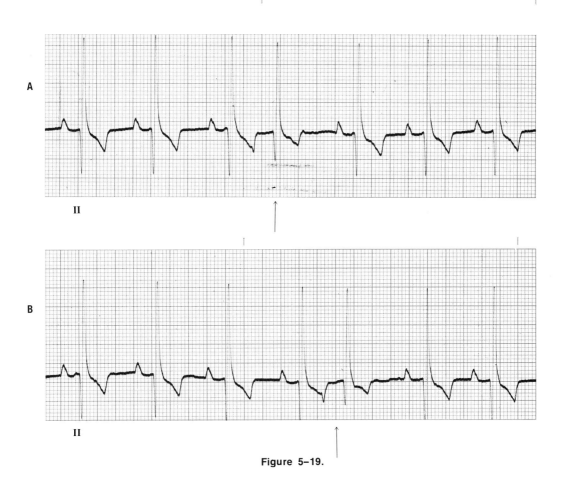

Figure 5–19.

Questions:

    a. There is a premature beat in the top strip (arrow), and one in the bottom strip (arrow). What type of premature beats are they?

b. What is their probable cause?

c. What is their treatment?

Answers:

a. These beats are supraventricular premature beats. They occur early, are followed by a pause, and the QRS complexes remain normal. Since the P wave is hidden in the preceding T wave, it cannot be evaluated to see whether they are atrial or junctional (nodal) premature beats. Since both types of supraventricular premature beats are treated the same, the diagnosis is sufficient (refer to Figures 4–13, 4–14, and 4–15).

b. They are probably caused by enlargement and stretching of the left atrium secondary to the insufficiency of the left atrioventricular valve.

c. The dog should be digitalized even though the usual signs of congestive heart failure are absent. An occasional premature beat would not cause syncope, but the bursts of tachycardia could cause it. The digitalis would control the tachycardia by prolonging conduction through the atrioventricular node.

20. This lead II recording is also from the schnauzer in the previous figure. There is a premature beat (arrow), followed by a pause, and then another abnormal beat.

Paper speed = 50 mm./sec., 1 cm. = 1 mv.
(Tracing courtesy of Dr. L. Tilley, New York, N.Y.)

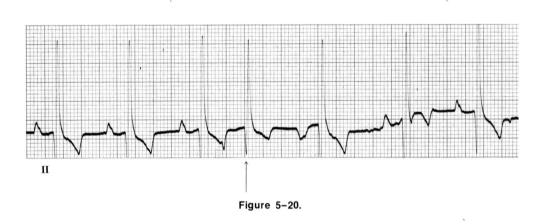

II

Figure 5–20.

Questions:

a. What type of premature beat is this?

b. What is the beat following the premature beat called?

Answers:

a. This is also a supraventricular premature beat.

b. This is a junctional (nodal) escape beat. It occurs after a pause, and has a negative P wave, which means that the impulse originated in the area of the atrioventricular node and spread backward through the atria (refer to Figures 4–44 and 4–45). Junctional or ventricular escape beats will occasionally be seen to punctuate a pause that follows a premature beat, as in this instance.

21. These lead II tracings are also from the same schnauzer as in the previous two figures. There is a premature beat in the top tracing (arrow) and one in the bottom tracing (arrow).

Paper speed = 50 mm./sec., 1 cm. = 1 mv.
(Tracings courtesy of Dr. L. Tilley, New York, N.Y.)

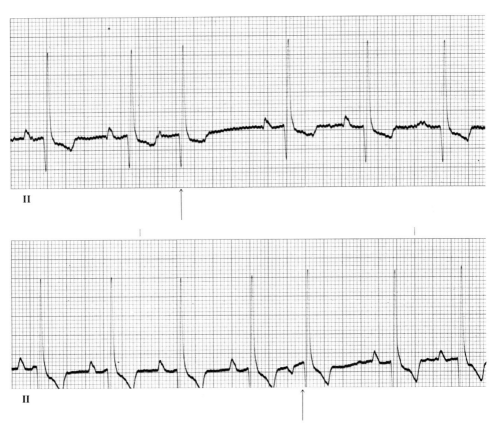

Figure 5–21.

Questions:

a. What type of premature beat is in the top tracing?

b. What type of premature beat is in the bottom tracing?

c. What is their significance?

Answers:

a. This is an atrial premature beat. It occurs early and is followed by a pause, the QRS complex is normal, and the P wave can be seen to be positive but different from the normal P waves (refer to Figure 4–13).

b. This is a junctional (nodal) premature beat. It occurs early and is followed by a pause, the QRS complex is normal, and the P wave is negative (refer to Figure 4–14).

c. Both tracings indicate the atrial disease that is occurring secondary to the mitral insufficiency. If they did not occur until after digitalis therapy was given, they would be due to digitalis intoxication.

22. This lead II recording is also from the same 11-year-old schnauzer as in the three previous figures. There is a burst of tachycardia at the beginning of the tracing, which terminates about the middle of the tracing.

Paper speed = 50 mm./sec., 1 cm. = 1 mv.
(Tracing courtesy of Dr. L. Tilley, New York, N.Y.)

Questions:

a. What is the type of tachycardia?

b. What is its significance?

Answers:

a. It is an atrial tachycardia. The heart rate during the tachycardia is about 230 beats per minute, the QRS complexes remain normal, and the P waves are positive, but different from the normal P waves (refer to Figure 4–18).

b. It is a sign that the atrial disease occurring secondary to the mitral insufficiency is severe. If it were to grow worse, atrial fibrillation could develop. On thoracic radiography of this dog the left atrium was markedly enlarged, even though the electrocardiogram does not demonstrate wide P waves.

23. This lead II electrocardiogram was recorded from a 1-year-old mixed breed dog that was suspected of having a pulmonic stenosis. He was uncooperative, so was given piperacetazine (Psymod) to quiet him down. There were no arrhythmias prior to the tranquilization.

Paper speed = 50 mm./sec., 1 cm. = 1 mv.

Questions:

a. What are the two premature beats that occur (second and fifth beats from the left)?

b. Why are they unusual for this type of premature beat?

c. What is their significance?

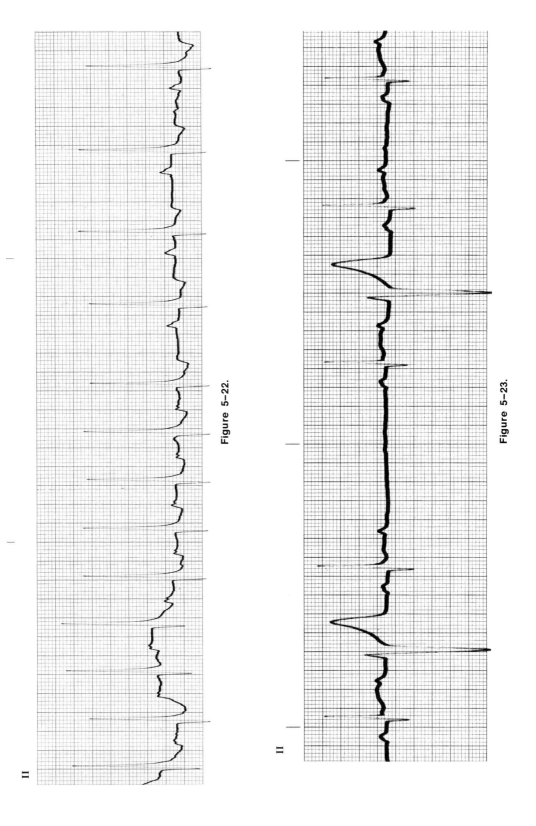

Figure 5–22.

Figure 5–23.

Answers:

a. Ventricular premature beats. They occur early, are not associated with a P wave (the T waves of the preceding beats falsely resemble P waves), and are bizarre in configuration (refer to Figure 4–24). The Q-T interval is 0.23 second (11½ boxes), which is just slightly prolonged beyond normal.

b. They are interpolated. They do not break the natural rhythm. They occur between two normal beats, and are not followed by a pause. This is seen occasionally when ventricular premature beats occur (refer to Figure 4–32). They would still be detected by auscultation on physical examination, and could cause a pulse deficit.

c. Since they followed tranquilization and are not very frequent, they are probably insignificant. The fact that they are interpolated is of interest but of no practical importance.

24. This lead II tracing was recorded from a mixed breed dog that had been given xylazine (Rompun) for radiographic examination. The electrocardiogram was recorded when bradycardia was detected.

Paper speed = 50 mm./sec., 1 cm. = 1 mv.

Questions:

a. What arrhythmias are present?

b. What is their significance?

c. How should he be treated?

Answers:

a. Sinus arrest, sinus bradycardia, and wandering pacemaker (refer to Figures 4–5, 4–10, and 4–12). Sinus arrest is diagnosed, because the long pause is greater than twice the normal R-R interval. If the R-R interval of the first two beats is measured, it can be seen that the pause is more than double that measurement, indicating sinus arrest rather than sinus arrhythmia (refer to Figures 4–5 and 4–9). The heart rate varies between 35 and 69 beats per minute, which is an average of about 50 beats per minute. The P waves vary slightly in height, indicating that wandering pacemaker is also present.

b. The arrhythmias are probably a result of tranquilization, since they were not present before the dog was tranquilized.

c. If atropine had been given with the tranquilizer, much of this would have been prevented. Atropine could be given now to increase the heart rate, although it probably is unnecessary since the dog is in no danger. He does not need much cardiac output when he is just lying still under the sedation.

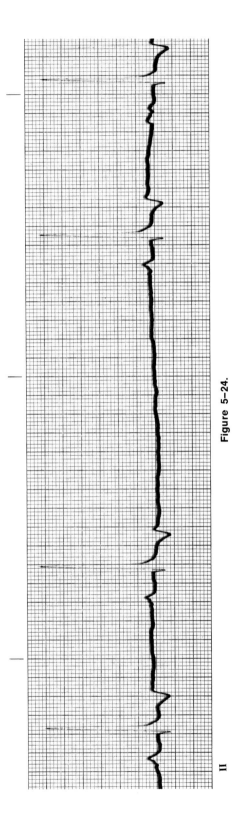

Figure 5-24.

25. This electrocardiogram was also recorded from the dog in the previous figure that had been given xylazine. A burst of tachycardia is seen in the middle of this tracing.

Paper speed = 50 mm./sec., 1 cm. = 1 mv.

Question:

What type of tachycardia is it?

Answer:

It is a supraventricular tachycardia. There is a burst of four premature beats in which the QRS complex remains normal, indicating supraventricular origin. The P waves of these complexes are hidden in the T waves of the preceding beats, so it cannot be determined whether they are atrial or junctional (nodal) in origin (refer to Figures 4–11, 4–18, and 4–19).

26. This lead II electrocardiogram was recorded from an 11-year-old beagle that had received tranquilization (Tranvet) for electrocardiography. This tracing was taken at slow speed to give a better indication of the regularity of the irregularity.

Paper speed = 25 mm./sec., 1 cm. = 1 mv.
(Tracing courtesy of Dr. A. Beck, New City, N. Y.)

Questions:

a. What arrhythmias are present?

b. What is the probable cause?

Answers:

a. Sinus arrest, second degree heart block, and junctional or ventricular escape beat. If two of the normal R-R intervals are measured, the pauses in the rhythm are still longer than two normal R-R intervals, indicating sinus arrest (refer to Figures 4–5 and 4–9). A P wave occurs (between the last two groups of beats) that has no QRS complex, indicating second degree heart block (refer to Figure 4–50). Following that P wave a pause, and then an escape beat, occur. The escape beat has no P wave preceding it, and the shape of its QRS complex is slightly different from the others. It is probably a ventricular escape beat that has arisen in the bundle of His; the QRS complex is almost normal (refer to Figure 4–31). It may also be a junctional escape beat in which the P wave became hidden in the QRS complex. It really does not matter, since an escape beat that occurs only occasionally is of little significance whether it is junctional or ventricular in origin.

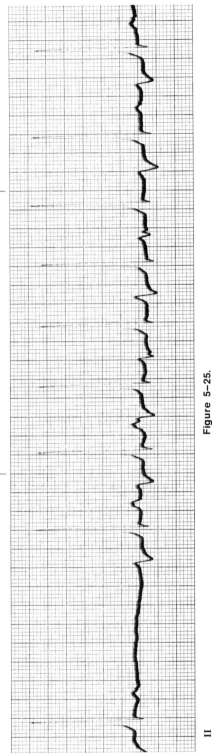

Figure 5–25.

II

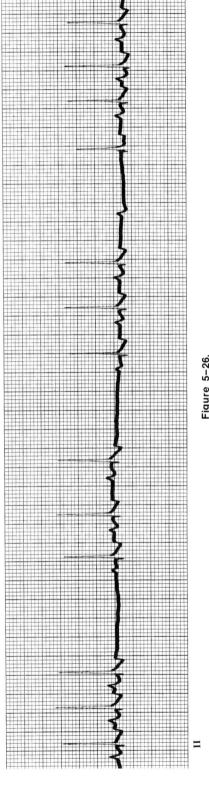

Figure 5–26.

II

b. These arrhythmias are probably vagal in origin. The "regular ir-regularity" is a clue that they are associated with respiration. The beats occur during inspiration and the pauses occur during expiration. This may be verified by watching the dog's respirations while recording the electrocardiogram. Atropine would alleviate these arrhythmias (refer to Figure 4–10).

27.   This lead II electrocardiogram was recorded from an 11-year-old beagle that had received tranquilization (Tranvet).

Paper speed = 50 mm./sec., 1 cm. = 1 mv.
(Tracing courtesy of Dr. A. Beck, New City, N. Y.)

Questions:

a. What arrhythmias are present?

b. Is there any evidence of hypertrophy of one of the cardiac chambers?

Answers:

a. Sinus arrest, ventricular escape beat, and wandering pace-maker. This is a sinus rhythm, and it is irregular. The pauses are more than twice the normal R-R interval, indicating sinus arrest rather than sinus arrhythmia (refer to Figures 4–5 and 4–9). Wandering pacemaker is seen as the slight fluctuation in the size of the P waves. After the long pause in the middle of the tracing, a P wave occurs, followed by an abnormal QRS complex. That P wave and that QRS complex are not related; note that the P-R interval is shorter than the others. This is a ventricular escape beat that depolarized the ventricles before the P wave could traverse the atrioventricular node.

b. Right atrial hypertrophy is diagnosed by the presence of "T_a" (T sub a) waves. Notice how the P-R segment dips below the baseline after each P wave (refer to Figure 3–18).

28.   These lead II tracings were recorded from an 11-year-old beagle that had had a hemangiosarcoma removed from the spleen two years previously. Metastasis had been seen to involve the kidney. On physical examination at this time, bouts of tachycardia were detected by auscultation.

Paper speed = 50 mm./sec., 1 cm. = 1 mv.
(Tracings courtesy of Dr. A. Beck, New City, N. Y.)

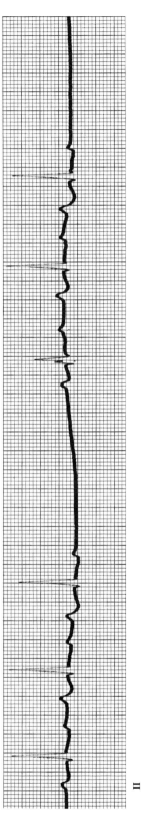

Figure 5–27.

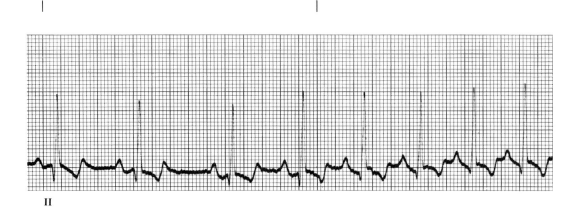

II

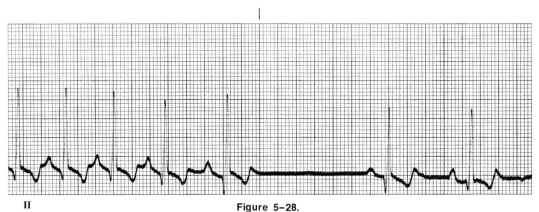

II   Figure 5–28.

Questions:

   a. The tachycardia begins in the top tracing and terminates in the bottom tracing. What type of tachycardia is it?

   b. In which atrium did it originate?

   c. What might be the cause here?

Answers:

   a. This is an instance of atrial tachycardia. The QRS complexes are normal, and the P waves during the tachycardia are positive but slightly different from the P waves when the rate is normal (refer to Figure 4–18). The tachycardia ends abruptly and is followed by a pause. When a pacemaker drives the heart more rapidly than the sinoatrial node and then abruptly quits, a pause of about 1 second will occur if the sinoatrial node is normal. This is called overdrive suppression (Hamlin, 1972). The pause in this tracing is about 0.9 second long.

   b. It probably originated in the right atrium. There is evidence of right atrial hypertrophy on the tracing. Notice that the P-R segment dips below the baseline after each P wave when the normal beats occur. This is a "T_a" (T sub a) wave and indicates right atrial hypertrophy (refer to Figure 3–18).

c. Hemangiosarcomas have a predilection for the right atrium (Kleine, 1970). These atrial arrhythmias may indicate that the tumor has metastasized there, or even that the original site was the right atrium.

29.   This is an electrocardiogram recorded from a middle-aged German Shepherd.

Paper speed = 50 mm./sec., 1 cm. = 1 mv.

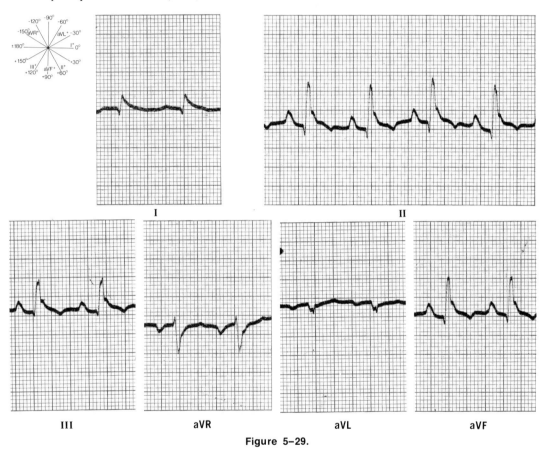

Figure 5–29.

Questions:

Read and interpret the electrocardiogram.

Answers:

Heart rate = 175 beats per minute
Heart rhythm: normal sinus rhythm (NSR)
Mean electrical axis = +70°
Measuring and multiplying:
  P wave = 0.04 second (2 boxes) by 0.3 mv. (3 boxes)
  P-R interval = 0.09 second (4½ boxes)
  QRS width = 0.07 to 0.08 second (3½ to 4 boxes)

R wave height = 1.2 mv. (12 boxes)
S-T segment and T wave: normal (slightly elevated S-T segment?)
Q-T interval = 0.17 second (8½ boxes)
Miscellaneous criteria: none
Electrocardiographic diagnosis: left ventricular hypertrophy and left bundle branch block.

The diagnosis may not be correct in this case. The notch that occurs on the downslope of the R wave in the QRS complex is called the "J" point. It signifies the end of depolarization and the beginning of repolarization. This means that the apparent delay in the terminal forces is really an elevation of the S-T segment. This may falsely make the QRS complexes look too wide. The abnormality in the S-T segment is suggestive of myocarditis. The dog showed no signs of cardiac disease, and thoracic radiographs were normal.

Lead aVL is the closest to being isoelectric. Lead II is perpendicular to lead aVL, and lead II is positive in this tracing. Lead II's positive pole is at +60°. Since aVL is not perfectly isoelectric, the axis is not perfectly +60°. Lead aVL is slightly more negative, so if the axis is shifted from +60° a little toward aVL's negative pole, it would be about +70°.

30. The top tracing is a lead II recording. It is inverted because the polarity is reversed by the recording machine. The fourth beat from the left is a ventricular premature beat. When it occurs, the blood pressure drops, as indicated by the recording of the aortic pressure below.

Paper speed = 50 mm./sec., 1 cm. = 1 mv.

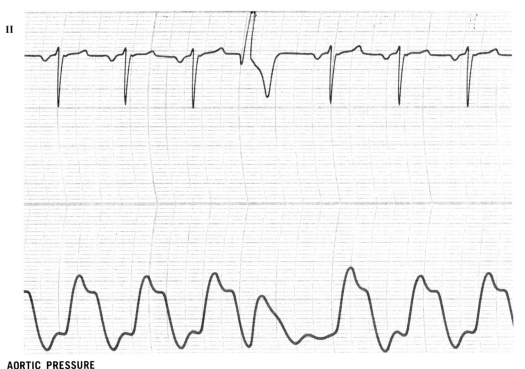

AORTIC PRESSURE

Figure 5–30.

Question:

How does the ventricular premature beat cause the fall in blood pressure?

Answer:

It caused the ventricles to depolarize again before they had a chance to fill completely with blood. As a result, stroke output decreased, and the pressure in the aorta fell (refer to Figure 4–1).

31. Paper speed = 50 mm./sec., 1 cm. = 1 mv.

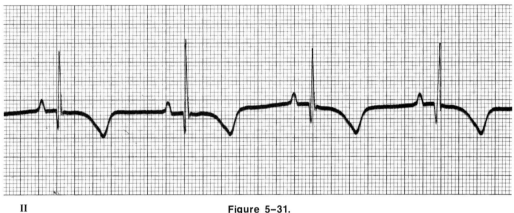

II   Figure 5–31.

Question:

Is this normal sinus rhythm or sinus arrhythmia?

Answer:

This is normal sinus rhythm; the R-R intervals are exactly alike. If they had been even slightly variable, this would have indicated sinus arrhythmia (refer to Figure 4–3).

32. This electrocardiogram was recorded during a cardiac catheterization proceedure.

Paper speed = 25 mm./sec., 1 cm. = 1 mv.

Question:

What arrhythmias are occurring?

Answer:

Transient complete right bundle branch block begins in the top tracing, and reverts to sinus rhythm by the end of the bottom tracing. Three

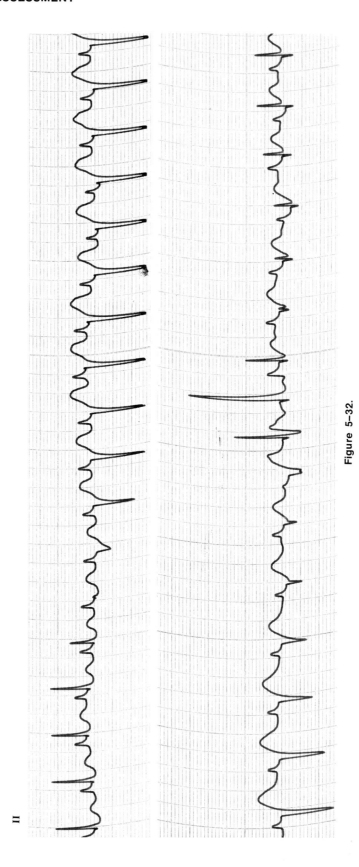

Figure 5–32.

II

ventricular premature beats occur in the middle of the bottom tracing. The right bundle branch complexes are bizarre and resemble ventricular tachycardia, but it can be seen that even when they occur, sinus rhythm is present (refer to Figure 4–55). The ventricular premature beats in the bottom tracing are bizarre and are not associated with P waves.

33. This lead II electrocardiogram was taken of a 5-year-old boxer that was on digitalis, and was anorectic, depressed, and vomiting.

Paper speed = 50 mm./sec., 1 cm. = 1 mv.

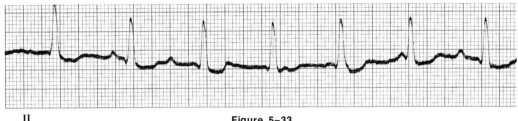

II   Figure 5–33.

Questions:

a. What is the arrhythmia?

b. What is its cause?

Answers:

a. Atrioventricular dissociation. The P waves, when they can be seen, occur at varying distances from the QRS complexes. The P wave can be seen to occur behind the QRS complex in the fourth beat from the left. When the P wave moves in and out of the QRS complexes, it is called accrochage (refer to Figures 4–37 and 4–38). This is really a form of ventricular tachycardia in which the rates of the P waves and of the QRS complexes are nearly equal. The QRS complexes look fairly normal because they arise near the bundle of His, which is common in atrioventricular dissociation.

b. The dog shows both physical and electrocardiographic signs of digitalis intoxication. He was on 0.375 mg. of digoxin b.i.d. The digoxin was discontinued until the dog's overall condition and heart rhythm improved. Then, 48 hours later, the digoxin was resumed at 0.25 mg. in the morning and 0.375 mg. at night.

34. These lead II electrocardiograms were recorded from a 5-year-old standard poodle. He had a history of profound weakness, lethargy, vague gastrointestinal signs, and urinary incontinence. On physical examination he had a heart rate of about 60 beats per minute, and adrenal insufficiency was suspected.

Paper speed = 50 mm./sec., 1 cm. = 1 mv.

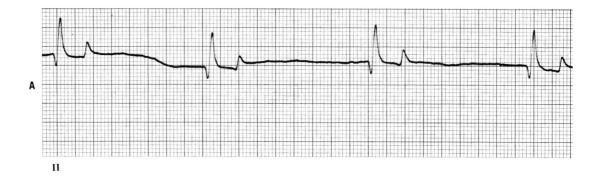

A

II

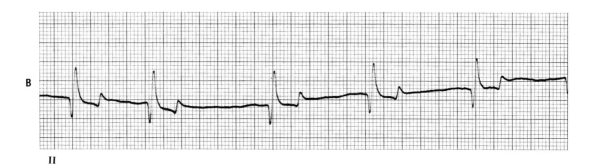

B

II

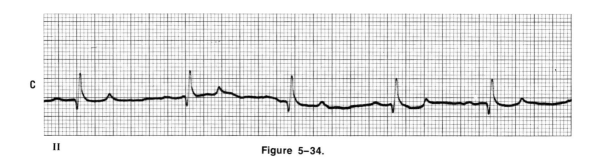

C

II

Figure 5–34.

Questions:

a. The top tracing is his initial electrocardiogram. Is there any indication of adrenal insufficiency?

b. Tracings B and C were recorded during treatment. What treatment was given?

Answers:

a. There is evidence of hyperkalemia on the tracing. The heart rate is about 66 beats per minute, the QRS complexes are prolonged to 0.07 second (3½ boxes), and atrial standstill is indicated by the absence of P waves and the straight, steady baseline between QRS complexes (refer to Figure 3–32). The serum K^+ was highly elevated (10.1 meq./l) at this time. Note that the Q-T interval is normal. It may or may not be prolonged with hyperkalemia.

b. Treatment was instituted with intravenous 5 per cent dextrose and saline, intravenous hydrocortisone, and intramuscular desoxycorticosterone acetate (DOCA). Tracing B was recorded 2 hours after tracing A, and the serum K^+ was 7.5 meq./l. The heart rate is increasing, but no P waves can be seen yet. The final tracing was recorded 3 hours after the initial one. At this point, the dog had received 500 cc. dextrose and saline, 100 mg. hydrocortisone intravenously, 25 mg. hydrocortisone intramuscularly, and 2.5 mg. DOCA intramuscularly, and his serum K^+ was 6.0 meq./l. Note that the heart rate is about 100 beats per minute, P waves are present, the QRS complexes are normal, and the T wave has returned to its normal appearance. The dog was also much improved. He was converted to oral mineralocorticoids and salt in his food, and is normal after 3½ years of treatment. The urinary incontinence also was resolved.

35. This electrocardiogram was recorded from a 1-year-old male Shetland sheepdog.

Paper speed = 50 mm./sec., 1 cm. = 1 mv.

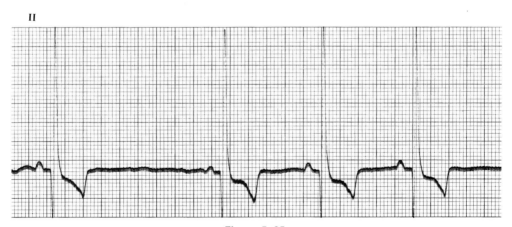

Figure 5–35.

Questions:

a. What abnormalities are present?

b. What two conditions can cause the electrocardiogram to look like this?

c. Which of those two conditions does this dog have?

Answers:

a. The R waves are 3.8 mv. (38 boxes) tall, indicating left ventricular hypertrophy. The QRS complexes are 0.06 second (3 boxes) wide. That is too wide for this small dog, and also indicates left ventricular hypertrophy. The S-T segment is depressed 2.5 mv. (2½ boxes), which is further evidence of left ventricular hypertrophy. The deep Q waves are suggestive of right ventricular hypertrophy (refer to Figures 3–19, 3–20, 3–22, and 3–25).

b. Patent ductus arteriosus and severe mitral insufficiency are the two conditions that can make the complexes so large that they go off the top and the bottom of the tracing.

c. This dog had a patent ductus arteriosus, which was corrected surgically. This would be expected because of his breed and his age.

36. These tracings were recorded from a 2-year-old Irish wolfhound with a history of weakness, lethargy, fever, lameness, and edema of the right front leg. Blood cultures were positive for *Pasteurella multocida.*

Paper speed = 50 mm./sec., 1 cm. = 1 mv.

Questions:

a. What arrhythmias are present?

b. What is their cause?

c. How should this dog be treated?

Answers:

a. In the top tracing, every third beat occurs early and is followed by a pause. They are diagnosed as supraventricular premature beats, because their QRS complexes remain normal. Their P waves are hidden in the T waves of the preceding beats, so it cannot be determined whether they are atrial or junctional (nodal) premature beats, but they are definitely supraventricular. When every third beat is a premature beat, it is termed a trigeminy. This is, therefore, a supraventricular trigeminal rhythm. The second complex from the left in the bottom tracing is a ventricular premature beat. It is not associated with a P wave and is obviously very bizarre. Another supraventricular premature beat occurs three beats later (refer to Figures 4–13, 4–14, 4–15, 4–17, and 4–24).

b. The dog has bacterial endocarditis, which is also causing myocarditis. The supraventricular premature beats are evidence that the atria are involved and the ventricular premature beat indicates the involvement of the ventricles. This is an ominous sign when such a wide area of the heart is affected.

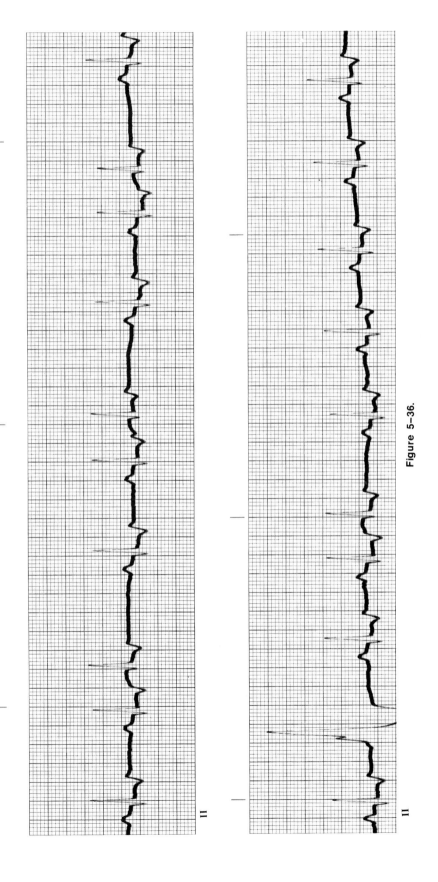

Figure 5–36.

c. In this instance, quinidine therapy is indicated. It is very effective at controlling both ventricular and supraventricular arrhythmias. Usually it is contraindicated for supraventricular types of arrhythmias because they are usually secondary to severe mitral insufficiency, and the dog is either in congestive heart failure or prone to it. Quinidine depresses myocardial contractility and would aggravate a congestive heart failure state. In this instance, however, the dog does not have severe mitral insufficiency and is not prone to congestive heart failure. The premature beats are in response to the inflammatory changes in both the atria and ventricles, and quinidine is the drug of choice to suppress them. When quinidine was given, the arrhythmias were gone within hours, but the next day the dog died suddenly. An autopsy showed that he had severe vegetative endocarditis and multiple infarcts in many areas of the body.

37. This electrocardiogram was run on a dog that was under anesthesia with thiamylal sodium. A pulse deficit was discovered and an electrocardiogram was recorded.

Paper speed = 50 mm./sec., 1 cm. = 1 mv.

Question:

There are three ventricular ectopic beats on this tracing. Can you find them?

Answer:

They are the second, sixth, and tenth beats from the left. Notice that their P-R intervals are shorter than those of the normal beats, and that they have shorter QRS complexes that have a notch in them on the upstroke of the R wave. Of interest is the fact that they occur so regularly. The distance between R waves of the abnormal beats is everywhere the same. This is called ventricular parasystole. The ventricular pacemaker fires at its own very slow rate, and the abnormal QRS complexes fall right on time. This arrhythmia disappeared within 5 minutes, and the anesthesia was otherwise uneventful.

38. These lead II electrocardiograms were recorded from a 13-year-old Irish setter that had an irregular heart beat.

Paper speed = 50 mm./sec., 1 cm. = 1 mv.

Questions:

a. What arrhythmias are present?

b. How should they be treated?

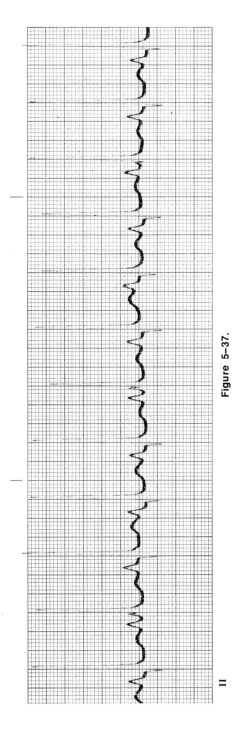

Figure 5–37.

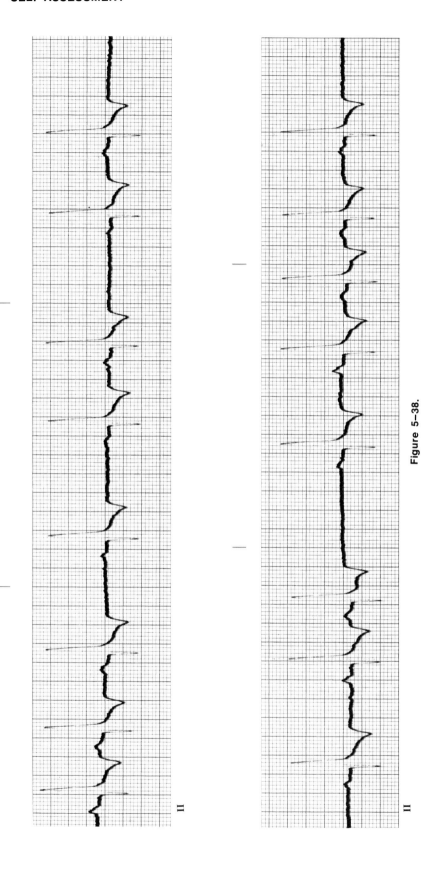

Figure 5-38.

Answers:

a. Sinus arrhythmia and sinus arrest are present. The "regular irregularity" is a clue that the irregularity is associated with respiration. The pauses that occur in the top tracing are shorter than two normal R-R intervals, and the pause in the bottom tracing is longer than two normal R-R intervals. Sinus arrhythmia is diagnosed in the top tracing, and sinus arrest is present below (refer to Figures 4–5 and 4–9).

b. No treatment is necessary.

39. Paper speed = 50 mm./sec., 1 cm. = 1 mv.

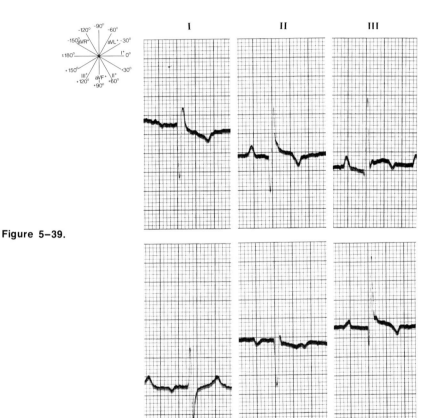

Figure 5–39.

Question:

What is the mean electrical axis?

Answer:

The axis is +135°. Lead II and lead aVR are both equally isoelectric. If lead II is used, the perpendicular lead on the axis chart is lead aVL, and lead aVL is negative on this tracing. Lead aVL's negative pole is at +150°. If lead aVR is used as isoelectric, the perpendicular is lead III, which is positive. Lead III's positive pole is +120°. If we average the difference between +120° and +150° we arrive at +135°. This is right axis deviation and indicates right ventricular hypertrophy.

40. This is a lead II electrocardiogram of the same 13-year-old Irish setter as in Figure 5–38.

Paper speed = 50 mm./sec., 1 cm. = 1 mv.

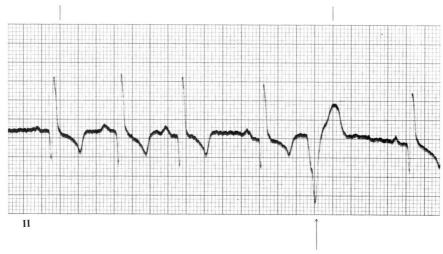

II

Figure 5–40.

Questions:

   a. What type of premature beat is this (arrow)?

   b. What is its significance?

Answers:

   a. It is a ventricular premature beat, as indicated by its obviously bizarre conformation (refer to Figure 4–24).

   b. There may be a few ventricular premature beats seen on electrocardiograms of older dogs. They are due to microscopic intramural myocardial infarcts, which may be normal aging changes in the dog. The ventricular premature beats are clinically insignificant in these old dogs as long as they do not become too frequent.

41. This electrocardiogram was recorded from a 16-year-old golden retriever. She was having seizures and was mentally confused.

Paper speed = 50 mm./sec., 1 cm. = 1 mv.

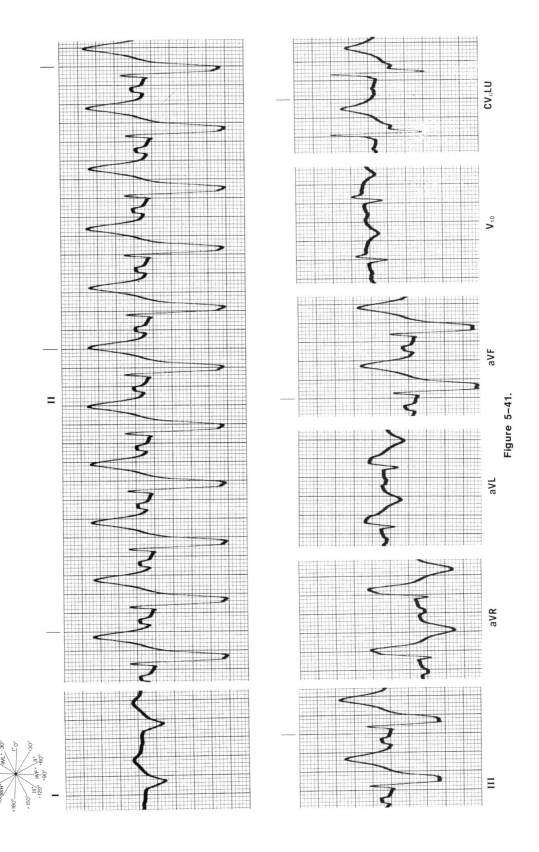

Figure 5-41.

Questions:

a. What is the electrocardiographic diagnosis?

b. What is its significance?

Answers:

a. This is complete right bundle branch block. The complexes look bizarre and could be mistaken for ventricular tachycardia, except that this is a sinus rhythm. The large negative S waves in leads I, II, III, and aVF, together with the axis of −120°, could be suggestive of right ventricular hypertrophy, but with right ventricular hypertrophy, the terminal deflections are not usually this wide (refer to Figure 4–55 for the differentiation of right bundle branch block, right ventricular hypertrophy, and ventricular tachycardia). There is usually an S wave present in lead V_{10} but there is none in this tracing.

b. This conduction disturbance is insignificant clinically other than that it can mimic, and thus must be differentiated from, other conditions. This tracing was recorded on 6/25/74. We first diagnosed complete right bundle branch block in this dog on 1/11/72, so she has had it for about 2½ years.

42. This electrocardiogram was taken of an aged standard poodle. He had asymptomatic mitral insufficiency and his respirations were embarrassed by a large nasal tumor.

Paper speed = 50 mm./sec., 1 cm. = 1 mv.

Question:

Please read his electrocardiogram and render an interpretation.

Answer:

Heart rate = 180 beats per minute
Heart rhythm = sinus tachycardia
Mean electrical axis = +75°
Measuring and multiplying:
   P wave = 0.05 second (2½ boxes) by 0.5 mv. (5 boxes)
   P-R interval = 0.12 second (6 boxes)
   QRS width = 0.06 second (3 boxes)
   R wave height = 3.3 mv. (33 boxes average)
   S-T segment and T wave: S-T slurring, large T waves
   Q-T interval = 0.20 to 0.22 second (10 to 11 boxes)
Miscellaneous criteria: positive T wave in lead V_{10}
   Electrocardiographic diagnosis: biventricular hypertrophy and biatrial hypertrophy

The P waves are too wide and too tall (refer to Figure 3–18), indicating hypertrophy of both atria. The R wave is too tall, and the S-T

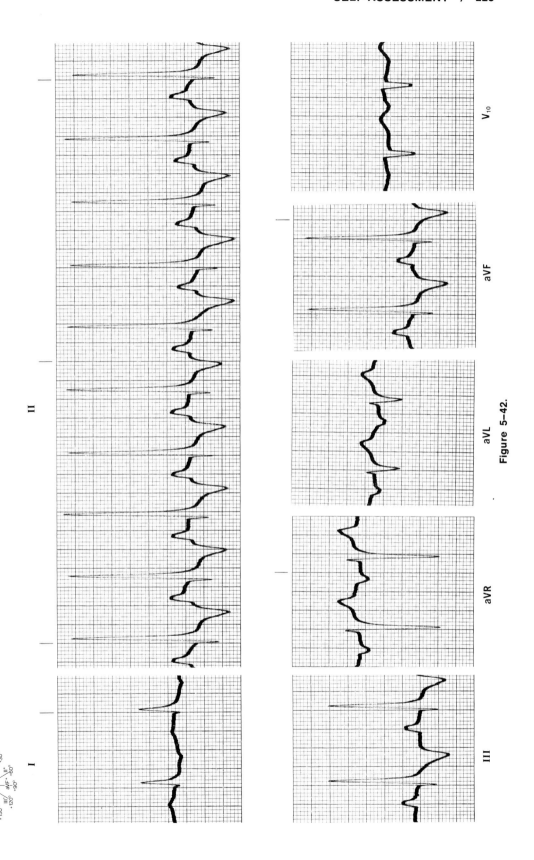

Figure 5–42.

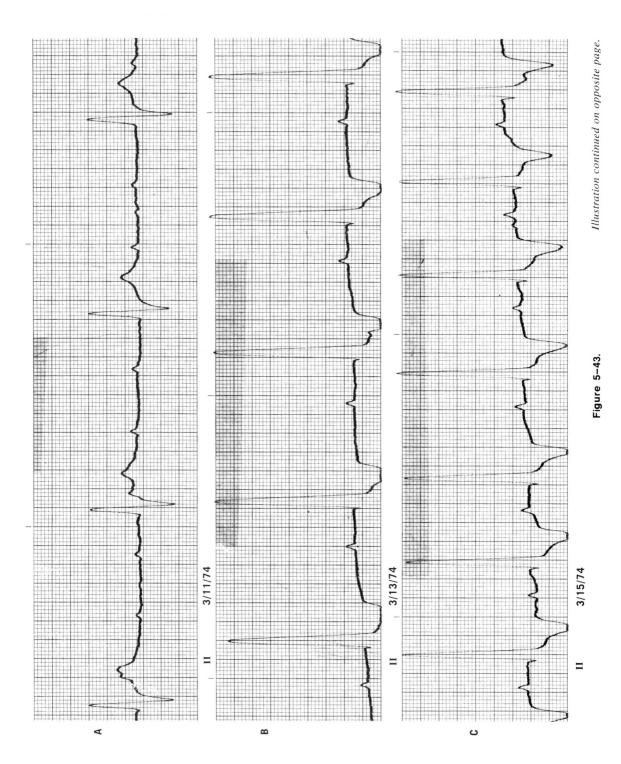

A

3/11/74

II B

3/13/74

II C

3/15/74

II

Illustration continued on opposite page.

Figure 5–43.

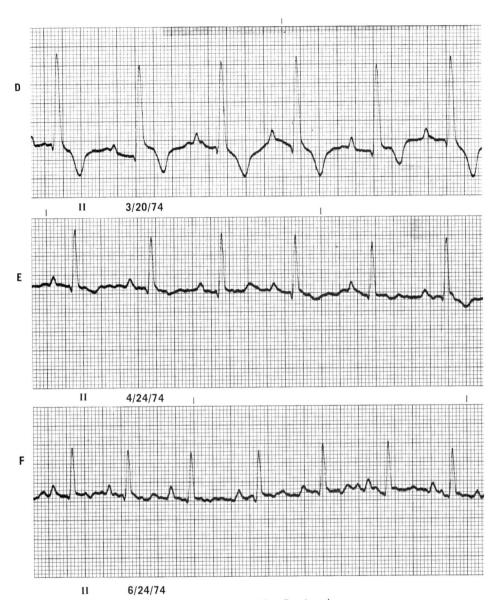

D

II   3/20/74

E

II   4/24/74

F

II   6/24/74

Figure 5-43. *Continued.*

segment is slurred, indicating left ventricular hypertrophy. The positive T wave in V_{10} indicates right ventricular hypertrophy. The axis remains normal, as would be expected with biventricular hypertrophy. Lead I and lead aVL are equally close to being isoelectric. If lead I is used, the perpendicular is aVF, which is positive on this tracing. Lead aVF's positive pole is at +90° (see the axis chart). If lead aVL were used as isoelectric, lead II would be perpendicular and positive. Lead II's positive pole is at +60°. If +60° and +90° are averaged, the result is +75°.

The sinus tachycardia and the large T waves may indicate that he is somewhat hypoxic as a result of interference with respiration by the nasal tumor.

43. Tracing A was recorded from a 4½-year-old female boxer. She was depressed, lethargic, weak, and had an elevated temperature. On physical examination, the heart rate was slow, so an electrocardiogram was taken. She had a white blood cell count of 30,800 with a regenerative left shift. Blood culture was negative. She was begun on penicillin therapy (Pen-Vee K) and tracings B, C, D, E, and F were recorded as treatment progressed.

Paper speed = 50 mm./sec., 1 cm. = 1 mv.
(Tracings courtesy of Dr. R. Lynk, Delmar, N. Y.)

Questions:

a. What arrhythmia is present in tracing A?

b. What arrhythmia is present in tracings B and C?

c. There is a conduction disturbance in tracings B, C, and D that is resolved in tracings E and F. What is this conduction disturbance?

d. What was the probable cause of these arrhythmias and conduction disturbances?

Answers:

a. Complete (third degree) heart block is seen in tracing A. There is no consistent association between the P waves and the QRS complexes (refer to Figure 4–53). The ventricular rate is 57 beats per minute, and the atrial rate is 176 beats per minute.

b. In tracings B and C, first degree heart block is present; note that in both tracings the P-R interval is greater than 0.13 second (6½ boxes) (refer to Figure 4–49). In tracing B the P-R interval averages 0.22 second (11 boxes), and in tracing C, recorded 2 days later, the P-R interval has decreased to 0.16 second (8 boxes). Notice now that, since the atrial impulses are stimulating ventricular depolarization, the QRS complexes are markedly different from those seen in tracing A.

c. Even though the complete heart block is abolished in tracing B, the dog is left with complete left bundle branch block, as indicated by the tall R waves and the QRS complexes of 0.08 to 0.09 second (4 to 4½ boxes) in width (refer to Figure 4–58). The bundle branch block also gradually resolves itself in tracings C and D, and is completely resolved in tracings E and F.

d. It appears that the dog had an episode of bacterial endomyocarditis with transient edema or inflammation in the area of the atrioventricular node and bundle of His; possibly both complications were present. At first, complete heart block occurred and was resolved within two days on penicillin therapy, but blockage involving the left branch of the bundle of His persisted. Eventually, the inflammation was completely resolved, and both the dog and her electrocardiogram have returned to normal. This is unusual, because complete heart block is usually a permanent conduction disturbance when it occurs, and carries a grave prognosis.

44. This electrocardiogram was recorded from a 3-year-old English pointer.

Paper speed = 50 mm./sec., 1 cm. = 1 mv.

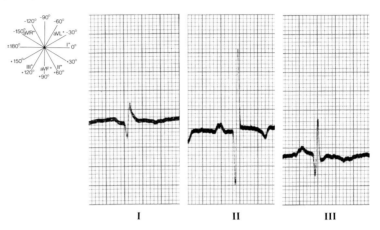

I   II   III

Figure 5–44.

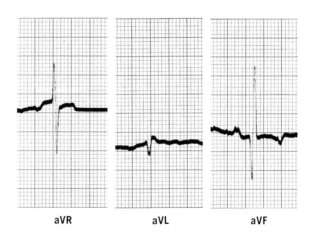

aVR   aVL   aVF

Questions:

    a. What is the mean electrical axis?

    b. Are there any signs of cardiac hypertrophy?

Answers:

    a. The axis is +90°. Lead I is isoelectric. Lead aVF is perpendicular to lead I, and aVF is positive in this tracing. Lead aVF's positive pole is at +90°.

b. The P wave in lead II is too wide (0.05 second or 2½ boxes), and is notched, indicating "P mitrale" or left atrial hypertrophy. The deep Q waves in II, III, and aVF are probably not significant in this breed of dog.

45. This is a lead II electrocardiogram.

Paper speed = 25 mm./sec., 1 cm. = 1 mv.

Questions:

a. What is the arrhythmia?

b. What is its cause?

Answers:

a. Sinus arrhythmia and sinus arrest are present. It is a "regularly irregular" sinus rhythm, and some of the pauses are greater than twice the normal R-R interval while others are not (refer to Figures 4–5 and 4–9 for the differentiation of sinus arrhythmia and sinus arrest).

b. It is associated with respirations. The baseline can be seen to fluctuate upward when the dog inhales and downward upon exhalation. During inspiration vagal tone diminishes and the heart rate increases, and during expiration the baseline dips and the rate slows as vagal tone returns. These are normal arrhythmias for the dog.

46. This electrocardiogram was recorded from a clinically normal 2½-year-old golden retriever male.

Paper speed = 50 mm./sec., 1 cm. = 1 mv.

Question:

Please read and interpret this electrocardiogram.

Answer:

Heart rate = 63 to 75 beats per minute
Heart rhythm = sinus arrhythmia
Mean electrical axis = +80°
Measuring and multiplying:
  P wave = 0.04 second (2 boxes) by 0.2 mv. (2 boxes)
  P-R interval = 0.10 second (5 boxes)
  QRS width = 0.04 second (2 boxes)
  R wave height = 2.2 mv. (22 boxes average)
  S-T seg. and T wave: normal
  Q-T interval = 0.21 second (10½ boxes)
Miscellaneous criteria: none
Electrocardiographic diagnosis: normal

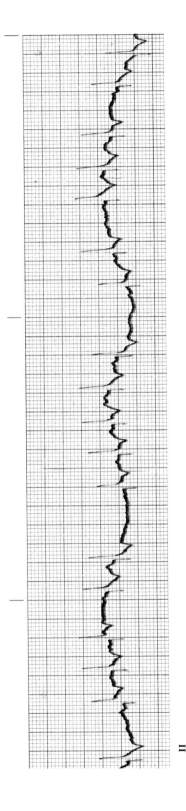

Figure 5–45.

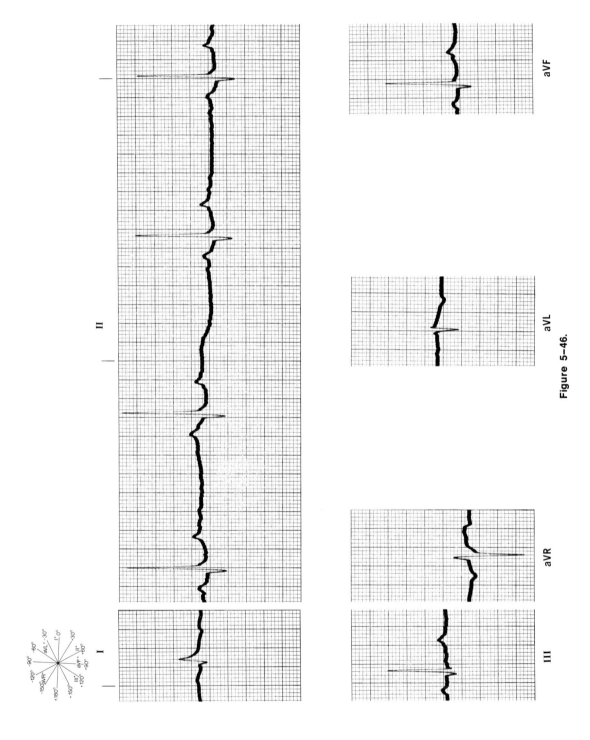

Figure 5-46.

The heart rate averages low-normal, and sinus arrhythmia is present, as indicated by the variation in R-R intervals (refer to Figure 4–5). Lead I is the lead closest to isoelectric. Lead aVF is perpendicular to lead I (use the axis chart), and lead aVF is positive in this tracing. Lead aVF's positive pole is at +90°. Since lead I is not perfectly isoelectric, +90° is not the exact axis. Lead I is slightly more positive than negative, so the axis is shifted a little from +90° toward lead I's positive pole, to +80°.

47. This lead II electrocardiogram was recorded from the same 4½-year-old female boxer as in Figure 5–43. She had a high fever and was in complete heart block at one time. When this tracing was recorded she was responding to penicillin therapy.

Paper speed = 50 mm./sec., 1 cm. = 1 mv.
(Tracing courtesy of Dr. R. Lynk, Delmar, N. Y.)

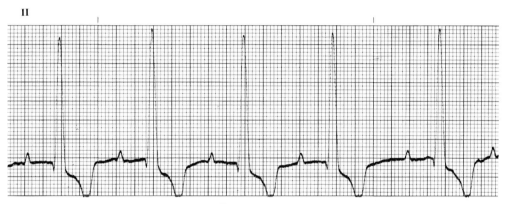

Figure 5–47.

Questions:

    a. What abnormalities are present?

    b. Are they significant?

Answers:

    a. First degree heart block and left ventricular hypertrophy or left bundle branch block are present. The P-R interval is 0.15 second (7½ boxes), indicating first degree heart block (refer to Figure 4–49). The S-T segment is depressed 0.35 mv. (3½ boxes) below the baseline, the R waves average 3.4 mv. (34 boxes) in height, and the QRS complexes are 0.07 second (3½ boxes) wide, suggesting left ventricular hypertrophy or left bundle branch block (refer to Figures 3–20, 3–21, 3–22, and 4–58).

    b. These changes may represent a result of bacterial endocarditis, myocarditis, or both. An inflammatory lesion in the area of the atrioventricular node or the bundle of His may have caused the temporary complete heart block, which is now responding to penicillin therapy. S-T segment depression can result from myocarditis or from left ventricular hypertrophy (refer to Figure 3–22). Nonspecific cardiac enlargement may occur with both endocarditis and myocarditis. In this case, the R waves were in the process of returning to normal. The dog was recovering from complete left bundle branch block (Figure 5–43).

48. This is a lead II electrocardiogram recorded from a 4-month-old female mixed breed dog weighing 7.3 kg., 24 hours after surgical correction of a patent ductus arteriosus.

Paper speed = 50 mm./sec., 1 cm. = ½ mv.

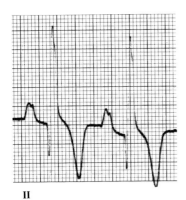

Figure 5–48.

II

Questions:

a. Keeping in mind that this is recorded at one-half sensitivity, what are the true measurements of these complexes?

b. What is the electrocardiographic diagnosis?

Answers:

a. Since this was recorded at 50 mm./sec. paper speed as usual, the width measurements do not change, but at one-half sensitivity, all height measurements must be doubled. Therefore, the measurements are:

P wave = 0.06 second (3 boxes) by 0.8 mv. (4 boxes).
P-R interval = 0.12 second (6 boxes)
QRS width = 0.08 second (4 boxes)
R wave height = 5.2 mv. (26 boxes)
S-T segment and T wave: S-T slurring, large T waves
Q-T interval = 0.22 second (11 boxes)
Miscellaneous criteria: "T_a" (T sub a) waves present, Q waves are 1.6 mv. (8 boxes) deep.

b. The electrocardiographic diagnosis is biatrial hypertrophy, biventricular hypertrophy, and left bundle branch block. The changes are severe. The wide notched P waves indicate left atrial hypertrophy and the tall P waves and "T$_a$" waves indicate right atrial hypertrophy (refer to Figures 3–15, 3–16, 3–17, and 3–18). Left ventricular hypertrophy is indicated by the tall R waves, the wide QRS complexes, and the slurring of the S-T segment (refer to Figures 3–18, 3–20, and 3–21). Left bundle branch block is present, note that the QRS complex is positive and wider than 0.07 second (3½ boxes) (refer to Figure 4–58). Right ventricular hypertrophy is diagnosed because the Q waves are so large (refer to Figure 3–25). The T waves are large because when there are large depolarization forces, as in this tracing, the repolarization forces are also large.

49. This full electrocardiogram was recorded from a 4-year-old female German shepherd with an abdominal mass. She was vomiting, and the electrocardiogram was taken presurgically to screen for electrolyte disturbances.

Paper speed = 50 mm./sec., 1 cm. = 1 mv.

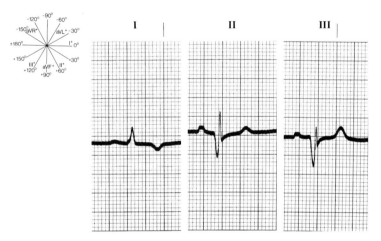

Figure 5–49.

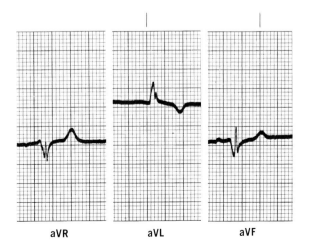

Questions:

    a. What is the mean electrical axis?

    b. Is there any evidence of electrolyte imbalance?

Answers:

    a. The mean electrical axis is −15°. Lead II and lead aVF are equally close to being isoelectric. If lead II is used, aVL is perpendicular to lead II on the axis chart, and lead aVL is positive on this tracing. Lead aVL's positive pole is at −30°. If lead aVF is used as isoelectric, lead I is perpendicular to aVF and in this tracing lead I is positive. Lead I's positive pole is at 0°. If 0° and −30° are averaged, the axis is −15°. This is a left axis deviation and indicates left ventricular hypertrophy.

    b. There are no alterations in the Q-T interval, the S-T segment, or the T wave to indicate electrolyte imbalances.

50. These electrocardiograms were recorded from a 5-year-old Newfoundland female. She had a rapid, irregular heart rate and a pulse deficit.

    Paper speed = 50 mm./sec., 1 cm. = 1 mv.

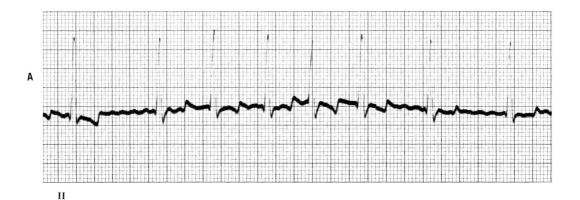

Figure 5–50.

Questions:

    a. What arrhythmia is recorded in tracing A?

    b. What is the heart rhythm in tracing B?

    c. What treatment produced the change?

Answers:

    a. Atrial fibrillation is present in tracing A. An irregular supraventricular tachycardia is seen, and there are no P waves when pauses occur. The P waves are replaced by fine baseline undulations termed "f" waves (refer to Figures 4–20 and 4–21).

    b. Normal sinus rhythm is present. There are P waves consistently related to every QRS complex, and the R-R intervals are exactly the same (refer to Figure 4–3).

    c. Digitalis and then digitalis and quinidine in combination were used to convert her to sinus rhythm at one time, but she reverted to atrial fibrillation when the therapy was discontinued. This time she would not convert with medical therapy, so D.C. cardioversion was used successfully. Tracing B was recorded within 1 hour of tracing A. The electrocardiogram in Figure 4–21 is of the same dog.

51. This tracing was recorded from a 1-year-old Newfoundland female with aortic stenosis.

    Paper speed = 50 mm./sec., 1 cm. = 1 mv.

Question:

    Read and interpret her electrocardiogram.

Answer:

    Heart rate = 160 beats per minute
    Heart rhythm: sinus arrhythmia, ventricular premature beat in leads
       I, II, and aVL
    Mean electrical axis = +90°
    Measuring and multiplying:
       P wave = 0.045 second (slightly over 2 boxes) by 0.25 mv. (2½
boxes)
         P-R interval = 0.10 second (5 boxes)
         QRS width = 0.04 second (2 boxes)
         R wave height = 2.2 mv. (22 boxes)
         S-T segment and T wave: S-T slurring
         Q-T interval = 0.16 second (8 boxes)
    Miscellaneous criteria: none
    Electrocardiographic diagnosis: left ventricular hypertrophy, left
       atrial hypertrophy, and ventricular premature beats

    The S-T segment slurring is a judgement call in this case, since most of the beats show it but some others (e.g., the third from the left) do not

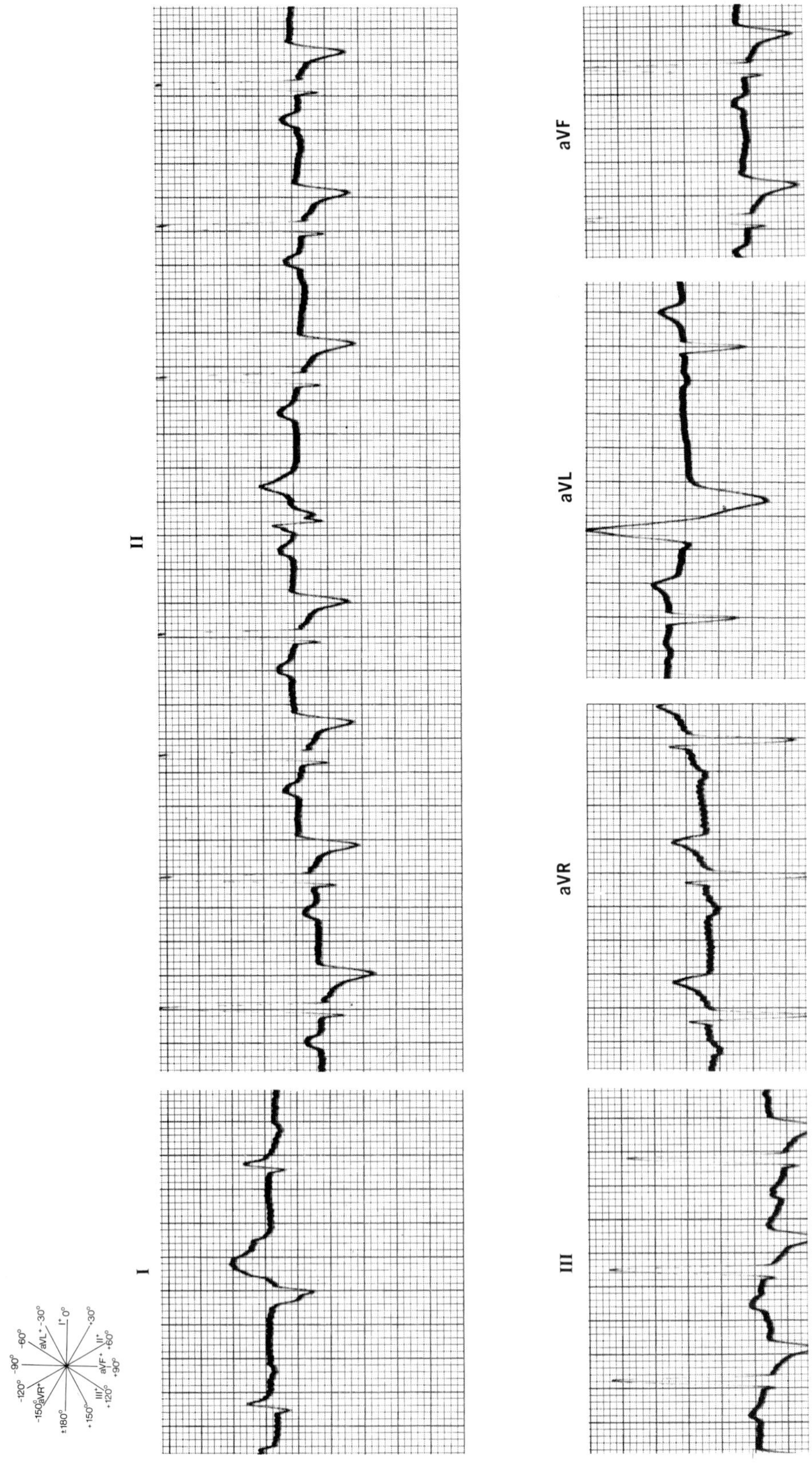

I

II

III

aVR

aVL

aVF

Figure 5–51.

show it well. The slurring of the S-T segment is the basis for diagnosing left ventricular hypertrophy (refer to Figure 3–21). The thoracic radiographs may be helpful in this case. Ventricular premature beats are associated with aortic stenosis and are probably due to microscopic infarctions in the left ventricular wall (Ettinger and Suter, 1970; Flickenger and Patterson, 1967). The wide P waves indicate left atrial hypertrophy (refer to Figure 3–16).

52. These tracings were taken of a 9-year-old male miniature poodle. He had a Grade 5 of 6 mitral insufficiency murmur and a collapsed trachea. He had been placed on digoxin, 0.125 mg. b.i.d. These tracings were recorded on 6/26/72 at 4 P.M., 6/28/72 at 8 A.M., and 6/28/72 at 5 P.M.

Paper speed = 50 mm./sec., 1 cm. = 1 mv.
(Tracings courtesy of Dr. L. Tilley, New York, N.Y.)

Questions:

a. What arrhythmia is present in tracing A?

b. What arrhythmia is present in tracing B?

c. Tracing C is normal. What was done to resolve the arrhythmias?

Answers:

a. Atrioventricular dissociation is present in tracing A. Notice how at the beginning of the strip the P waves move into the QRS complexes. This is termed accrochage (refer to Figure 4–38). For a sustained period of time the P waves and QRS complexes occur simultaneously. This is called synchrony (refer to Figure 4–37). Synchrony and accrochage are characteristic of atrioventricular dissociation.

b. Now the P waves and QRS complexes are consistently related to each other but the P-R interval averages 0.14 second (7 boxes), indicating first degree heart block (refer to Figure 4–49).

c. Atrioventricular dissociation and first degree heart block are both signs of digitalis intoxication. The poodle was also anorexic and was vomiting. Digoxin was withdrawn on 6/26/72 when he was admitted, and the electrocardiogram finally returned to normal about 2 days later. The dog felt much better at this time. No more digoxin was given, since the dog's clinical signs were reated to the collapsed trachea.

53. This full electrocardiogram was recorded from a 7-year-old Vizla that had a leiomyosarcoma of the small bowel and was 8 per cent dehydrated. Left ventricular enlargement was seen on thoracic radiographs. The serum K^+ was 5.3 meq./l. and the serum Na^+ was 132 meq./l. At one time adrenal insufficiency was suspected, and this electrocardiogram was taken.

Paper speed = 50 mm./sec., 1 cm. = 1 mv.

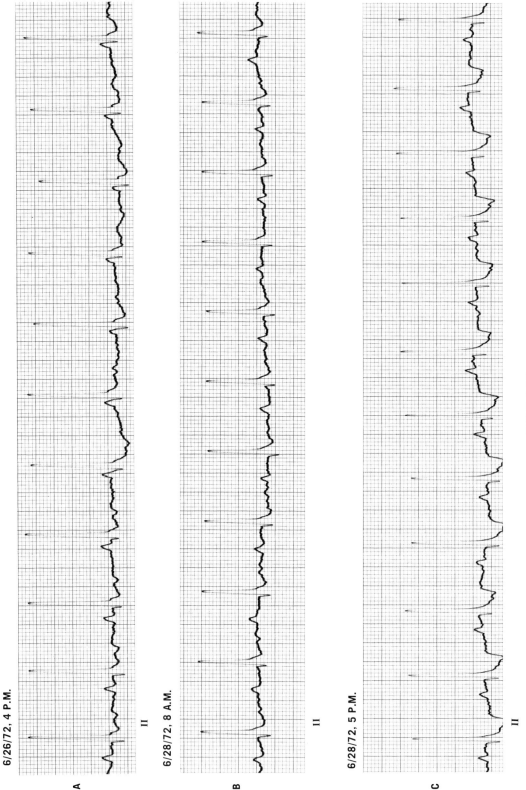

6/26/72, 4 P.M.

II

A

6/28/72, 8 A.M.

II

B

6/28/72, 5 P.M.

II

C

Figure 5–52.

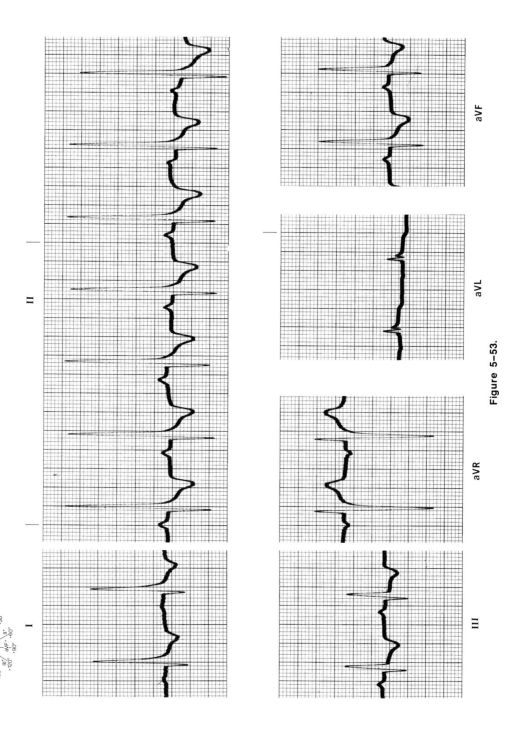

Figure 5-53.

Question:

Read and interpret this electrocardiogram.

Answer:

Heart rate = about 150 beats per minute
Heart rhythm: normal sinus rhythm
Mean electrical axis = +50°
Measuring and multiplying:
  P wave = 0.04 second (2 boxes) by 0.3 mv. (3 boxes)
  P-R interval = 0.09 second (4½ boxes)
  QRS width = 0.06 second (3 boxes)
  R wave height = 2.8 mv. (28 boxes average)
  S-T segment and T wave: S-T slurring
  Q-T interval = 0.185 second (9½ boxes)
Miscellaneous criteria: none

Electrocardiographic diagnosis: left ventricular hypertrophy. The slurring of the S-T segment indicates left ventricular hypertrophy, although the height and width of the QRS complexes are within normal limits (refer to Figure 3–21). The Q waves are quite deep but may be normal in a dog of this body type.

Lead aVL is closest to isoelectric. Lead II is perpendicular to lead aVL on the axis chart and is positive in this tracing. Lead II's positive pole is at +60°. Since lead aVL is not perfectly isoelectric, the axis is not perfectly +60°. Lead aVL is slightly more positive than negative, so the axis is shifted a little from +60° toward aVL's positive pole and is about +50°.

54. These are continuous lead II recordings from a 6-year-old female mixed breed dog with diabetes mellitus. She had experienced a hyperthermic episode during surgery for cataract removal and subsequently developed disseminated intravascular coagulation with petechiae and hemoptysis. The platelet count was 8,000/cu. mm., fibrinogen was 0, and fibrinogen degradation products were greater than 40 (very elevated). An arrhythmia and a pulse deficit were detected.

Paper speed = 50 mm./sec., 1 cm. = 1 mv.

Questions:

a. What arrhythmia is present?

b. What is the probable cause?

Answers:

a. Ventricular tachycardia is present. The first and fourth beats from the left side of the top tracing are capture beats, in which a PQRST occurs normally. The rest of the QRS complexes are bizarre and are not associated with P waves. When four or more ventricular ectopic beats occur in a row, it is a ventricular tachycardia; the presence of capture

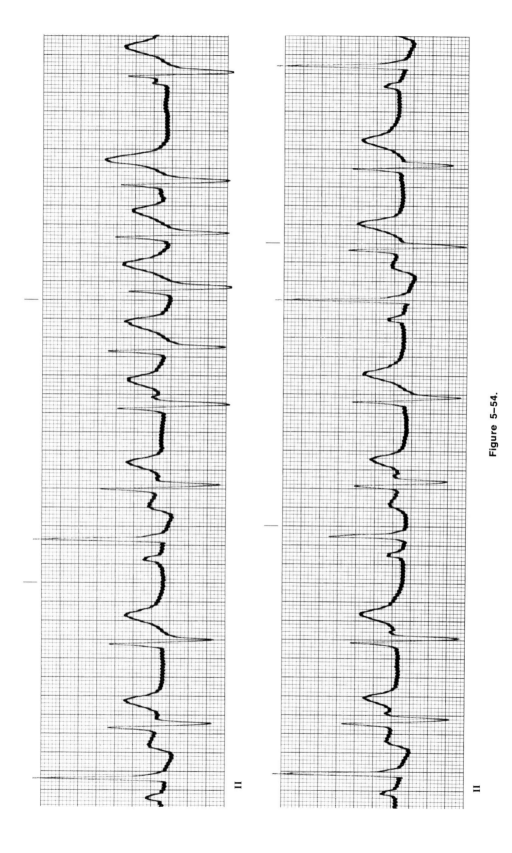

Figure 5-54.

beats also assists in the diagnosis (refer to Figures 4–33 to 4–35). In the bottom tracing, capture beats and ventricular ectopic beats also occur, and the fourth beat from the left may be a fusion beat, with a P wave, a normal P-R interval, and a QRS complex that is different from both the normal and the abnormal ones (refer to Figures 4–34 and 4–35).

b. It may be that myocarditis is occurring as a result of either infarction of or bleeding into the myocardium which is in turn a result of disseminated intravascular coagulation.

55. This is of the same dog as in the previous figure, and these three tracings demonstrate the dramatic response to treatment. These are continuous lead II recordings, and treatment was begun when the top strip was recorded. Fewer ventricular ectopic beats occur in the middle strip, and the ventricular arrhythmias are abolished toward the end of the bottom lead II tracing. This occurred within less than 1 minute.

Paper speed = 50 mm./sec., 1 cm. = ½ mv.

Question:

What drug was used to abolish the ventricular tachycardia?

Answer:

The dog was collapsed and unable to rise, so an intravenous drip of 2 mg./cc. lidocaine was prepared by adding 20 cc. of 2 per cent lidocaine without epinephrine to 200 cc. of 5 per cent dextrose in water. The drip was given rapidly until conversion occurred. The dog was begun on 5 mg./lb. of quinidine sulfate orally every 6 hours. The lidocaine drip was used as needed to maintain control of the arrhythmia until the oral quinidine became effective. The lidocaine drip was discontinued altogether within 12 hours, and the rhythm remained converted when the dog was switched to the longer-acting forms of quinidine (Quinaglut tablets) every 12 hours. Heparin and blood transfusions were also given and the dog survived the episode of disseminated intravascular coagulation but died several days later of acute hemorrhagic pancreatitis and acute hepatic necrosis.

56. This lead II electrocardiogram was recorded from a 7-year-old male Chihuahua that was in congestive heart failure as a result of mitral insufficiency. Skipped beats were heard during physical examination.

Paper speed = 50 mm./sec., 1 cm. = 1 mv.
(Tracing courtesy of Dr. L. Tilley, New York, N.Y.)

Question:

What arrhythmia is present?

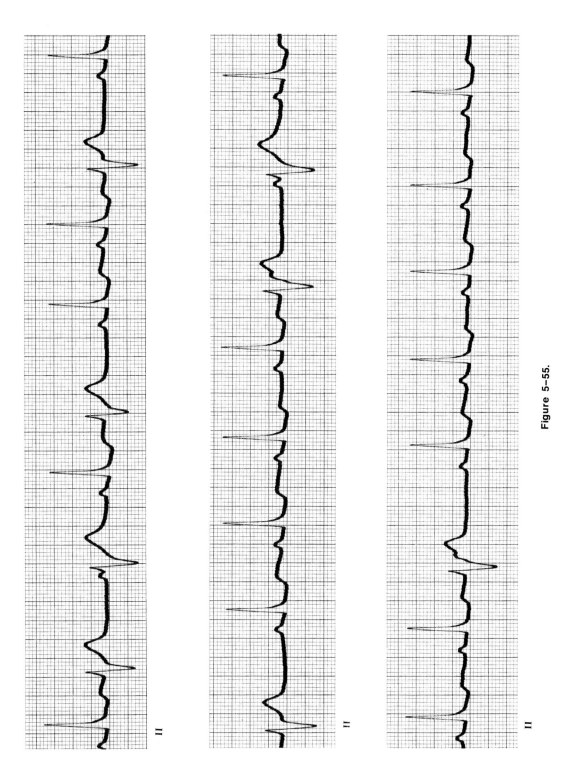

Figure 5–55.

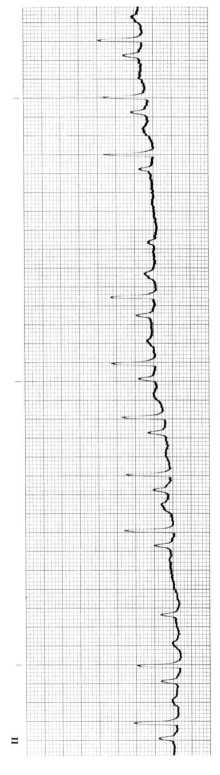

Figure 5–56.

Answer:

Second degree heart block is present, as indicated by the two P waves that occur without an accompanying QRS complex (refer to Figures 4–50 and 4–52). This dog had not been given digitalis, so this was probably associated with the congestive heart failure. The heart rate is 200 beats per minute between episodes of second degree heart block, so sinus tachycardia is also present.

57. These continuous lead II recordings were taken from a 10-year-old mixed breed male dog that was in Phase 4 congestive heart failure due to mitral insufficiency.

Paper speed = 50 mm./sec., 1 cm. = 1 mv. (middle of lower tracing recorded at 25 mm./sec)
(Tracings courtesy of Dr. L. Tilley, New York, N.Y.)

Question:

What is occurring in these tracings?

Answer:

Wandering pacemaker is present (refer to Figure 4–7). The P wave is large and positive at first but changes with each beat until it actually becomes negative as the pacemaker site wanders all the way down to the area of the atrioventricular node (junctional area). The pacemaker remains junctional for a short time, and then, during the period in the bottom tracing when the paper is run at half-speed, the pacemaker site gradually wanders back up in the atria until the P wave is again positive. This cycle repeated itself many times in this tracing and was associated with the congestive heart failure.

58. Two premature beats occur on this tracing (arrows).

Paper speed = 50 mm./sec., 1 cm. = 1 mv.
(Tracing courtesy of Dr. L. Tilley, New York, N.Y.)

Questions:

a. What type of premature beats are they?

b. What is their usual significance?

Answers:

a. The first one is a junctional (nodal) premature beat; it occurs early, is followed by a pause, the QRS complex remains normal, and the P wave is negative (refer to Figure 4–14). The second premature beat is a supraventricular premature beat. It also occurs early, is followed by a

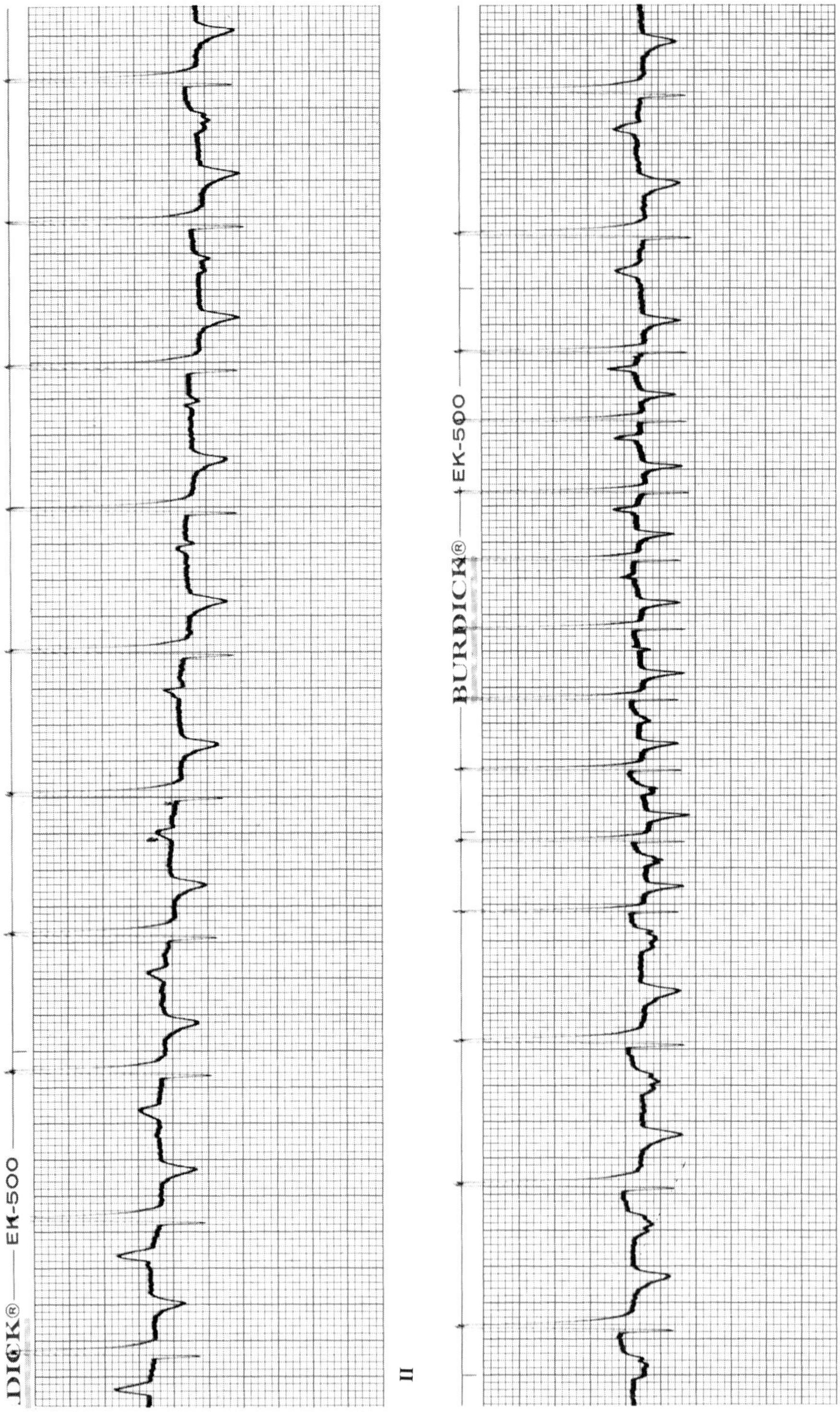

Figure 5–57.

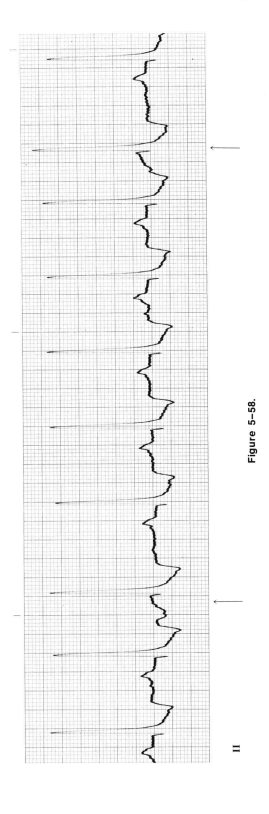

Figure 5–58.

pause, and has a normal QRS complex, but this time the P wave is hidden in the T wave of the previous beat. This makes it impossible to differentiate whether it is junctional or atrial in origin. This, however, is unimportant; its significance is that it is supraventricular (refer to Figures 4–13, 4–14, 4–15, and 4–24).

b. These supraventricular premature beats are usually caused by atrial enlargement and strain secondary to severe insufficiency of one or both of the atrioventricular valves. They should be treated with digitalis. If they were to occur while a dog is on digitalis, however, they should be considered to be due to digitalis intoxication.

59. These lead II electrocardiograms were recorded from a dog with digitalis intoxication.

Paper speed = 50 mm./sec., 1 cm. = $\frac{1}{2}$ mv.
(Tracings courtesy of Dr. L. Tilley, New York, N.Y.)

Question:

What arrhythmias are present?

Answer:

Wandering pacemaker, junctional and ventricular escape beats, and second degree heart block are all present. These may all be due to the vagal effects of digitalis. In the upper tracing, from left, three beats occur in which the P wave height varies, indicating wandering pacemaker (refer to Figure 4–6). After a pause, a junctional escape beat occurs with a negative P wave (refer to Figures 4–44 and 4–45), then a negative P wave occurs without a QRS complex indicating second degree heart block (refer to Figure 4–50). After the isolated P wave, a bizarre QRS complex occurs without a P wave. This is a ventricular escape beat (refer to Figure 4–47). Then another negative P wave occurs, followed by another bizarre ventricular beat, but they are not related, as indicated by the abnormally long P-R interval.

In the bottom tracing, three ventricular escape beats occur in a row. The last one appears at first to be associated with a P wave but is not, because that P-R interval is abnormally short. The tracing finishes with three junctional (nodal) beats in a row. These disturbances disappeared when digitalis was discontinued temporarily. The dosage was then reduced.

60. This lead II tracing also was recorded from a dog with digitalis intoxication.

Paper speed = 50 mm./sec., 1 cm. = 1 mv.
(Tracing courtesy of Dr. L. Tilley, New York, N.Y.)

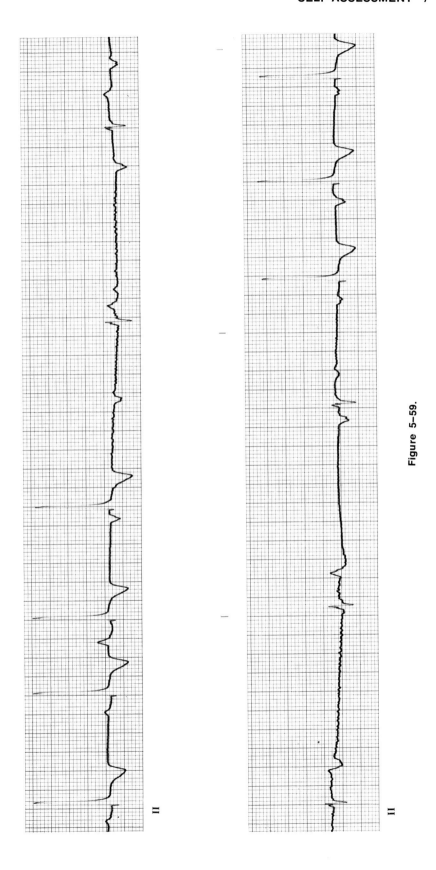

Figure 5–59.

II

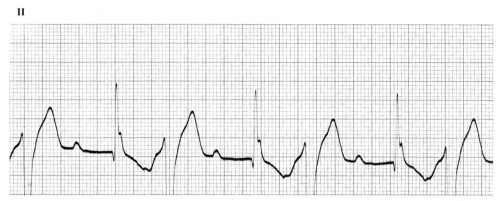

Figure 5–60.

Question:

What arrhythmias are present?

Answer:

Ventricular premature beats and first degree heart block are present. In this tracing every other beat is a bizarre ventricular premature beat. This is called ventricular bigeminy (refer to Figures 4–28 and 4–30). The P-R interval of the normal beats is consistently prolonged to 0.21 second (10½ boxes), indicating first degree heart block (refer to Figure 4–49). Since the P waves of the normal beats occur so soon after the ventricular ectopic beats, the first degree heart block may be caused by the atrioventricular node with the ventricles remaining refractory to impulse conduction, so that a delay occurs before the next impulse can be conducted.

It can also be seen that the Q-T intervals of the normal beats are consistently prolonged, to 0.24 second (12 boxes). This could be caused by hypokalemia (refer to Figure 3–34). Hypokalemia predisposes the dog to digitalis intoxication, so this dog's serum K^+ level should be checked.

61.   Two premature beats occur on this lead II electrocardiogram.

Paper speed = 50 mm./sec., 1 cm. = 1 mv.
(Tracings courtesy of Dr. L. Tilley, New York, N.Y.)

Questions:

a. These are ventricular premature beats. What criteria are used to determine this?

b. What do these beats signify?

Answers:

a. They occur early, are followed by a pause, their QRS complexes are distorted, and they are not associated with P waves. These are single, unifocal ventricular premature beats (refer to Figure 4–25). They

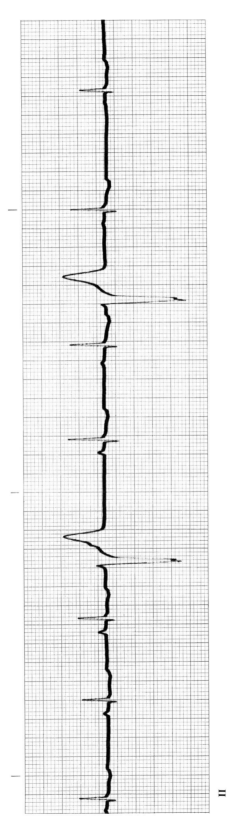

Figure 5–61.

are slightly different than usual. Most often, ventricular premature beats are coupled to the previous beat, as in Figure 5–60, indicating that they always have the same relationship to the previous beat. In this tracing, however, it can be seen that the second ventricular premature beat is closer to the previous beat than is the first one. When they vary in their relationship to the previous beat, as in this tracing, it is called ventricular parasystole. If more of the tracing were examined, it would also be seen that they tend to occur at their own regular R-R intervals, and the distance from premature beat to premature beat would be exactly regular (refer to Figure 5–37). There is no particular clinical significance in differentiating between coupling and parasystole, but it is interesting.

b. These beats signify that myocarditis is present. There is an inflammatory focus in the ventricular myocardium. A complete search for the cause must be done.

62.   Tracings A, B, C, D, and E were recorded from the same dog. A, B, and C are pretreatment recordings, and D and E are post-treatment.

Paper speed for A and B = 50 mm./sec., 1 cm. = 1 mv.
Paper speed for C, D, and E = 50 mm./sec., 1 cm. = 1/2 mv.
(Tracing courtesy of Dr. L. Tilley, New York, N.Y.)

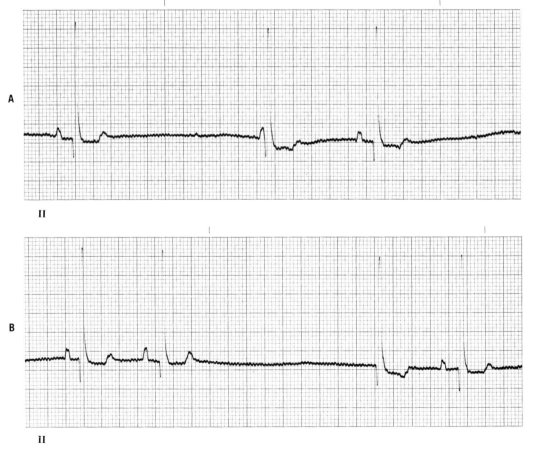

A

II

B

II

Figure 5–62.   Illustration continued on opposite page.

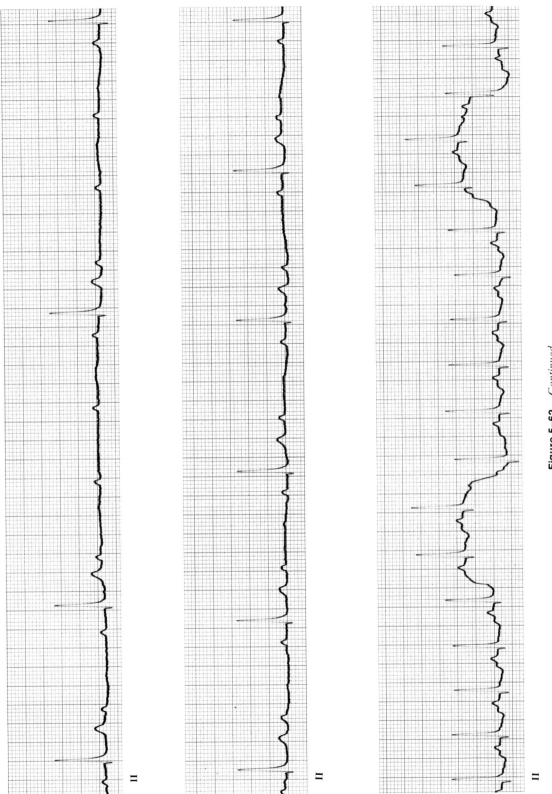

Figure 5–62, *Continued.*

Questions:

  a. What arrhythmia is present in tracings A and B?

  b. What arrhythmia is present in tracing C?

  c. What drug was used to abolish the arrhythmias?

Answers:

a. The middle beat in tracing A and the third beat from the left in tracing B are ventricular escape beats. They occur after a long pause and are not associated with a P wave (refer to Figure 4–47). In tracing A, a P wave can be seen just at the beginning of the escaped QRS complex. Since the QRS complex of the escape beat is normal in appearance, the beat probably originated in the bundle of His (refer to Figure 4–31). Occasionally, when a junctional premature beat occurs, its P wave may be hidden in the QRS complex, but in tracing A, a positive P wave that is not associated with that QRS complex can be seen. The pauses are caused by sinus arrhythmia in tracing A and by sinus arrest in tracing B (refer to Figures 4–5 and 4–9).

b. Tracing C reveals advanced second degree heart block. There are several P waves with no QRS complexes, but the PQRS complexes that do occur all have consistent P-R intervals, which indicates that some of the P waves are able to traverse the atrioventricular node and stimulate ventricular depolarization. A period of 2:1 block occurs, followed by two periods of 4:1 block (refer to Figures 4–50, 4–51, and 4–52).

c. Atropine was given subcutaneously (0.02 mg./lb.), and tracings D and E show the response to atropine therapy. In tracing D, 2:1 second degree heart block is still present, but later, in tracing E, the arrhythmias are completely abolished by atropine. This proves that these arrhythmias were vagal in origin (refer to Figure 4–10). There is some respiratory artifact in tracing E.

63. Tracings A and B are of a dog suspected of having digitalis intoxication.

  Paper speed = 50 mm./sec., 1 cm. = 1 mv.
  (Tracings courtesy of Dr. L. Tilley, New York, N.Y.)

Question:

  Is there any evidence of digitalis intoxication in these tracings?

Answer:

  Yes. In tracing A, the rhythm is junctional (nodal) in origin, as indicated by the negative P waves in lead II. The heart rate is about 100 beats per minute, which technically makes this a junctional tachycardia

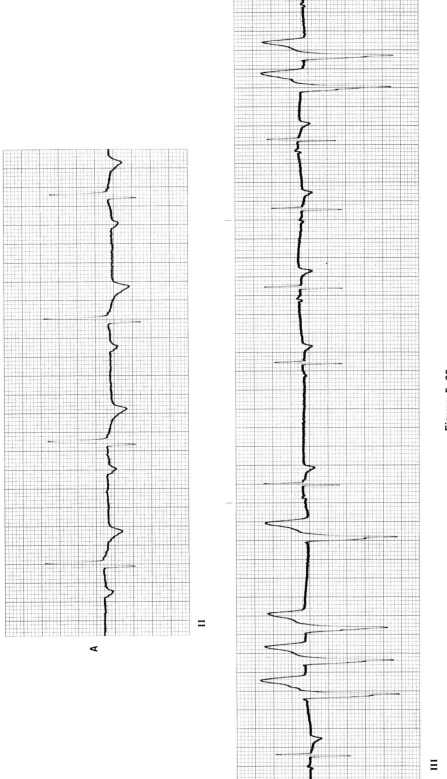

Figure 5–63.

(refer to Figures 4–23 and 4–46). Junctional arrhythmias are commonly associated with digitalis intoxication.

Tracing B is recorded from lead III, and the P waves are biphasic, but now ventricular premature beats are occurring, as further evidence of digitalis intoxication. In the beginning of this tracing, three ventricular premature beats occur in a row. This is called a run (refer to Figure 4–27). A pause follows, and then a ventricular escape beat occurs (refer to Figure 4–47). At the end of the tracing, two ventricular premature beats occur in succession. This is called a pair (refer to Figure 4–26). Ventricular premature beats should be considered a sign of serious digitalis intoxication.

64. This 13-year-old male miniature poodle was given 0.125 mg. digoxin t.i.d. for 3 days. Now he is vomiting, anorexic, and has bloody diarrhea. He is weak and ataxic. An irregular rhythm and a pulse deficit are present. Tracing A was recorded upon admission (7/4/72) and tracing B was recorded after 3 days treatment (7/7/72).

Paper speed = 50 mm./sec., 1 cm. = 1 mv.
(Tracing courtesy of Dr. L. Tilley, New York, N.Y.)

Questions:

a. What is the arrhythmia?

b. How would you treat it?

Answers:

a. This is a ventricular tachycardia of multifocal origin. Every beat is a ventricular premature beat, and all are of varying conformations (refer to Figure 4–36). This should be considered a dangerous prefibrillatory rhythm, especially since the dog shows signs of weakness and ataxia.

b. Digoxin was discontinued immediately and quinidine therapy was instituted to suppress the ventricular arrhythmias. Tracing B, recorded 3 days later, demonstrates that the ventricular arrhythmias are completely controlled. First degree heart block is still present, as indicated by the prolongation of the P-R interval to 0.17 second ($8\frac{1}{2}$ boxes) (refer to Figure 4–49). The dog was feeling much better at this time. The quinidine can be discontinued when the excessive levels of digoxin are eliminated from the system. This usually takes 1 to 3 days, but may take as long as 7 to 10 days.

65. Paper speed = 50 mm./sec., 1 cm. = 1 mv.
(Tracings courtesy of Dr. L. Tilley, New York, N.Y.)

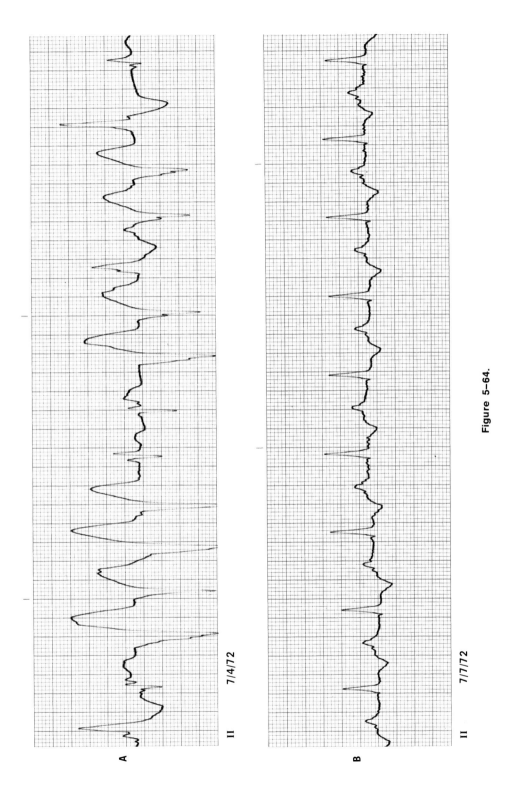

A   II   7/4/72

B   II   7/7/72

Figure 5–64.

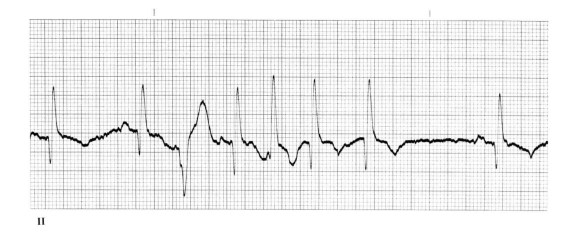

II

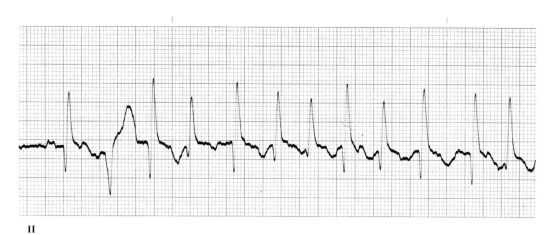

II

Figure 5–65.

Questions:

a. What arrhythmias are present in these continuous lead II electrocardiograms?

b. What is a likely cause?

Answers:

a. Two bursts of junctional (nodal) tachycardia occur. Each burst is preceded by a ventricular premature beat. The ventricular premature beats are bizarre in conformation, and each one is followed by a burst of tachycardia (about 250 to 300 beats per minute), which may be recognized as supraventricular because of the nearly normal QRS complexes. Negative P waves can be seen, which indicates that these are paroxysms of junctional (nodal) tachycardia (refer to Figures 4–23 and 4–46).

b. Junctional tachycardia is most often caused by digitalis intoxication, as was the case here. The ventricular premature beats provide additional evidence of digitalis intoxication.

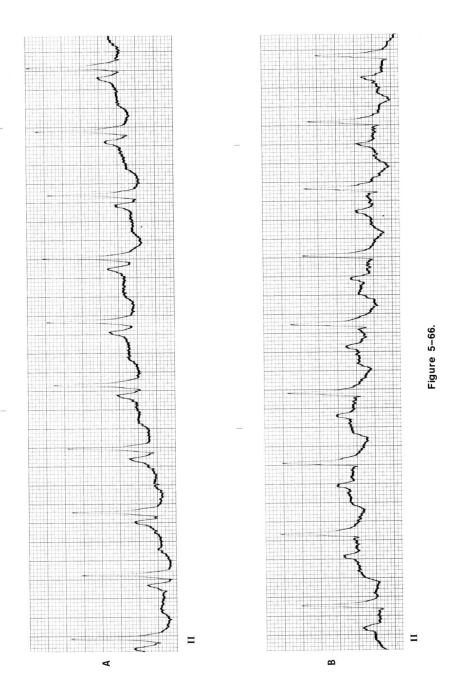

Figure 5–66.

66. Tracings A and B were recorded from the same dog as in Figure 5–65. They are "before" and "after" tracings.

Paper speed = 50 mm./sec., 1 cm. = 1 mv.
(Tracings courtesy of Dr. L. Tilley, New York, N.Y.)

Questions:

a. What is the arrhythmia on tracing A?

b. What drug is the most common cause of this arrhythmia?

c. Tracing B is the dog's normal rhythm. What was done to restore the rhythm to normal?

Answers:

a. This is atrioventricular dissociation with synchrony (refer to Figure 4–37). The P waves and QRS complexes are occurring at the same rate, and the P waves fall almost on top of the QRS complexes, which proves that the P's and QRS's are not associated. The abnormal QRS complexes are not very different from the normal ones in the bottom strip. This is often the case in atrioventricular dissociation, because the ventricular pacemaker is often in or near the bundle of His.

b. Atrioventricular dissociation is most often caused by digitalis intoxication, as it was here.

c. The bottom tracing was recorded 36 hours after discontinuing digitalis therapy.

67. Paper speed = 50 mm./sec., 1 cm. = 1 mv.
(Tracing courtesy of Dr. L. Tilley, New York, N.Y.)

Questions:

a. What arrhythmia is present?

b. What type is it?

Answers:

a. This is second degree heart block. An occasional P wave occurs without a QRS complex (refer to Figures 4–50 and 4–52).

b. This is the Wenkebach phenomenon, or Mobitz type I second degree heart block. The P-R interval becomes prolonged just before the QRS complex is dropped (refer to Figure 4–52). This is most often associated with digitalis intoxication.

68. This tracing was recorded from a 12-year-old male mixed breed dog that was suffering from smoke inhalation and had pulmonary edema.

Paper speed = 50 mm./sec., 1 cm. = 1 mv.
(Tracing courtesy of Dr. L. Tilley, New York, N.Y.)

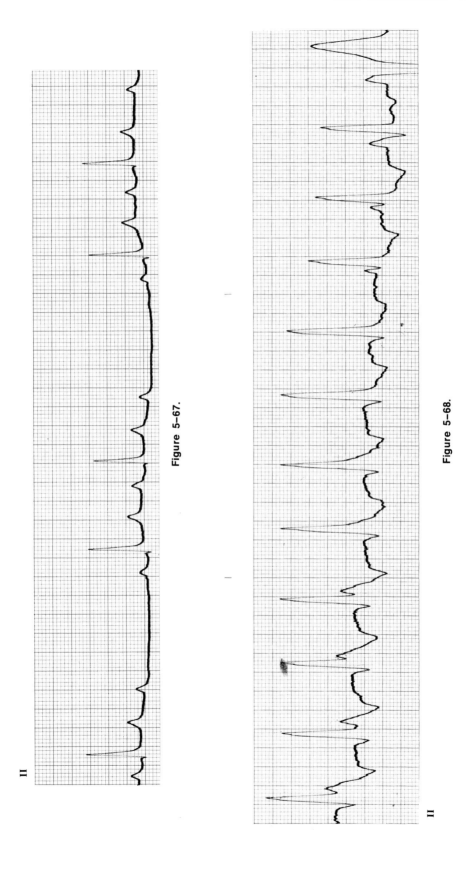

Figure 5–67.

Figure 5–68.

Questions:

  a. What arrhythmia is this?

  b. What is its significance?

Answers:

  a. This is ventricular tachycardia. At the beginning of the tracing, P waves can be seen to occur behind the QRS complexes; then they are lost in the QRS complexes for four beats, and at the end of the tracing they reappear in front of the QRS complexes. This demonstrates the lack of relationship between the P waves and the QRS complexes. This is a form of atrioventricular dissociation with accrochage (refer to Figure 4–38). The last four beats on the tracing demonstrate that this ventricular tachycardia is of multifocal origin, as can be noted from the fact that these ventricular beats are of different conformation than any of the others (refer to Figure 4–36).

  b. It signifies that the ventricular myocarditis is severe, and the multifocal origin is an even more ominous sign. It may have been caused by the poisonous gases in the fire or may be due to hypoxia from the pulmonary edema. The dog subsequently died.

69. This tracing was also recorded from the 12-year-old dog in Figure 5–68.

  Paper speed = 50 mm./sec., 1 cm. = 1 mv.
  (Tracing courtesy of Dr. L. Tilley, New York, N.Y.)

Question:

  This tracing demonstrates a capture beat and a fusion beat, both of which break the multifocal ventricular tachycardia. Which one is the capture beat and which is the fusion beat?

Answer:

  The capture beat is the first beat on the left. It has a P wave, a normal P-R interval, and a normal QRS complex. The fourth beat from the left has a P wave, a normal P-R interval, and then a QRS complex that is abnormal in form because the P wave and the abnormal ectopic focus both attempted to discharge the ventricles at the same time (refer to Figures 4–33, 4–34, and 4–35). Capture and fusion beats are diagnostic of ventricular tachycardia.

70. This tracing is also from the same 12-year-old dog as in the two previous figures. It was recorded after the ventricular tachycardia was abolished using 2 per cent lidocaine without epinephrine.

  Paper speed = 50 mm./sec., 1 cm. = 1 mv.
  (Tracing courtesy of Dr. L. Tilley, New York, N.Y.)

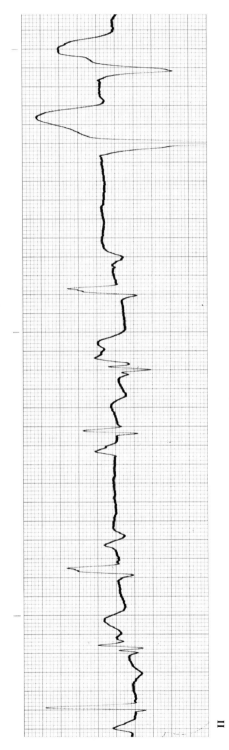

Figure 5–69.

II

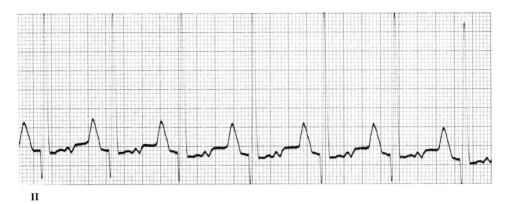

II

Figure 5–70.

Question:

Is there any evidence of cardiac enlargement?

Answer:

Yes. There is biatrial hypertrophy, left ventricular hypertrophy, and possibly right ventricular hypertrophy. The P waves are 0.07 second (3½ boxes) wide, which indicates left atrial hypertrophy (refer to Figures 3–16 and 3–17). The P waves average 0.6 mv (6 boxes) in height, and depression of the P-R segment (called "T_a" wave) are both evidence of right atrial hypertrophy (refer to Figures 3–15, 3–17, and 3–18). The R waves are 3.7 mv. (37 boxes) tall, which indicates left ventricular hypertrophy, and the Q waves are becoming quite deep as though biventricular hypertrophy were present (refer to Figures 3–20, 3–25, and 3–28).

71.   Paper speed = 50 mm./sec., 1 cm. = 1 mv.
      (Tracing courtesy of Dr. L. Tilley, New York, N.Y.)

Question:

Is this sinus arrhythmia or sinus arrest?

Answer:

This is sinus arrest. If the first two R-R intervals on the left are used as two normal R-R intervals, it can be seen that the long pause is greater than two normal R-R intervals. This differentiates sinus arrest from sinus arrhythmia (refer to Figures 4–5 and 4–9). It can also be seen that the QRS complex following the pause is abnormal, and its P-R interval is shorter than normal. This, then, is probably a ventricular escape beat, and that P wave is not associated with it. Since it is almost normal in shape, it probably arose somewhere near the bundle of His (refer to Figure 4–31).

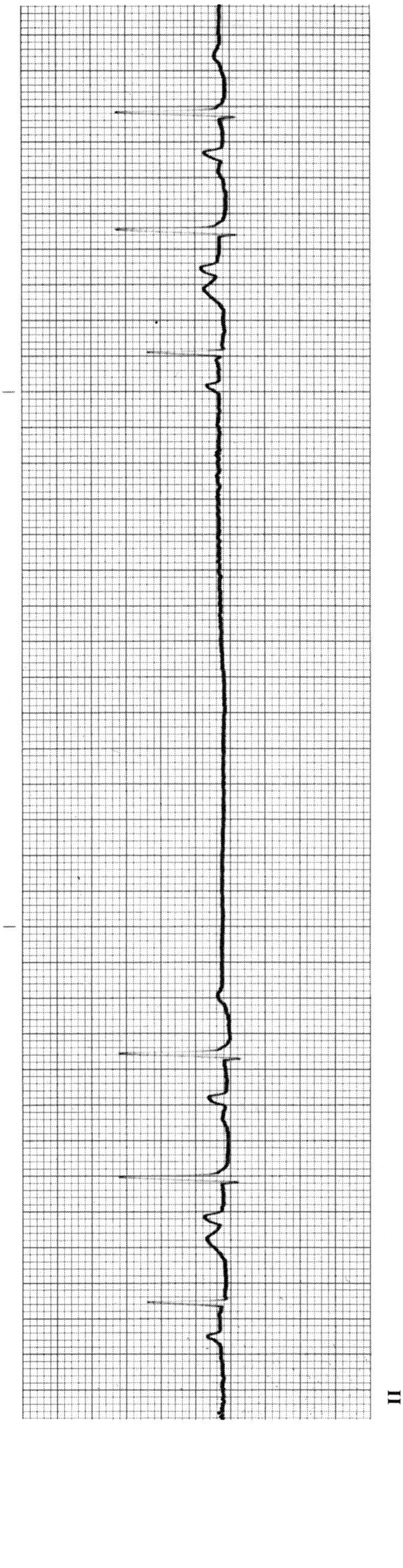

Figure 5–71.

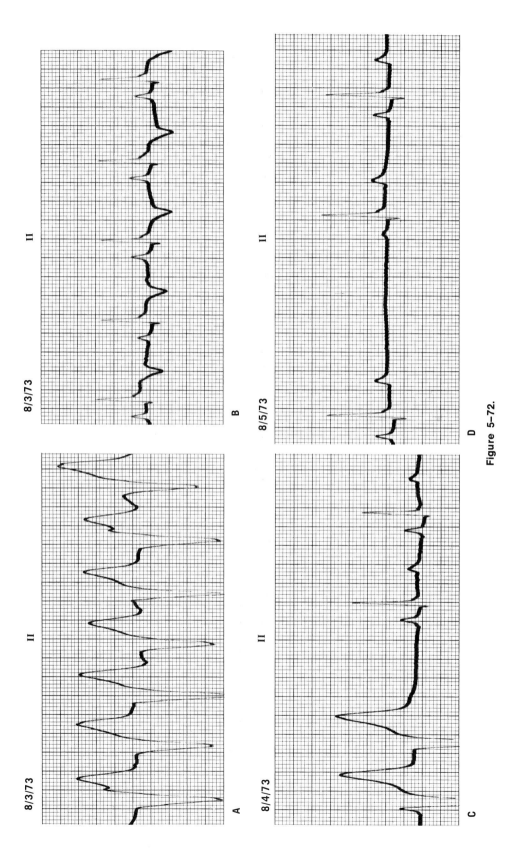

Figure 5-72.

72. Tracings A, B, C, and D were recorded from a dog that had been hit by a car and had traumatic myocarditis. Tracing A is the initial recording and tracing B was recorded after treatment with lidocaine intravenously. Tracing C was recorded the next day, when the dog was on oral quinidine. Tracing D was recorded 2 days after the original insult.

Paper speed = 50 mm./sec., 1 cm. = 1 mv.

Questions:

a. What rhythm is indicated in tracing A?

b. Is there any evidence of myocarditis in tracing B?

c. What rhythm is indicated in tracing C?

d. Is there any evidence of myocarditis in tracing D?

Answers:

a. Ventricular tachycardia is indicated by the series of bizarre ventricular beats that are not associated with P waves (refer to Figure 4–33).

b. The ventricular arrhythmias are well controlled, but the S-T segment shows significant elevation, which suggests that myocarditis is present (refer to Figure 3–23).

c. A pair of ventricular premature beats occur (refer to Figure 4–26). The S-T segment is not as elevated in the two normal beats as it was the previous day.

d. This recording, taken 2 days after the original insult, is within normal limits. The S-T segment is no longer significantly elevated. The dog was eventually withdrawn from quinidine therapy after several weeks. The arrhythmia did not return.

73. Paper speed = 50 mm./sec., 1 cm. = 1 mv.

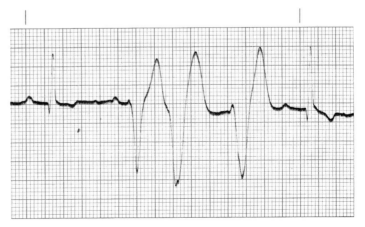

II

Figure 5–73.

Questions:

a. What is it called when three ventricular premature beats occur in a row, as in this tracing?

b. Are these of unifocal or multifocal origin?

Answers:

a. This is a ventricular run (refer to Figure 4–27). The first ventricular premature beat falsely appears to be associated with a P wave, but the P-R interval is obviously shorter than those of the normal beats, which proves that it is not associated with the P wave.

b. They are of multifocal origin; their conformations are slightly different. This is more worrisome than if they were of unifocal origin, because more than one area of ventricular myocardium must be irritable (refer to Figures 4–27 and 4–30).

74. This lead II electrocardiogram was recorded from a 4-year-old male Doberman pinscher with idiopathic cardiomyopathy.

Paper speed = 50 mm./sec., 1 cm. = 1 mv.

Questions:

a. What two arrhythmias are present?
b. What is their significance?

Answers:

a. Atrial fibrillation is the dominant rhythm, and one ventricular premature beat occurs early in the tracing. The irregular heart rate, fairly normal QRS complexes and lack of P waves all indicate that atrial fibrillation is present (refer to Figures 4–20 and 4–21). One ventricular premature beat is called a single (refer to Figure 4–25).

b. Most dogs with idiopathic cardiomyopathy are presented in atrial fibrillation (Ettinger and Suter, 1970). With adequate medical care, dogs with atrial fibrillation live about 4 to 6 months although this Doberman lived for 2 years (Bolton and Ettinger, 1971).

Occasional ventricular premature beats are commonly seen in association with idiopathic cardiomyopathy. This dog was on treatment with digitalis at the time of this recording, but he felt well and ate well, so the ventricular premature beat was thought to be a part of the dog's primary condition. No treatment was given since the ventricular premature beats occurred infrequently.

75. This lead II electrocardiogram was recorded from a dog that had been hit by a car the previous day. He was under thiamylal sodium anesthesia when this electrocardiogram was taken.

Paper speed = 50 mm./sec., 1 cm. = 1 mv.

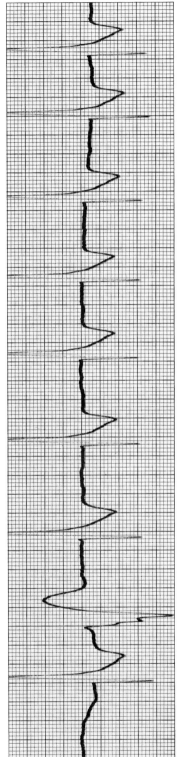

Figure 5-74.

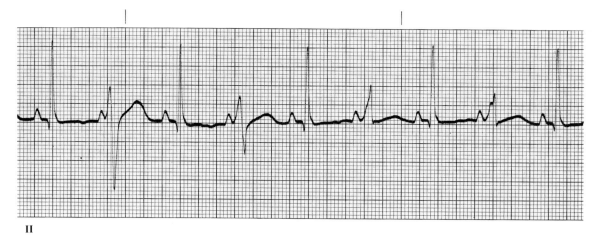

II

Figure 5–75.

Questions:

  a. What arrhythmia is present?

  b. Is there any cause for concern?

Answers:

  a. Every other beat is a ventricular premature beat, which indicates that this is a ventricular bigeminy (refer to Figure 4–28). Each abnormal beat is abnormal in form, and even though there are P waves in front of each one, the P-R intervals are obviously much shorter than the normals. This means that the P waves of the abnormal beats are not associated with the QRS complexes. The ventricular premature beats vary in form, so they are of multifocal origin (refer to Figure 4–30).

  b. Multifocal ventricular premature beats are always worrisome whenever they occur. It is a good idea to rest a dog that has been hit by a car for 3 or 4 days after the accident before giving general anesthesia. In our clinic we have observed several dogs that have developed severe ventricular arrhythmias under anesthesia when they were anesthetized too soon after the accident. The ventricular arrhythmias persisted in this dog, and anesthesia was discontinued. Three days later the dog was anesthetized for radiographs with no complications.

76. This lead II electrocardiogram was recorded from a St. Bernard following surgery for gastric torsion. The dog was recovering poorly from anesthesia, and a pulse deficit, as well as a jugular pulse, was noticed.

  Paper speed = 50 mm./sec., 1 cm. = 1 mv.

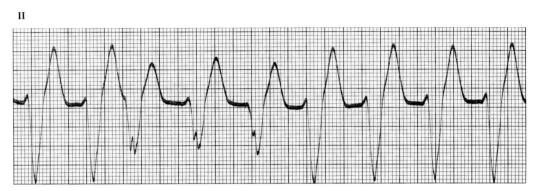

II

Figure 5-76.

Questions:

 a. What is the arrhythmia?

 b. How should it be treated?

 c. Why did the dog have a jugular pulse and a pulse deficit?

Answers:

 a. This is ventricular tachycardia of multifocal origin. All of the beats are bizarre, and none are associated with P waves. The third, fourth, and fifth beats from the left are of different configuration than the others, which indicates the multifocal nature of this arrhythmia (refer to Figures 4–33 and 4–36).

 b. This should be treated with 2 per cent lidocaine without epinephrine, since epinephrine is arrhythmogenic. A 2 mg./cc. intravenous drip was prepared by placing 20 cc. of 2 per cent lidocaine without epinephrine into 200 cc. of 5 per cent dextrose in water. The drip was run quickly until conversion to sinus rhythm was obtained (it took about 50 seconds). The dog was then begun on oral quinidine sulfate at 5 mg./lb. every 6 hours. The lidocaine drip was used as needed to control the arrhythmia until the oral preparation maintained control (about 9 hours later). The dog made an uneventful recovery, and quinidine therapy was discontinued about 4 weeks later with no problems.

 c. The pulse deficit occurs when the ventricular beat is either too rapid or too inefficient to propel enough blood to raise the aortic blood pressure high enough to in turn palpate a femoral pulse (refer to Figure 4–1). The jugular pulse occurs because the atria are also beating, although the P waves are hidden by the larger QRS complexes on the electrocardiogram. When the atria beat against the atrioventricular valves (which have been prematurely closed by an ectopic ventricular beat), the atrial contraction forces blood retrograde into the great veins, and a jugular pulse occurs.

77.   Paper speed = 50 mm./sec., 1 cm. = 1 mv.

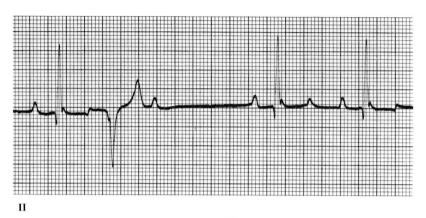

II

Figure 5–77.

Question:

What happened here?

Answer:

A ventricular premature beat occurred (second beat from left), and then a P wave occurred so soon that the ventricles were still refractory to another impulse. As a result, the P wave did not stimulate the ventricles because the ventricles had not yet recovered from the last beat, so an episode of second degree heart block can be seen (refer to Figure 4–50).

78.   This electrocardiogram was recorded from a 6-year-old male English pointer with aortic stenosis and a ventricular septal defect.

Paper speed = 50 mm./sec., 1 cm. = 1 mv.

Questions:

a. What is his mean electrical axis?

b. Are there any other signs of cardiac hypertrophy?

Answers:

a. The mean electrical axis is −30°. Only leads I, II, III, aVR, aVL, and aVF are used to determine axis. Lead II is the isoelectric lead,

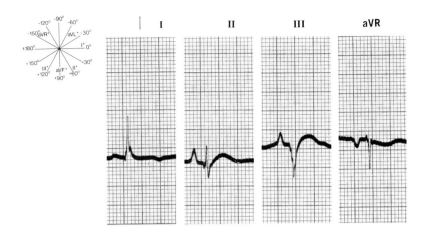

Figure 5–78.

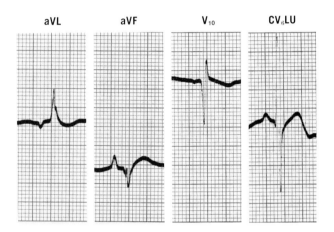

and on the axis chart, lead aVL is perpendicular to lead II. Lead aVL is positive in this tracing, and aVL's positive pole is located at −30°. This is a severe left axis deviation and indicates severe left ventricular hypertrophy. There was marked left ventricular enlargement on thoracic radiographs of this dog, and at necropsy there was remarkable left ventricular hypertrophy.

b. There is an S wave in lead CV_6LU that is deeper than 0.7 mv. (7 boxes), which indicates right ventricular hypertrophy (refer to Figure 3–26), which was also seen on radiographs and at necropsy.

79. This electrocardiogram was recorded from a 4-year-old German shepherd female as a routine part of a diagnostic work-up. She had a history of cardiac arrest when being spayed at 1 year of age.

Paper speed = 50 mm./sec., 1 cm. = 1 mv.

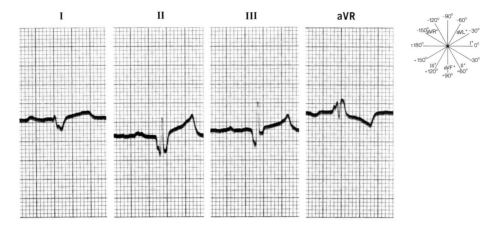

Figure 5–79.

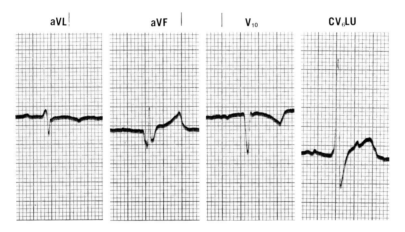

Questions:

a. What is your electrocardiographic diagnosis?

b. The heart was normal on thoracic radiographs. What would your diagnosis be now?

c. Can we anesthetize her?

Answers:

a. The axis is indeterminate; many of the leads are isoelectric. Since lead I is negative, the axis may be slightly rightward, because the negative half of lead I is on the right half of the axis chart. Right ventricular hypertrophy is suggested by the presence of an S wave in leads I, II, III, and aVF, and by the S wave in lead CV_6LU that is deeper than 0.7 mv. (7 boxes) (refer to Figures 3–24 and 3–26). One thought to keep in mind is that the terminal forces (S waves) of leads I, II, III, aVF, and CV_6LU are quite prolonged (wide). This should arouse suspicion that this might be incomplete right bundle branch block (refer to Figure 4–57).

b. Since the thoracic radiographs show no right ventricular enlargement, the diagnosis is incomplete right bundle branch block.

c. Anesthesia was accomplished without complications. Right bundle branch block is not associated with any cardiac dysfunction unless it accompanies right ventricular enlargement and congestive heart failure (Patterson et al., 1961). It is usually an insignificant finding (Bolton and Ettinger, 1972).

80. This lead II electrocardiogram was recorded from an old cocker spaniel that had severe mitral insufficiency and was being treated with digoxin.

Paper speed = 25 mm./sec., 1 cm. = 1 mv.
(Tracing courtesy of Dr. E. Grano, Briarcliff Manor, N. Y.)

Questions:

a. This is an unusual one. What kind of arrhythmia is present?

b. What is the probable cause?

Answers:

a. This is atrial tachycardia with block. Starting at the left, a normal beat occurs, followed by a supraventricular premature beat and a pause; then another normal beat occurs, also followed by a supraventricular premature beat and a pause. This is called supraventricular bigeminy (refer to Figure 4–17). Then a normal beat occurs, followed by an atrial premature beat and then a burst of eight P waves with no QRS complexes. Since other P waves are associated with QRS complexes, this is an advanced second degree heart block (refer to Figure 4–51). A QRS complex occurs with no related P wave (bundle of His beat?), then two normal P waves occur without QRS complexes, which also indicates second degree heart block. Another normal beat followed by an atrial premature beat occurs. Two normal beats are followed by a pause that is longer than two normal R-R intervals, which indicates sinus arrest (refer to Figures 4–5 and 4–9). Two normal beats end the tracing.

This is a complex set of arrhythmias. When the burst of P waves occurs, they are easily seen to be positive but different from the normal P waves, a hallmark of atrial tachycardia (refer to Figure 4–18).

b. Atrial tachycardia with block is unusual but is most often associated with digitalis intoxication. The dose of digoxin has been reduced and the dog is now doing well, although there are still a few paroxysms of tachycardia.

81. This electrocardiogram was recorded from a 1-year-old female English setter suspected of having pulmonic stenosis.

Paper speed = 50 mm./sec., 1 cm. = 1 mv.

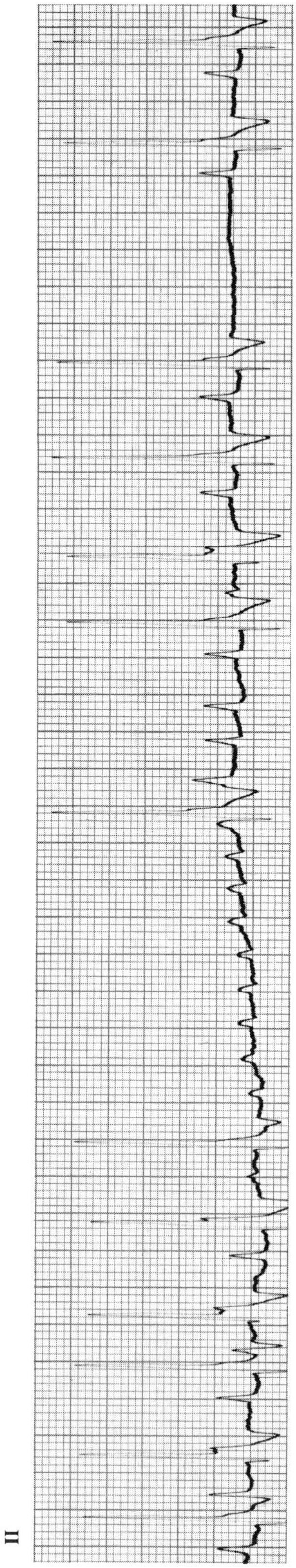

Figure 5–80.

II

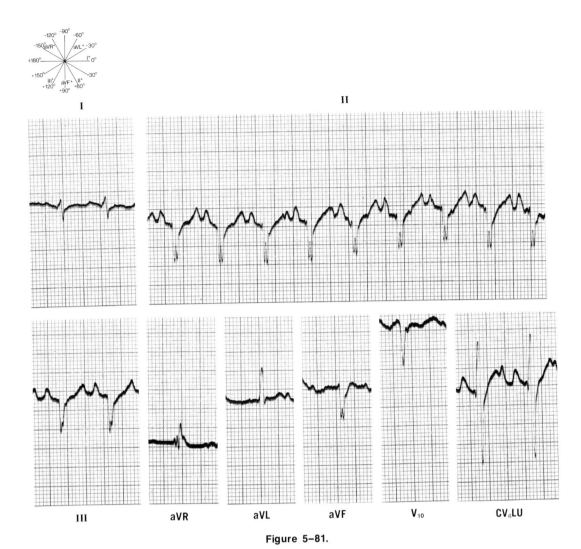

Figure 5–81.

Questions:

    a. Please read and interpret her electrocardiogram.

    b. Does the electrocardiogram support the clinical diagnosis?

Answers:

    a. Heart Rate = 250 beats per minute
       Heart rhythm: sinus tachycardia
       Mean electrical axis = $-90°$
       Measuring and multiplying:
         P wave = 0.04 second (2 boxes) by 0.3 mv. (3 boxes)
         P-R interval = 0.07 to 0.08 second (3½ to 4 boxes)
         QRS width = 0.05 second (2½ boxes)
         R wave height: no R wave

S-T segment and T wave: normal

Q-T interval = 0.16 second (8 boxes)

Miscellaneous criteria: S waves in leads I, II, and III, positive T wave in V_{10}, deep S wave in lead CV_6LU

Electrocardiographic diagnosis: sinus tachycardia and right ventricular hypertrophy

b. The electrocardiogram goes along well with the diagnosis of pulmonic stenosis. The thoracic radiographs also showed a markedly enlarged right ventricle and an enlarged main pulmonary artery segment. It is unusual to have an axis of $-90°$, but when it occurs, it is due to right ventricular hypertrophy. In this electrocardiogram, lead I is isoelectric, and lead aVF is the perpendicular lead on the axis chart. Lead aVF is negative, and aVF's negative pole is at $-90°$. The S_1, S_2, S_3 pattern, the positive T wave in V_{10}, and the deep S in CV_6LU all lend support to the diagnosis of right ventricular hypertrophy (refer to Figures 3–24, 3–26, and 3–27). The dog showed no clinical signs, and the sinus tachycardia was thought to be due to nervousness.

82. In this tracing every third beat is a ventricular premature beat.

Paper speed = 50 mm./sec., 1 cm. = 1 mv.

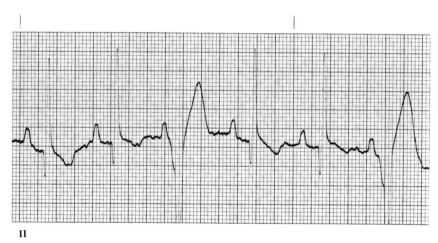

II

Figure 5–82.

Question:

What is the term used to describe this rhythm?

Answer:

Ventricular trigeminy (refer to Figure 4–29). If these were atrial premature beats it would be an atrial trigeminy (refer to Figure 5–36). It is also a trigeminy if there are two premature beats for every normal beat (refer to Figure 4–29).

83. Paper speed = 50 mm./sec., 1 cm. = 1 mv.

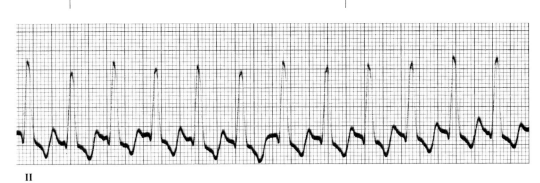

Figure 5-83.

Question:

Is this atrial tachycardia or sinus tachycardia?

Answer:

It may be impossible to differentiate between atrial and sinus tachycardia using only the electrocardiogram. In this tracing, the heart rate is about 250 beats per minute, and at this rate the P waves are hidden in the T waves of the preceding beats. The R-R intervals vary from 0.22 to 0.24 second (11 to 12 boxes). This suggests that there is some sinus arrhythmia present, which would favor a diagnosis of sinus tachycardia (refer to Table 4-4 and Figures 4-11, 4-18, and 4-19). In this case, the electrocardiogram was taken after atropine and acepromazine were given to a 4-year-old Great Dane. Since the dog did not have this arrhythmia before the drugs were given, this is probably a sinus tachycardia in response to the atropine.

84. Paper speed for A = 50 mm./sec., 1 cm. = 1 mv.

Paper speed for B = 50 mm./sec., 1 cm. = 1/2 mv.

Questions:

a. What two conditions can make the R waves so tall and the Q waves so deep that the complex becomes too large for the paper? The bottom strip was run at one-half sensitivity to get the entire tracing on the paper.

b. This is the electrocardiogram of a 10-year-old male coonhound. Which of the two conditions does he probably have?

Answers:

a. Patent ductus arteriosus and severe mitral insufficiency are two conditions that can cause this (refer to Figure 5-35).

II

A

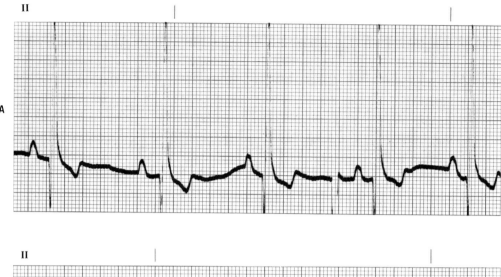

II

B

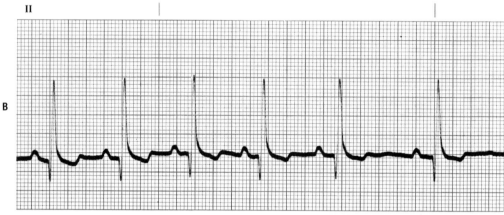

Figure 5-84.

b. This was an older dog; he had severe mitral and tricuspid insufficiency.

85. Paper speed = 50 mm./sec., 1 cm. = 1 mv.

Question:

What is the mean electrical axis in this tracing?

Answer:

It cannot be determined, because all of the leads are isoelectric. This is termed an electrically vertical heart (refer to Figure 3-13).

86. This electrocardiogram was recorded from a 5-year-old male Shetland sheepdog that had severe dyspnea due to a chylothorax.

Paper speed 50 mm./sec., 1 cm. = 1 mv.

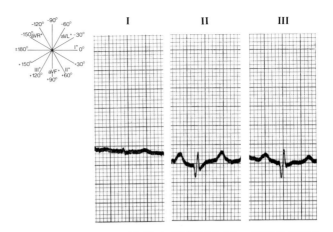

Figure 5–85.

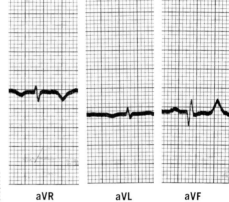

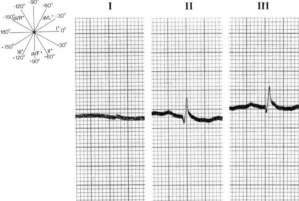

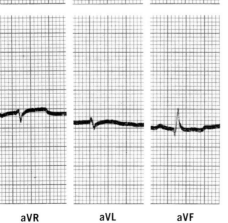

Figure 5–86.

Question:

What does the electrocardiogram show in this case?

Answer:

When there is a greater amount of tissue or fluid surrounding the heart, the electrocardiographic complexes are not conducted to the surface as well, and so they become attenuated or dampened. This may happen with pleural or pericardial effusion, or with thoracic masses such as neoplasms or diaphragmatic hernias. The small amplitude complexes indicate that the chest should at least be carefully examined and x-rayed if necessary.

87. This electrocardiogram was recorded from a 4-year-old borzoi.

Paper speed = 50 mm./sec., 1 cm. = 1 mv.

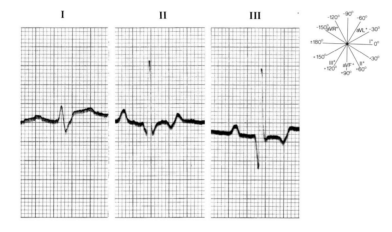

Figure 5–87.

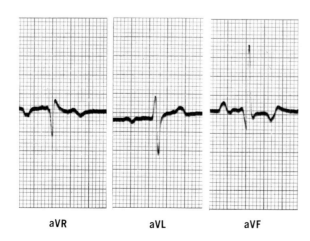

Questions:

 a. What is the mean electrical axis?

 b. Are there any signs to indicate cardiac hypertrophy?

Answers:

 a. The axis is +90°. Lead I is isoelectric. Lead aVF is perpendicular to lead I on the axis chart, and aVF is positive in this tracing. Lead aVF's positive pole is at +90°.

 b. There is an S wave present in leads I, II, and III, indicating right ventricular hypertrophy (refer to Figure 3–24). A test for heartworm and a chest x-ray would be indicated.

88. Tracings A, B, C, D, and E were recorded from a dog that had been hit by a car. He had hemothorax and pulmonary hemorrhage as well as hemoperitoneum, and was in severe respiratory distress.

 Paper speed = 50 mm./sec., 1 cm. = 1 mv.

Question:

 What is happening in each tracing?

Answer:

 In tracing A, the heart rate is 63 to 75 beats per minute, the T waves are large, and the Q-T interval is greatly prolonged, to 0.38 second (19 boxes). This probably indicates myocardial hypoxia. In tracing B, the hypoxia is worsening. The S-T segment is depressed now, and the T waves are even larger. In tracing C, the heart rate is very slow, the T waves are huge, and the P waves are depressed as atrial standstill is beginning to occur. In tracing D, an idioventricular rhythm is seen as bizarre QRS complexes occur at their own slow rate, and the lack of P waves indicates atrial standstill. In tracing E, one more bizarre ventricular beat occurs, and then cardiac standstill occurs (refer to Figures 3–22, 3–32, and 4–48).

89. These are continuous lead II recordings taken from a Great Dane that had acute hemolytic anemia and marked thrombocytopenia.

 Paper speed = 50 mm./sec., 1 cm. = 1 mv.

Questions:

 a. What arrhythmia is present?

 b. Should we worry?

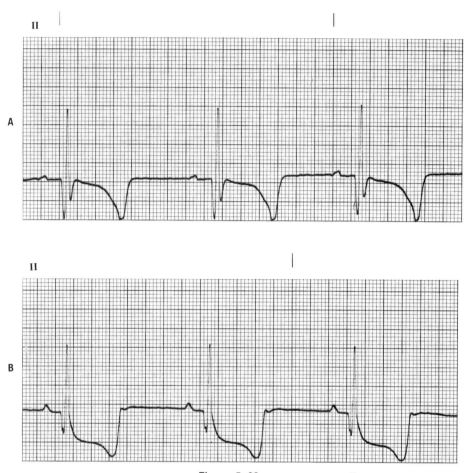

Figure 5–88.
Illustration continued on opposite page.

Answers:

a. Ventricular tachycardia is present. In the top tracing, all of the beats are bizarre, and are not associated with P waves. In the bottom tracing, the first beat is a normal capture beat, then four more bizarre ventricular beats occur before another capture beat occurs. The last complex on the lower tracing is a fusion beat, in which there is a P wave, a normal P-R interval, and then a QRS complex that is halfway between the normal QRS complexes and the bizarre ventricular ectopic complexes. Capture and fusion beats are diagnostic of ventricular tachycardia. This is the same Great Dane as in Figures 4–33, 4–34, and 4–35 (q.v.).

b. We should be very worried. The dog could die at any moment. In the top tracing, one ventricular beat occurs almost on top of the previous one (fifth and sixth beats from left). This is extremely dangerous when it occurs; the dog could have fibrillated at that point. In this instance, 2 per cent lidocaine without epinephrine would be indicated, stat.

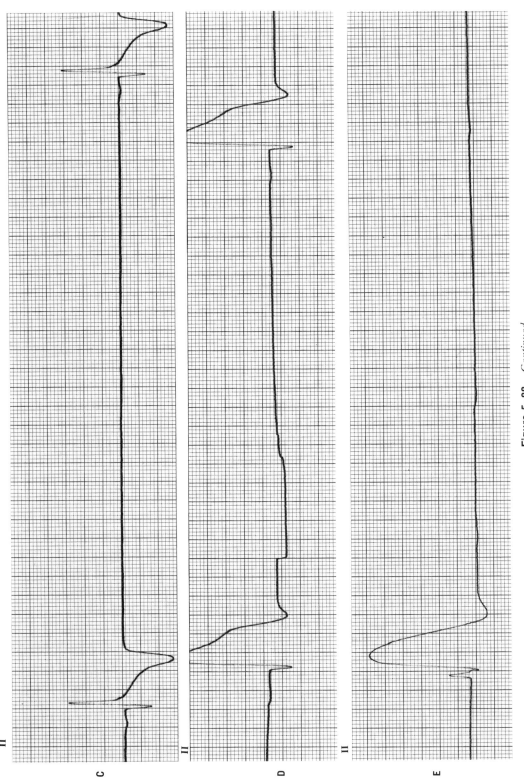

Figure 5–88. *Continued.*

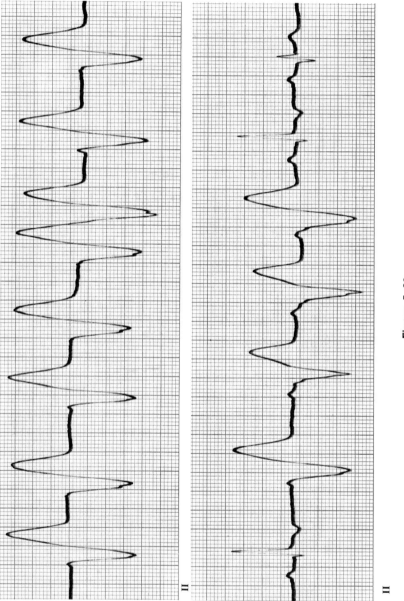

Figure 5–89.

II

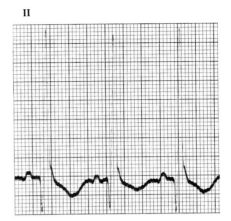

Figure 5-90.

90. This is a lead II electrocardiogram recorded from a 2-year-old English pointer.

Paper speed = 50 mm./sec., 1 cm. = 1 mv.

Question:

Is there any evidence of cardiac hypertrophy?

Answer:

The R waves average 3.8 mv. (38 boxes) in height, and the Q waves are about 0.9 mv. (9 boxes) deep. In any other dog, one might think about biventricular hypertrophy. In the pointer, however, one should withhold this diagnosis until seeing thoracic radiographs of the dog. The pointer is one breed that seems to be able to break the rules. Occasionally, a normal pointer will have tall R waves and deep Q waves. If there is any question, thoracic radiography should be done. This pointer's thoracic radiographs were normal.

91. This lead II electrocardiogram was recorded from a diabetic, ketoacidotic dog that was comatose.

Paper speed = 50 mm./sec., 1 cm. = 1 mv.

II

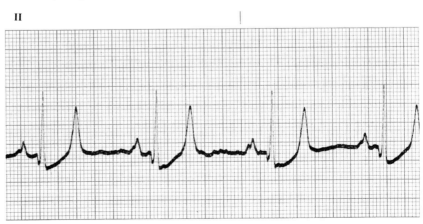

Figure 5-91.

Question:

Is there any evidence for electrolyte imbalance?

Answer:

The tall T waves suggest that the animal may be hyperkalemic. The heart rate is still normal, and the P waves are not depressed yet, so one might expect a mild elevation of serum K^+ to 6.0 to 6.5 meq./l. (refer to Figure 3–32). The Q-T interval is prolonged to 0.26 second (13 boxes). This may be seen with either hypokalemia, hyperkalemia, or hypocalcemia (refer to Figures 3–32, 3–34, and 3–35). There is S-T segment depression, which might suggest myocardial hypoxia and acidosis, or might indicate myocarditis (refer to Figure 3–22). The serum K^+ at the time of this tracing was 2.8 meq./l. Usually, with hypokalemia, the T waves are smaller and may be biphasic (refer to Figures 3–34 and 5–111).

It is interesting to note that the electrocardiogram does not always correlate with the serum K^+. The electrocardiogram is a better representative of the cellular metabolism changes, and it tends to make one wonder about the validity of measuring serum electrolytes.

92. This lead II electrocardiogram was recorded from the same Great Dane as in Figure 5–89.

Paper speed = 50 mm./sec., 1 cm. = 1 mv.

Question:

There are three abnormal beats here. Can you find them?

Answer:

Two of them are obvious. They are ventricular premature beats. They occur early, are bizarre in form, and are not associated with P waves. They are single, unifocal, ventricular premature beats (refer to Figure 4–25). The third abnormal beat is the fourth beat from the left. It has a normal P wave and a normal P-R interval, but the QRS complex is altered. The P wave occurred, traversed the atrioventricular node, and began to depolarize the ventricles. At the same time that the P wave initiated ventricular depolarization, the ectopic focus also fired and tried to discharge the ventricles. This is a fusion beat (refer to Figure 4–34).

93. This lead II electrocardiogram was recorded from a miniature poodle with a collapsed trachea of 2 years' duration and Grade 4 of 6 mitral insufficiency.

Paper speed = 50 mm./sec., 1 cm. = 1 mv.

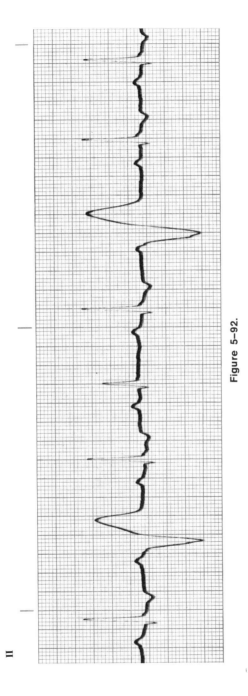

Figure 5–92.

II

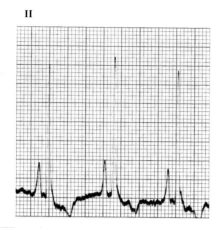

Figure 5-93.

Question:

What are the electrocardiographic abnormalities?

Answer:

Tall peaked P waves indicate right atrial hypertrophy (P pulmonale) (refer to Figures 3–15 and 3–17). Tall R waves and S-T segment depression are indicative of left ventricular hypertrophy (refer to Figures 3–20 and 3–22).

If the only electrocardiographic abnormality seen is P pulmonale, a respiratory system disease should be suspected. This has been a frequent finding in dogs with collapsed trachea.

94. This lead II electrocardiogram was recorded from a 5-year-old Belgian shepherd female that had terminal renal insufficiency due to renal amyloidosis.

Paper speed = 50 mm./sec., 1 cm. = 1 mv.

II

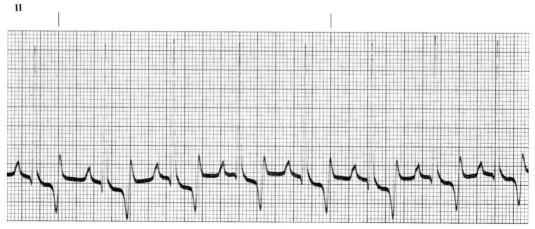

Figure 5-94.

Question:

Is there any evidence for hyperkalemia?

Answer:

The T waves are quite large, although the heart rate, the P waves, and the Q-T intervals are all normal. This could be compatible with a mild elevation of serum K^+ (refer to Figure 3-32).

95. Paper speed = 50 mm./sec., 1 cm. = 1 mv.

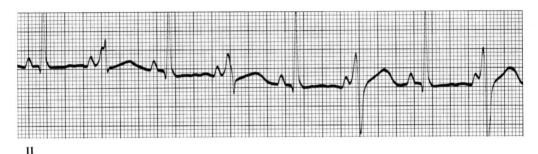

II

Figure 5-95.

Question:

What is the arrhythmia?

Answer:

This is a ventricular bigeminy of multifocal origin. Every other beat is a ventricular premature beat, and they vary in shape (refer to Figures 4-28 and 4-30). This is from the same dog as in Figure 5-75.

96. This electrocardiogram was recorded from an obese male mixed breed dog that was listless, anorexic, and profoundly weak. He had an irregular heart beat and a pulse deficit.

Paper speed = 50 mm./sec., 1 cm. = 1 mv.

Question:

a. What is the arrhythmia?

b. Could this cause weakness?

Answers:

a. This is another example of ventricular tachycardia. From the left a bizarre ventricular ectopic beat occurs, followed by a fusion beat,

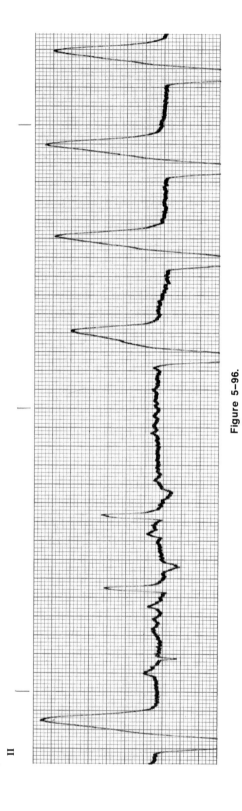

Figure 5–96.

two capture beats, and then the ventricular tachycardia resumes (refer to Figures 4–34 and 4–35).

b. This could definitely cause weakness because cardiac output decreases when the ventricular ectopic beats occur. He could also collapse or suffer a seizure, or both.

97. This lead II electrocardiogram was recorded from an old mixed breed dog with digitalis intoxication.

Paper speed = 50 mm./sec., 1 cm. = 1 mv.

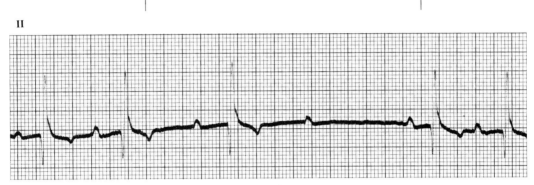

Figure 5–97.

Questions:

a. What arrhythmia is present?

b. The dog is on 0.25 mg. digoxin b.i.d. What would you do?

Answers:

a. Second degree heart block is present and the P-R interval becomes prolonged before the QRS complex is dropped. This is the Wenkebach phenomenon, or a Mobitz type I second degree heart block (refer to Figures 4–50 and 4–52).

b. The digitalis should be discontinued until the arrhythmia is abolished. It should then be resumed at 0.25 mg. in the morning and 0.125 mg. in the evening.

98. Tracings A and B were recorded from another dog with severe Coombs' positive hemolytic anemia.

Paper speed = 50 mm./sec., 1 cm. = 1 mv.

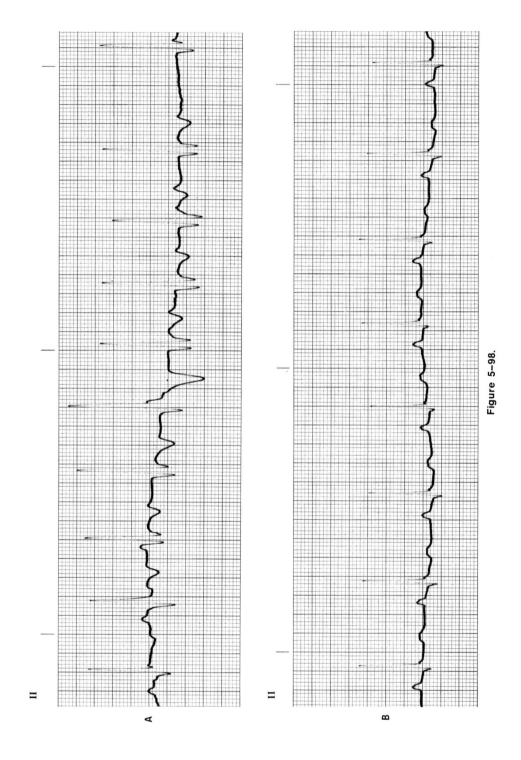

II

A

II

B

Figure 5–98.

Questions:

    a. What is the arrhythmia in tracing A?

    b. The dog was collapsed. What drug was used to produce tracing B?

Answers:

    a. Ventricular tachycardia is present. Two normal capture beats begin the tracing, and are followed by a series of beats in which the QRS complexes are altered and not associated with P waves (refer to Figure 4–33). One of the abnormal QRS complexes is different in appearance from the others, so there is a multifocal origin. The QRS complexes are not terribly bizarre, which indicates that they probably arose somewhere near the bundle of His (refer to Figure 4–31).

    b. Since the dog was collapsed, an intravenous drip of 2 mg./cc. lidocaine without epinephrine was prepared. This was given rapidly until conversion occurred, in strip B. The lidocaine was then used as needed and oral quinidine was begun, but the dog died. Both dogs observed by us that had hemolytic anemia and myocarditis subsequently died.

99. This electrocardiogram was recorded from an Old English sheepdog that was in for a diagnostic workup.

    Paper speed = 50 mm./sec., 1 cm. = 1 mv.

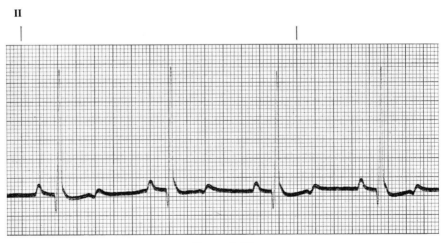

Figure 5–99.

Question:

    Is there any abnormality?

Answer:

The R waves average 3.2 mv. (32 boxes) in height. This is slightly over the limit, although thoracic radiographs did not reveal any left ventricular enlargement. The Q-T interval is 0.26 second (13 boxes), and the T waves are small and biphasic. This might occur with either hypokalemia or hypocalcemia. The dog had reticulosis. His serum K^+ was 4.5 meq./l. and serum calcium was not done.

100. These tracings represent continuous lead II recordings from a 2-year-old St. Bernard.

Paper speed = 50 mm./sec., 1 cm. = 1 mv.

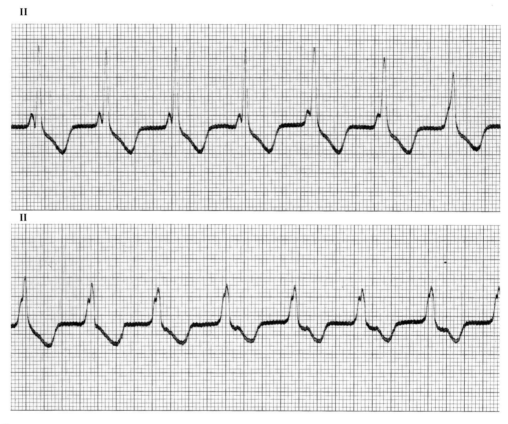

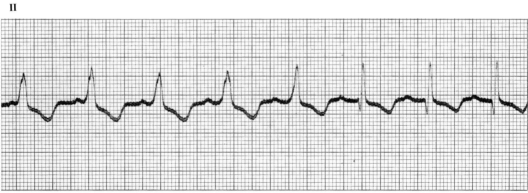

Figure 5–100.

Questions:

a. What arrhythmia is present?

b. What is the most common cause?

Answers:

a. Atrioventricular dissociation with accrochage is occurring. In the top tracing, the P waves can be seen to move into the QRS complexes. Toward the end of the middle tracing, the P waves actually appear behind the QRS complexes and make a bump in the S-T segment. In the last tracing, the P waves move out of the QRS complexes. The last three beats are capture beats. They all have the same P-R intervals, and notice that the QRS complexes are more normal (they have a Q wave and are not as wide as the others). When the P waves are not associated with the QRS complexes, and they move in and out and even behind, as in this tracing, it is atrioventricular dissociation with accrochage (refer to Figure 4–38). The three capture beats establish that this is a form of ventricular tachycardia.

b. Digitalis intoxication is the most common cause of atrioventricular dissociation.

101. This is a continuous lead II electrocardiogram recorded from a 10-year-old female beagle with mitral and tricuspid insufficiency and congestive heart failure. Premature beats were detected on auscultation. She is not on any medication.

Paper speed = 50 mm./sec., 1 cm. = 1 mv.

Questions:

a. What type of premature beats would you expect this particular dog to have?

b. What type does she have on this electrocardiogram (arrows)?

Answers:

a. Since she has atrioventricular valvular insufficiencies, it might be expected that she would have atrial enlargement and stretching. This could irritate the atria and cause atrial or junctional premature beats to occur.

b. In the top tracing, three junctional (nodal) premature beats occur. These beats are followed by a pause, and their P waves are negative (refer to Figure 4–14). In the lower tracing several premature beats occur, and they are supraventricular in origin, because their QRS complexes remain normal. Since their P waves are hidden in the T waves of the preceding beats, it cannot be determined whether they are junctional or atrial. It is most important, however, to recognize that they

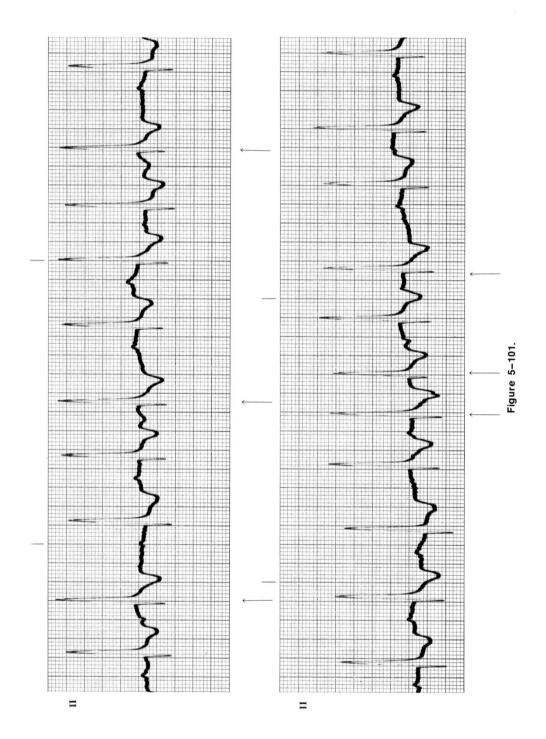

Figure 5–101.

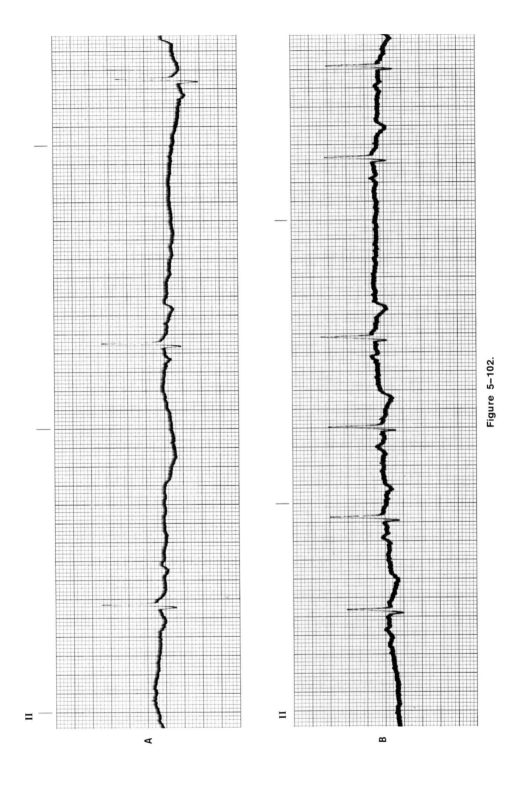

Figure 5–102.

are supraventricular in origin. They indicate that the dog should be placed on digitalis therapy.

102. Paper speed = 50 mm./sec., 1 cm. = 1 mv.

Questions:

    a. What is the rhythm in strip A?

    b. What drug was given to produce strip B?

Answers:

    a. This is a junctional escape rhythm. The P waves are negative, which indicates that the beats originate in the area of the atrioventricular node (junctional area), and the heart rate is about 42 beats per minute (refer to Figure 4–46).

    b. Atropine was given to determine whether this was a vagally-induced arrhythmia. The arrhythmia is much improved, but sinus arrhythmia and wandering pacemaker are still present (refer to Figures 4–5, 4–9, and 4–10).

103. This is a lead II electrocardiogram recorded from the same collie as in Figure 4–11. The dog had sinus tachycardia due to a high fever. This was from a later part of the same tracing as in Figure 4–11.

    Paper speed = 50 mm./sec., ½ cm. = 1 mv.

Question:

    What happens in this tracing?

Answer:

    An episode of second degree heart block suddenly occurs, which is unusual. Two P waves occur without a QRS complex, and the third P wave is delayed but finally provokes a QRS complex. Another P wave can be seen to occur, causing a bump in the downstroke of the T wave, then another PQRS complex occurs and the heart rate gradually increases again. This is an unusual case of sinus tachycardia with block (refer also to Figures 5–56 and 5–80).

104. This electrocardiogram was recorded from a German shepherd with pleural effusion, pericardial effusion, and ascites.

    Paper speed = 50 mm./sec., 1 cm. = 1 mv.

Question:

    What abnormality is present?

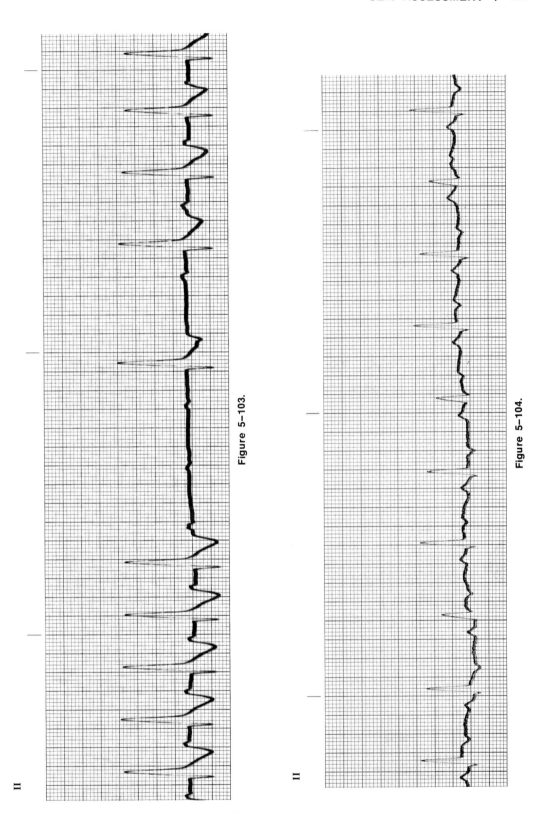

Figure 5–103.

Figure 5–104.

Answer:

This electrocardiogram demonstrates electrical alternation of the heart (electrical alternans). The height of the QRS complex varies in the presence of normal sinus rhythm. In man, this usually indicates the presence of myocardial disease and often suggests a poor prognosis (Bellet, 1972). It has been associated with coronary artery disease, aortic insufficiency, aortic stenosis, hypertension, myocarditis, congestive heart failure, and digitalis intoxication, and is frequently seen with pericardial disease in man (Bellet, 1972; Friedberg, 1966). Although the exact mechanism is not known, it has been suggested that various portions of the heart possess a lower excitability than other portions when this condition occurs. As a result, fewer fibers respond in some ventricular beats, while they may all respond to another beat, which changes the millivoltage of the complex (Bellet, 1972). Another theory (among other theories that have been proposed) suggests that transient partial bundle branch block occurs (Bellet, 1972).

105. These lead II electrocardiograms were recorded from a 17-year-old German shepherd suspected of having ruptured chordae tendineae.

Paper speed = 50 mm./sec., 1 cm. = 1 mv.

Questions:

a. What arrhythmia is present in tracing A?

b. What arrhythmia is present in tracings B and C?

c. What treatment should be given?

Answers:

a. Atrial flutter is present. The ventricles respond in a regular manner to every third or fourth P wave. The P waves are of bizarre configuration (refer to Figure 4–22).

b. In tracings B and C, the rhythm varies from flutter to fibrillation, and back again. The ventricles now are responding in an irregular manner. This is termed a fibrillo-flutter rhythm.

c. The dog died of acute congestive heart failure, but the treatment of choice would have been digitalis. If the heart failure could have been controlled with digitalis, quinidine could then have been added in an attempt to restore sinus rhythm (Robertson, 1970).

106. Paper speed = 25 mm./sec., 1 cm. = 1 mv.

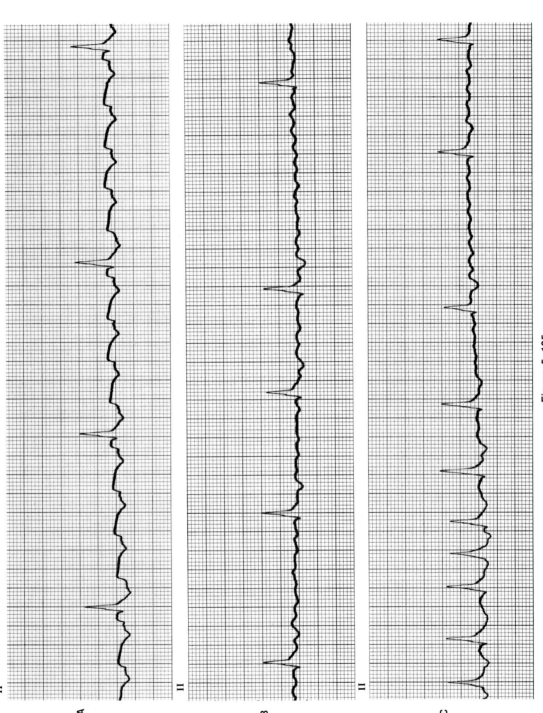

II

A

II

B

II

C

Figure 5–105.

II

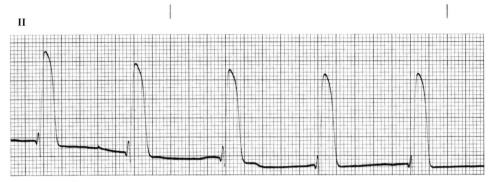

Figure 5–106.

Questions:

a. What is this arrhythmia?

b. What is its significance?

Answers:

a. This is an idioventricular rhythm, also known as a ventricular escape rhythm. No P waves occur because atrial standstill is present. Since the ventricles do not receive impulse stimulation from above, they beat at their own rate. They are beating at 60 beats per minute in this instance, which is slightly more rapid than usual (refer to Figures 2–5 and 4–48).

b. This is a preterminal rhythm. This could be due to hyperkalemia, or may be seen as a terminal rhythm in a dying dog, as in this case. This dog had already undergone cardiac arrest once.

107. These continuous lead II electrocardiograms were recorded from an old dog with a prostatic abscess. At the middle of the first tracing a burst of tachycardia occurs, which terminates toward the middle of the bottom tracing.

Paper speed = 50 mm./sec., 1 cm. = 1 mv.

Question:

What type of tachycardia is this?

Answer:

This is paroxysmal sinus tachycardia. The P waves during the burst of tachycardia are identical to those when the heart rate is normal, which indicates that this is a sinus tachycardia (refer to Table 4–4 and Figures 4–11 and 4–18). It is unusual for sinus tachycardia to occur in paroxysms; it is usually continuous.

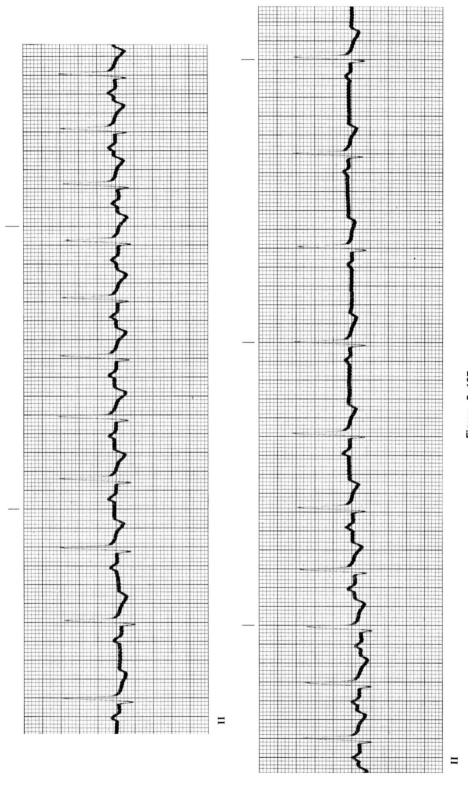

II

II

Figure 5–107.

The heart rate at the end of the lower tracing is 120 beats per minute, and during the tachycardia the heart rate is 200 beats per minute. The R-R intervals also vary slightly during the tachycardia, which favors the diagnosis of sinus tachycardia.

108. These are two different examples of ventricular fibrillation.

Paper speed = 50 mm./sec., 1 cm. = 1 mv.

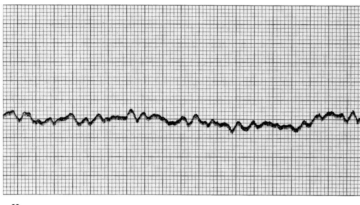

II

Figure 5–108.

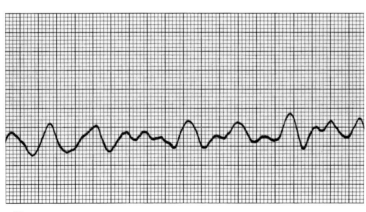

II

Question:

If you had a choice, which one would you rather treat, on the basis of these electrocardiograms?

Answer:

If one had a choice, it would be better to treat the dog in the lower tracing. This dog has coarse ventricular fibrillation, as opposed to fine fibrillation in the dog in the top tracing (refer to Figure 4–43). Coarse fibrillation is more likely to convert to sinus rhythm with D.C. shock than is fine fibrillation. Epinephrine could be used in the top tracing to attempt to produce more coarse fibrillations.

109. The top lead II tracing was recorded the morning before this 4-month-old miniature poodle underwent surgical correction of a patent ductus arteriosus. That evening, approximately 9 hours after surgery, the dog suffered acute left-sided congestive heart failure. The bottom electrocardiogram was taken at that time. The dog was severely dyspneic and was cyanotic due to pulmonary edema. She responded to treatment with diuretics, digoxin, aminophylline, morphine and oxygen. She made a complete recovery and was taken off all medication 3 weeks later.

Paper speed = 50 mm./sec., 1 cm. = 1 mv.

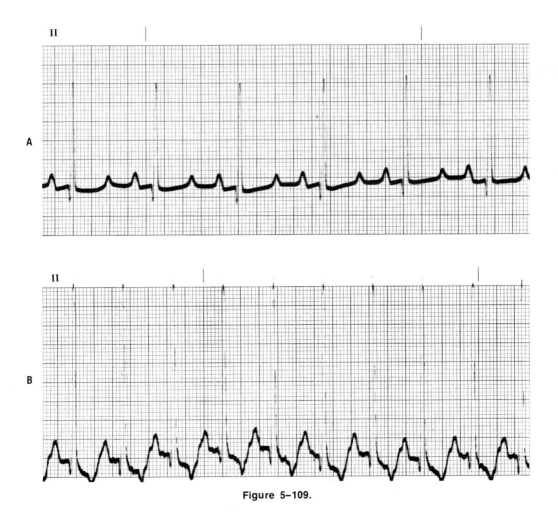

Figure 5–109.

Questions:

    a. What is the electrocardiographic diagnosis in tracing A?

    b. What has happened in tracing B?

Answers:

    a. A "T_a" (T sub a) wave indicates right atrial hypertrophy (refer to Figure 3–18). The R waves are 2.7 mv. (27 boxes) tall. This is slightly taller than normal for this breed of dog and suggests left ventricular hypertrophy (refer to Figure 3–20). The Q-T interval is slightly prolonged to 0.24 second (12 boxes).

    b. In tracing B, when the dog is in acute failure, sinus tachycardia is occurring at a heart rate of 215 beats per minute. Now the R waves are greater than 4.5 mv. (45 boxes) tall, and the S-T segment is depressed. The P waves are now 0.6 mv. (6 boxes) tall, and 0.05 mv. (2½ boxes) wide. It appears that the hemodynamic changes that occurred after closure of the ductus have caused dilatation of both atria and of the left ventricle (refer to Figures 3–18, 3–20, and 3–22). These changes would have to be a result of dilatation, since it is too soon for hypertrophy to occur. The S-T segment changes could accompany the left ventricular dilatation, or might be due to the hypoxia and cyanosis (refer to Figure 3–22).

110. This lead II electrocardiogram was recorded from an old dog with severe azotemia due to end stage kidney disease. A premature beat occurs on this tracing.

    Paper speed = 50 mm./sec., 1 cm. = 1 mv.

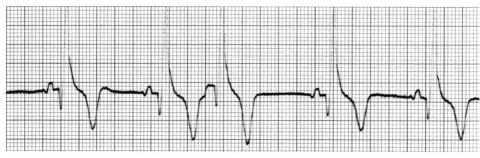

II   **Figure 5–110.**

Questions:

    a. What type of premature beat is this?

    b. What is its probable cause?

    c. Are there any other electrocardiographic changes that might indicate the severity of the renal condition?

Answers:

    a. This is a supraventricular premature beat. It occurs early and is followed by a pause, the QRS complex remains normal, and the P wave is obscured by the T wave of the preceding beat (refer to Figures 4–13, 4–14, and 4–15).

b. It probably represents atrial myocarditis secondary to the azotemia.

c. The T waves are becoming large, although the heart rate is still normal, and the P waves are still visible. The serum K^+ may be mildly elevated (refer to Figure 3–32). Also notice that the QRS complex is very wide (0.10 second or 5 boxes). This is difficult to interpret. Ordinarily, this would indicate left bundle branch block (refer to Figure 4–58). Notice, however, that on the downstroke of the R waves there is a definite notch. This may be the "J point," which signifies the end of depolarization and the beginning of repolarization. If that is true, then most of the QRS width is due to a delay in early repolarization (S-T segment), and this may indicate a ventricular myocarditis or an electrolyte imbalance. This part of the tracing is difficult to interpret.

111. These lead II electrocardiograms were recorded from a 6-year-old male Siberian husky. He was profoundly weak and had difficulty rising.

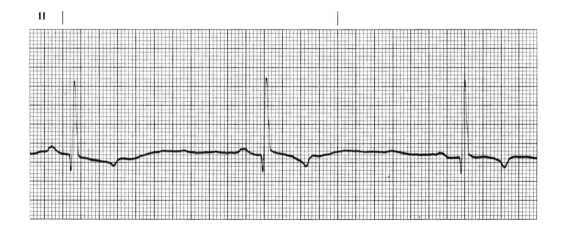

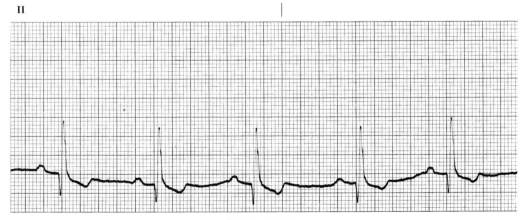

Figure 5–111.

There were no other clinical signs. The top tracing was recorded at the time of admission. The bottom tracing was recorded after 24 hours of treatment.

Paper speed = 50 mm./sec., 1 cm. = 1 mv.

Questions:

  a. What abnormalities are present in the top tracing?

  b. What treatment was given to produce the bottom tracing?

Answers:

  a. The heart rate is about 55 beats per minute, and the Q-T interval is prolonged to 0.28 second (14 boxes). The P waves seem flat and slightly wide (0.06 second or 3 boxes). The slow heart rate and prolonged Q-T interval suggest that hypokalemia or hyperkalemia is present (refer to Figures 3–32 and 3–34). Hyperkalemia does not consistently prolong the Q-T interval. Hypocalcemia can also prolong the Q-T interval, but does not tend to cause such bradycardia. The serum K^+ was 2.6 meq./l. at the time of this recording, and calcium was 10.0 mg. per cent (normal).

  b. Over a 24-hour period the dog was given 40 meq. of K^+ in an intravenous drip. The electrocardiogram has returned to normal now and the serum K^+ is 4.0 meq./l. The dog was normal and had good strength at this time. This was a case of idiopathic hypokalemia, as was that of the St. Bernard in Figure 3–34. Neither of these dogs suffered a reoccurrence of the condition.

112. Paper speed = 50 mm./sec., 1 cm. = 1 mv.

Questions:

  a. What is the mean electrical axis?

  b. Are there any other signs of cardiac enlargement?

Answers:

  a. The axis is +100°. Lead I is closest to being isoelectric, and lead aVF is perpendicular to lead I on the axis chart. Lead aVF is positive in this tracing, and lead aVF's positive pole is at +90°. Since lead I is not perfectly isoelectric, the axis is not exactly +90°. Lead I is a little more negative than positive, so the axis is shifted from +90° a little toward lead I's negative pole, and is interpolated to +100°. This was recorded from a large dog, so +100° is still within normal limits.

  b. There are no other indications of cardiac enlargement.

113. Paper speed = 50 mm./sec., 1 cm. = 1 mv.

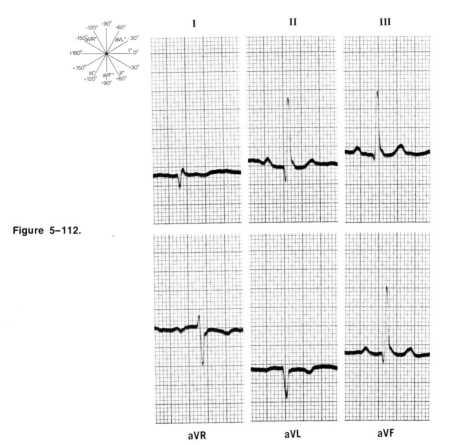

Figure 5–112.

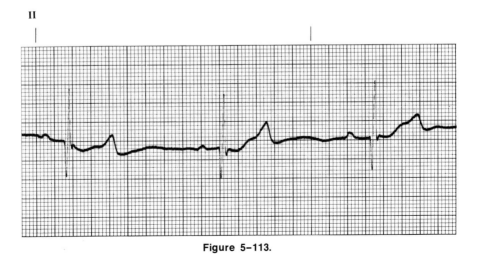

Figure 5–113.

Question:

What abnormality is present on this electrocardiogram?

Answer:

The Q-T interval is prolonged to 0.30 second (15 boxes). This indicates that the serum K^+ and Ca^{++} should be checked. This dog's serum K^+ was 4.7 meq./l. (normal), but his serum calcium level was low (8.0 mg. per cent).

REFERENCES

Bellet, S.: Essentials of Cardiac Arrhythmias: Diagnosis and Management. W. B. Saunders Co., Philadelphia, 1972.

Bolton, G. R., and Ettinger, S.: Paroxysmal Atrial Fibrillation in the Dog. J.A.V.M.A. 158 (1971):64.

Bolton, G. R., and Ettinger, S. J.: Right Bundle Branch Block in the Dog. J.A.V.M.A. 160 (1972):1104.

Ettinger, S. J. and Suter, P. F.: Canine Cardiology. W. B. Saunders Co., Philadelphia, 1970.

Flickenger, G. L., and Patterson, D. F.: Coronary Lesions Associated with Congenital Subaortic Stenosis in the Dog. J. Path. Bact., 93 (1967):133.

Friedberg, C. K.: Diseases of the Heart. 3rd ed. W. B. Saunders Co., Philadelphia, 1966.

Hamlin, R. L., Smetzer, D. L., and Breznock, E. M.: Sinoatrial Syncope in Miniature Schnauzers. J.A.V.M.A., 161 (1972):1022.

Kleine, L. J., Zook, B. C., and Munson, T. O.: Primary Cardiac Hemangiosarcomas in Dogs. J.A.V.M.A., 157 (1970):326.

Patterson, D. F., Detweiler, D. K., Hubben, K., and Botts, R. P.: Spontaneous Abnormal Cardiac Arrhythmias and Conduction Disturbances in the Dog. A Clinical and Pathologic Study of 3,000 Dogs. Am. J. Vet. Res., 22 (1961):355.

Robertson, B. T.: Correction of Atrial Flutter With Quinidine and Digitalis. J. Small Anim. Pract., 11 (1970):251

APPENDIX OF TYPICAL CANINE ELECTROCARDIOGRAMS

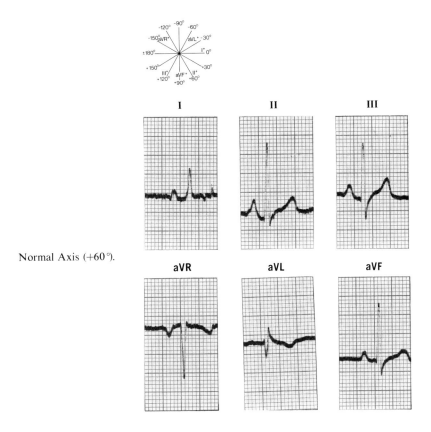

Normal Axis (+60°).

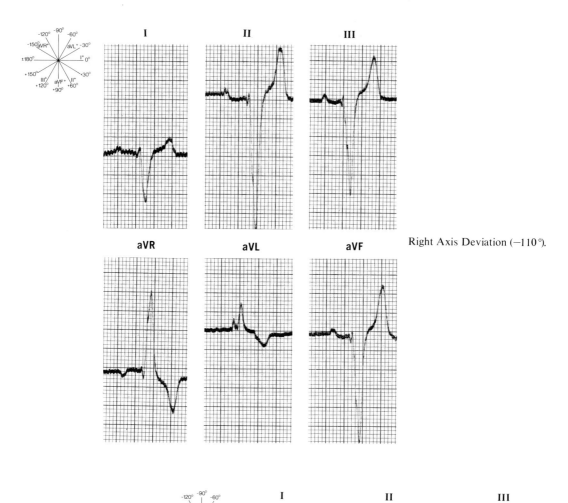

Right Axis Deviation (−110°).

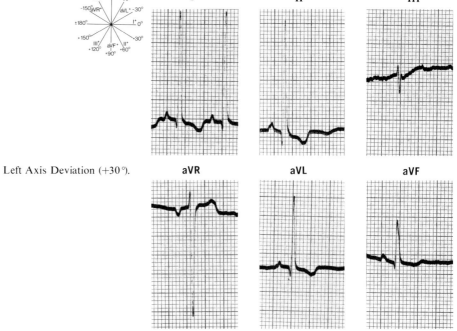

Left Axis Deviation (+30°).

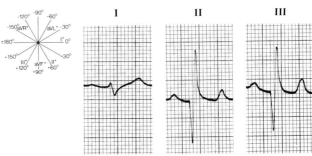

Electrically Vertical Heart (All Leads Isoelectric; Axis Indeterminate).

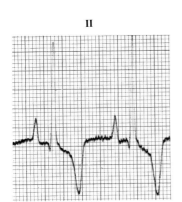

Right Atrial Hypertrophy (P pulmonale).

Left Atrial Hypertrophy (P mitrale).

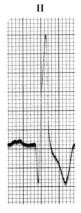

II

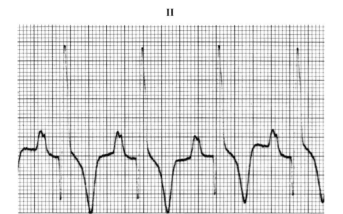

Biatrial Hypertrophy.

Left Ventricular Hypertrophy (Tall R Waves).

II

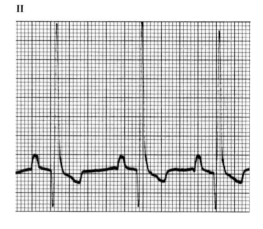

II

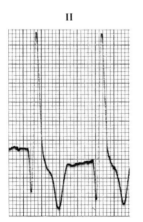

II

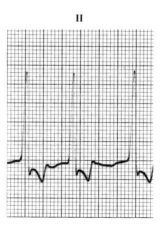

Left Ventricular Hypertrophy (Wide QRS Waves and S-T Slurring).

S-T Segment Depression.

II

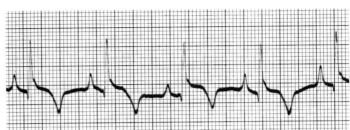

S-T Segment Elevation.

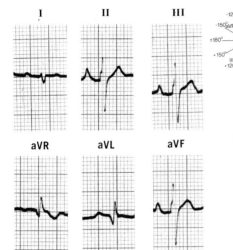

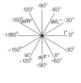

Right Ventricular Hypertrophy (S₁, S₂, S₃ Pattern).

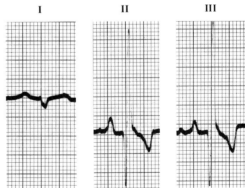

Right Ventricular Hypertrophy (Deep Q Waves in II, III, and aVF.).

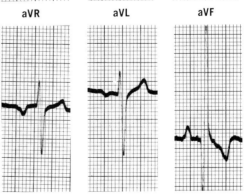

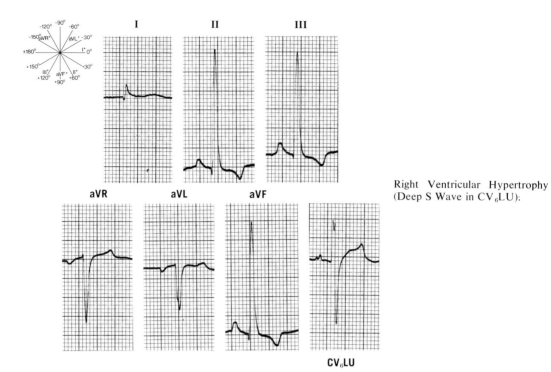

Right Ventricular Hypertrophy (Deep S Wave in CV$_6$LU):

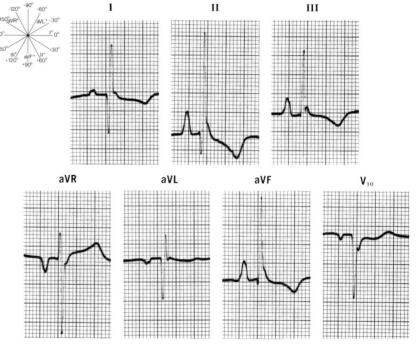

Right Ventricular Hypertrophy (Positive T Wave in V$_{10}$).

II

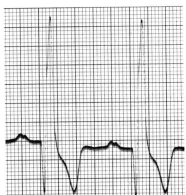

Biventricular Hypertrophy (tall R Wave, Wide QRS Wave, Deep Q Wave, and S-T Slurring).

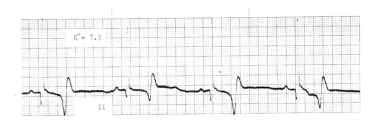

Hyperkalemia (Bradycardia, Large T Waves, and Q-T Interval Prolongation).

II

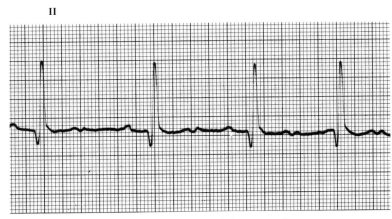

Hypokalemia (Prolonged Q-T Interval).

II

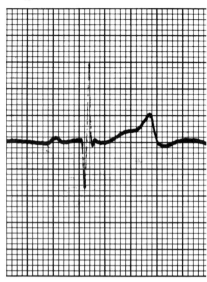

Hypocalcemia (Prolonged Q-T Interval).

II

Hypercalcemia (S-T Segment Elevation).

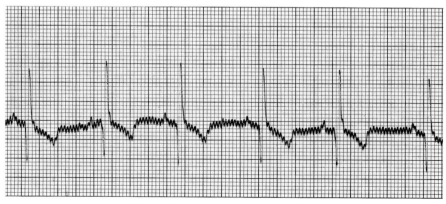

60-Cycle Electrical Interference Artifact.

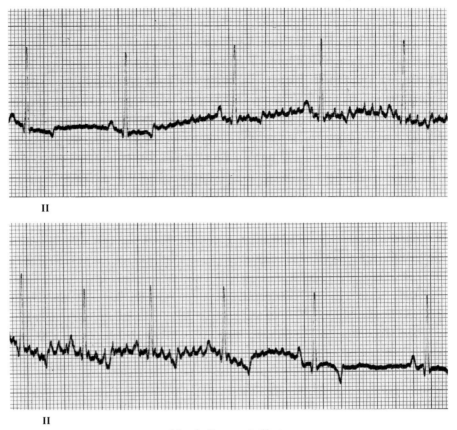

II

II

Muscle Tremor Artifact.

II

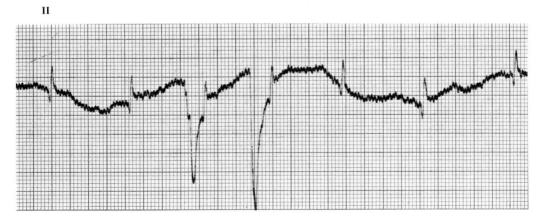

Muscle Twitch Artifact.

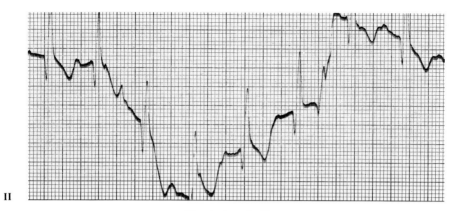

II

Respiratory Artifact.

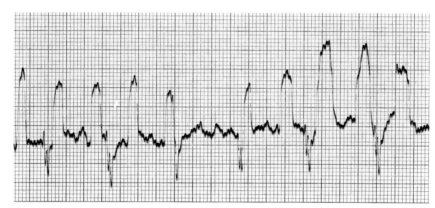

II

Panting Artifact.

II

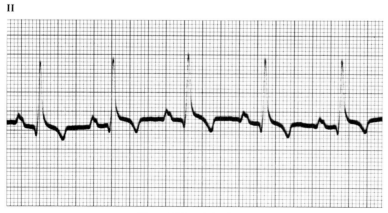

Normal Sinus Rhythm.

II

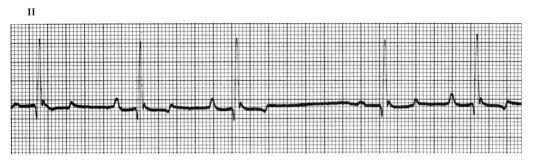

Sinus Arrhythmia and Wandering Pacemaker.

II

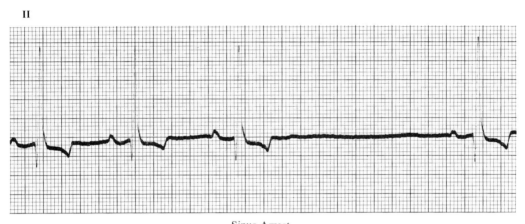

Sinus Arrest.

II   T = 105.0

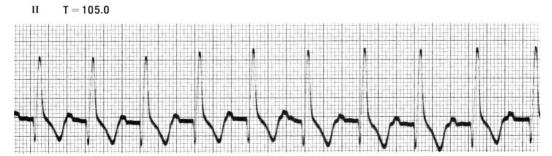

Sinus Tachycardia.

Sinus Tachycardia with Block.

Sinus Bradycardia.

II

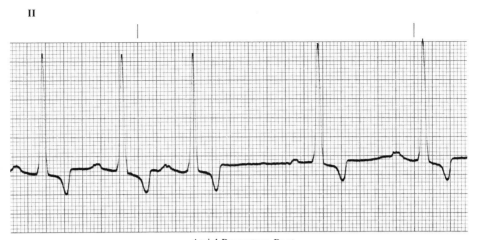

Atrial Premature Beat.

II

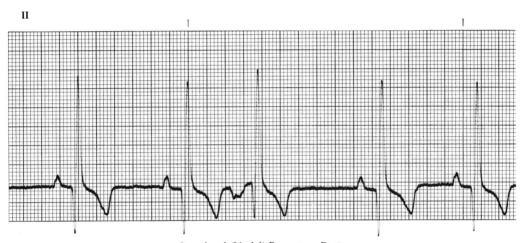

Junctional (Nodal) Premature Beat.

II

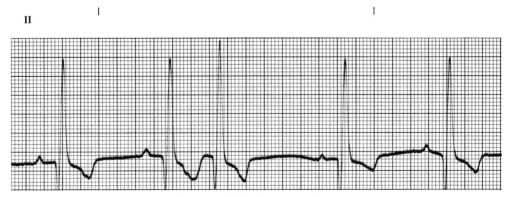

Supraventricular Premature Beat.

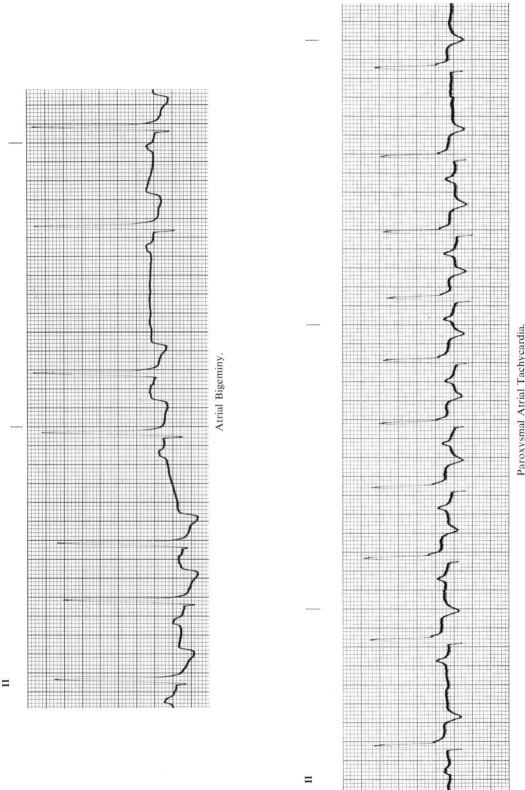

Atrial Bigeminy.

Paroxysmal Atrial Tachycardia.

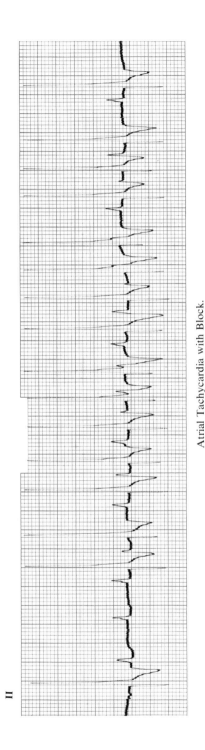

Atrial Tachycardia with Block.

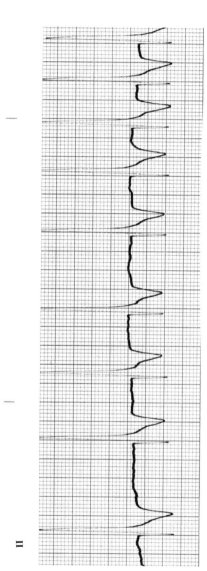

Atrial Fibrillation.

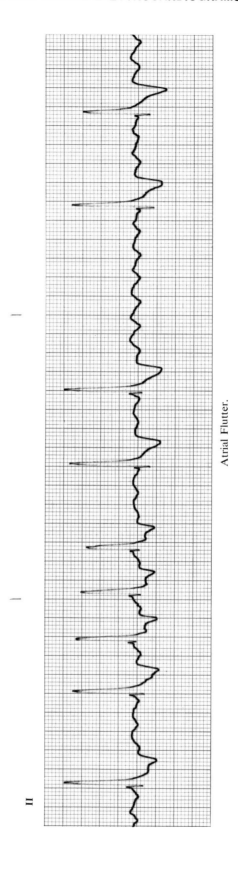

Atrial Flutter.

II

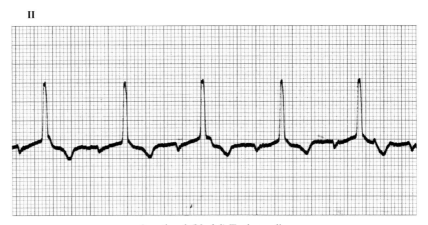

Junctional (Nodal) Tachycardia.

II

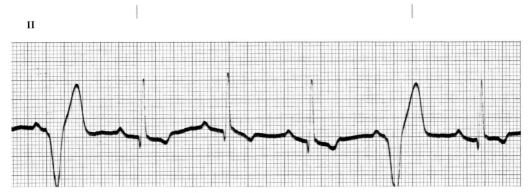

Unifocal Ventricular Premature Beats.

II

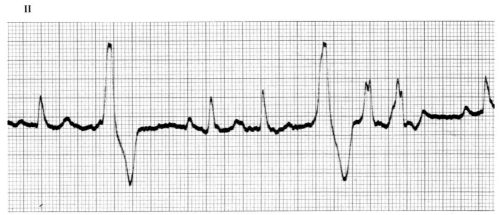

Multifocal Ventricular Premature Beats.

II

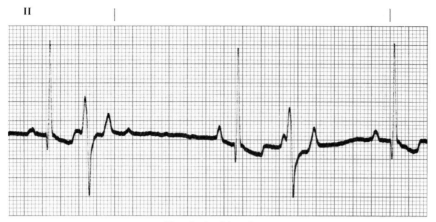

Ventricular Bigeminy.

II

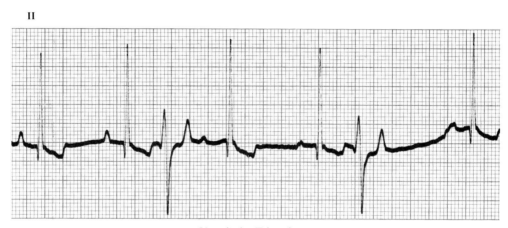

Ventricular Trigeminy.

II

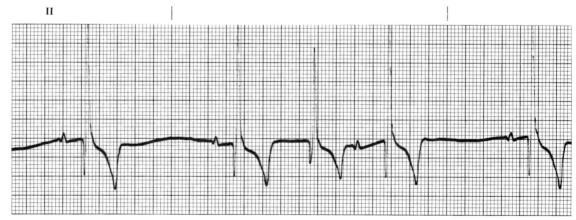

Interpolated Ventricular Premature Beat.

II

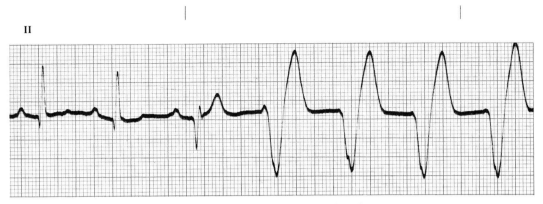

Ventricular Tachycardia with Capture and Fusion Beats.

II

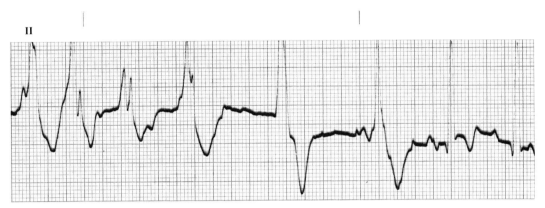

Multifocal Ventricular Tachycardia.

II

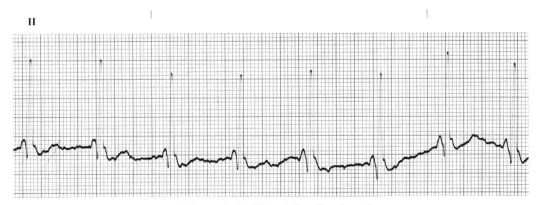

Atrioventricular Dissociation (Synchrony).

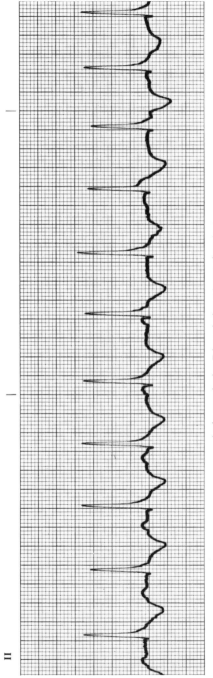

Atrioventricular Dissociation (Accrochage).

II

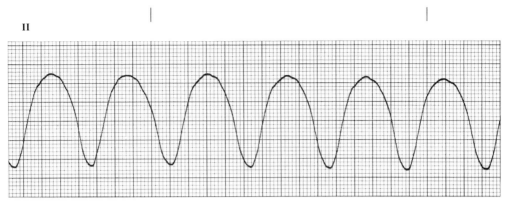

Ventricular Flutter.

II

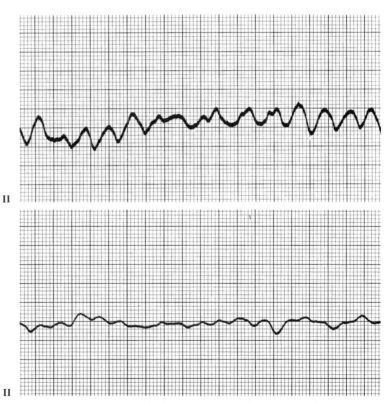

II

Coarse *(top)* and Fine *(bottom)* Ventricular Fibrillation.

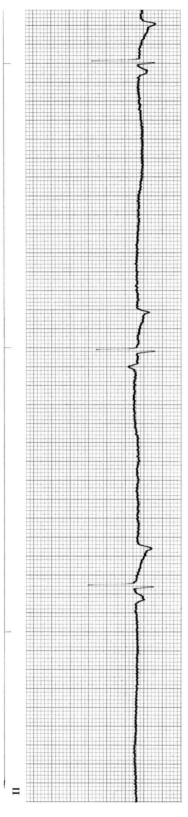

Junctional (Nodal) Escape Beats.

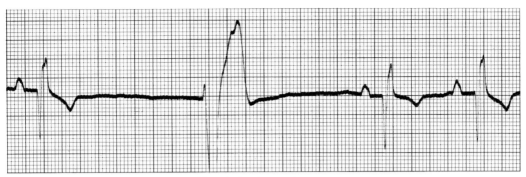

Ventricular Escape Beat.

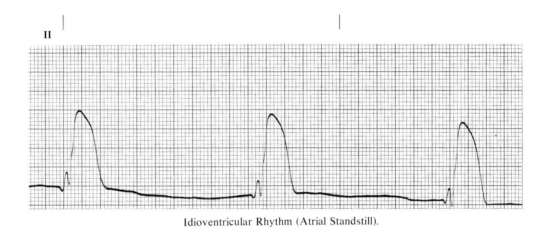

Idioventricular Rhythm (Atrial Standstill).

II

First Degree Heart Block.

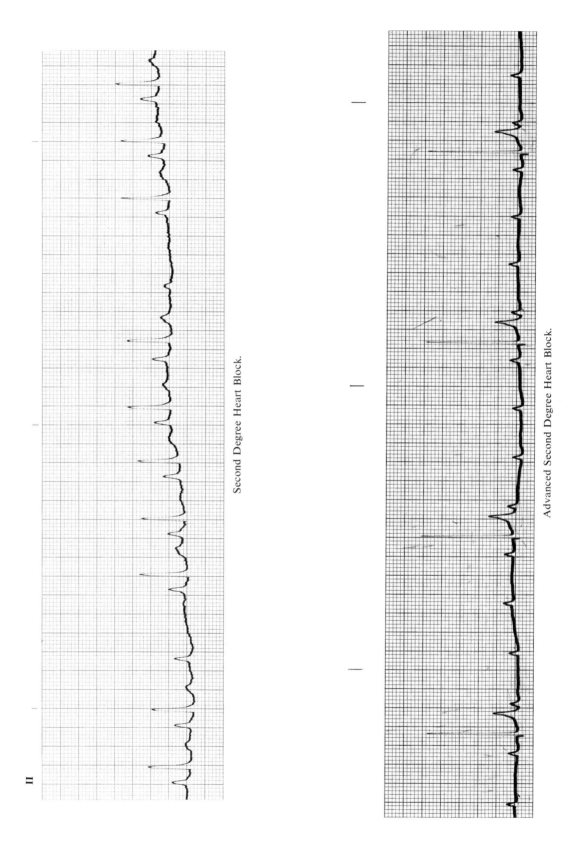

Second Degree Heart Block.

Advanced Second Degree Heart Block.

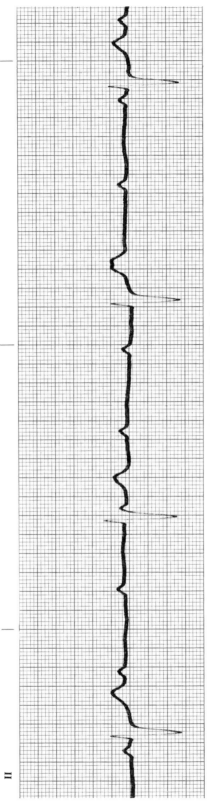

Complete (Third Degree) Heart Block.

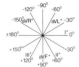

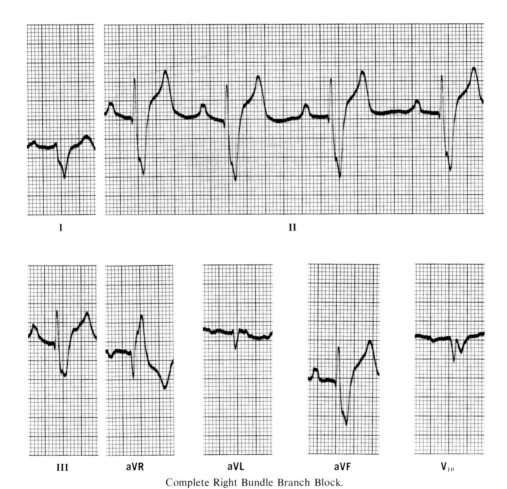

Complete Right Bundle Branch Block.

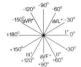

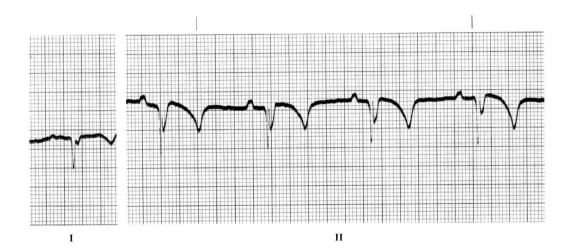

I   II

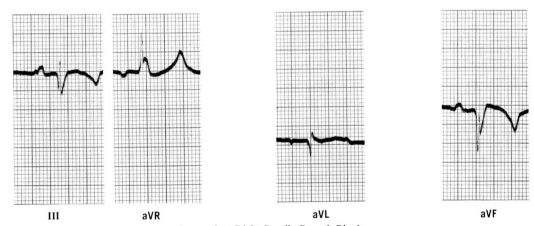

III   aVR   aVL   aVF

Incomplete Right Bundle Branch Block.

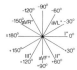

I II

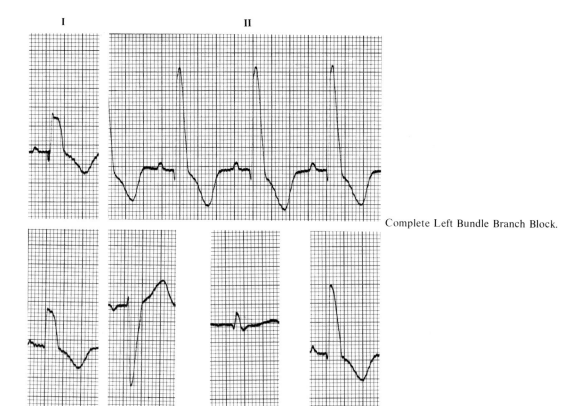

Complete Left Bundle Branch Block.

III aVR aVL aVF

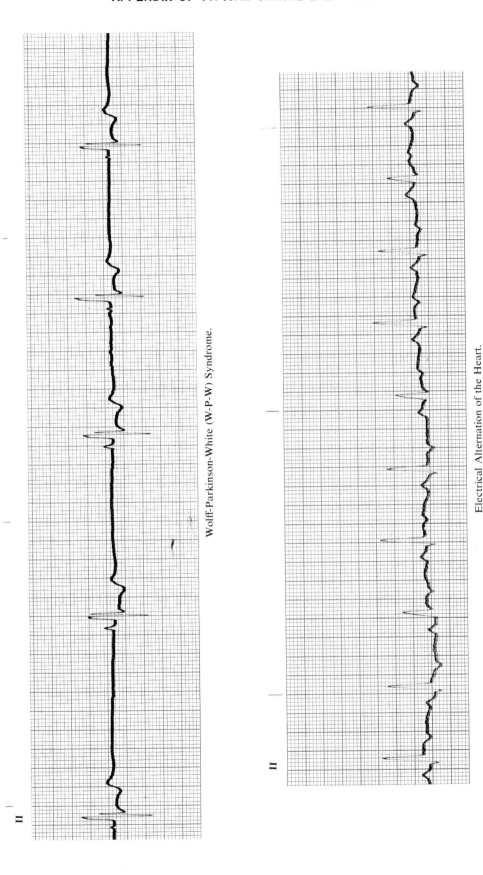

Wolff-Parkinson-White (W-P-W) Syndrome.

Electrical Alternation of the Heart.

GLOSSARY OF TERMS

aberrant conduction—abnormal spread of a supraventricular impulse through the ventricles, usually as a result of delayed activation of one of the bundles of His. It results in a QRS complex of slightly different conformation than normal. *Example:* if an atrial premature beat occurs and tries to depolarize the ventricles before they are completely repolarized from the previous beat, the beat may be aberrantly conducted through the ventricles, because some areas may still be refractory to stimulation.

accrochage—atrioventricular dissociation in which the rate of the P waves is nearly equal to but slightly slower than the rate of the ectopic ventricular impulses, so that the P wave moves into and out of the QRS complexes (see also atrioventricular dissociation).

all or none law—the fact that an impulse great enough to depolarize one fiber will depolarize all of the fibers and produce maximal contraction and, conversely, that an impulse will fail to produce a contraction during the absolute refractory period of the syncytium, regardless of the strength of the impulse.

anomalous complexes—all ventricular complexes that differ from the dominant normal sinus beats, including both aberrant beats and ectopic beats.

antegrade conduction—normal conduction of impulses from the sinoatrial node through the atria to the atrioventricular node and bundle of His to the bundle branches. This is in contrast to *retrograde conduction,* in which the impulse is conducted in reverse order through all or part of the conduction system.

antiarrhythmic agent—a drug that is used to suppress irritable foci and quell ectopic tachyarrhythmias. Among these are quinidine, procainamide, lidocaine, diphenylhydantoin, propranolol, and bretylium.

arrhythmia—any disturbance in the heart rate or rhythm, or in the normal rate and sequence of conduction.

artifact—any false electrocardiographic finding caused by motion or 60 cycle electrical interference.

artificial pacemaker—an electronic device that acts as an automatic fiber to initiate and sustain a regular cardiac rhythm at an acceptable heart rate. Pacemakers are used when bradycardia is profound, as in serious heart block situations.

atrial—pertaining to the main upper chambers of the heart. This adjective is used in preference to *auricular* when describing abnormalities of these chambers.

atrial bigeminy—a condition in which every other beat is an atrial premature beat.

345

atrial complex—that portion of the electrocardiogram that indicates atrial activity (the P wave).

atrial fibrillation—lack of effective atrial contraction due to the presence of very many chaotic, unorganized atrial impulses. It is almost always caused by severe atrial disease in the dog and is characterized electrocardiographically by a rapid, irregular ventricular response and the absence of P waves. The QRS complexes are normal, the P waves being replaced by baseline fasciculations called "f waves."

atrial flutter—a rapid rhythmic beating of the atria, often at a rate of about 300 per minute. Regular "F waves" replace the P waves, and the ventricles generally respond in a periodic manner at a slower rate. The QRS complexes remain normal.

atrial parasystole—a condition in which an ectopic atrial focus fires at a regular, uninterrupted rate at the same time that the normal sinus beats fire at their regular uninterrupted rate (see parasystole).

atrial premature beat—a type of supraventricular premature beat that arises spontaneously from an ectopic atrial focus. On the electrocardiogram, the P wave is positive but different from P waves of sinus origin. The QRS complex remains normal or may be slightly aberrant (see supraventricular premature beat).

atrial standstill—lack of atrial activity for three or more successive R-R intervals, producing a straight, steady baseline on the electrocardiogram. Idioventricular beats and rhythms occur (see idioventricular).

atrial tachycardia—four or more atrial premature beats in succession. On the electrocardiogram, the P waves are positive but different from those seen when the heart rate is normal. The QRS complexes remain normal. Atrial tachycardia usually occurs in paroxysms (see paroxysmal tachycardia).

atrial trigeminy—a condition in which every third beat is an atrial premature beat, or in which there are two atrial premature beats for every normal sinus beat.

atrioventricular dissociation—a form of ventricular tachycardia in which the rate of the P waves is nearly equal to, but slightly slower than, the rate of the ectopic ventricular complexes. There are two forms:
synchrony: the rate of the P waves is equal to that of the ventricular ectopic beats for a period of time, but a short P-R interval demonstrates their dissociation. Synchrony is also known as *isorhythmic dissociation.*
accrochage: the P wave rate is slightly slower than the rate of the ectopic ventricular beats, and the P waves are seen to move into and out of the QRS complexes.

atrioventricular heart block—an interference with the transmission of atrial impulses through the atrioventricular node to the ventricles. The degree of interruption of impulse transmission varies in severity as follows:
first degree heart block: all of the atrial impulses are conducted to the ventricles, but are delayed at the atrioventricular node. On the electrocardiogram, the P-R interval is prolonged beyond 0.13 second.

second degree heart block: some of the atrial impulses fail to stimulate the ventricles, while others are successfully transmitted. On the electrocardiogram, one or several P waves are not followed by a QRS complex, while other complexes are normal. Two types of second degree heart block may be differentiated by the electrocardiogram: (a) Mobitz I (Wenckebach phenomenon), in which the P-R interval becomes progressively longer until a QRS complex is dropped; and (b) Mobitz II, in which the P-R interval remains constant before the dropped beat.

third degree heart block: most severe form of heart block, in which all of the atrial impulses are blocked at the atrioventricular node. The atria beat at their own rate, and the ventricles beat at their own much slower rate. There is no association between the more rapid P waves and the slower idioventricular complexes.

atrioventricular junction—(see junction).

atrioventricular nodal beats—atrioventricular junctional beats. Since the tissues in the atrioventricular node are not capable of initiating impulses, beats arising in this area should be called *junctional* rather than *nodal* (see junction).

atrioventricular node—the structure over which the atrial impulses are conducted to the ventricles.

attenuation—a dampening of the electrocardiographic complexes, caused by fluids or masses or air in the thorax, pericardium, or lungs. The interference with the conduction of impulses to the body surface causes the complexes to be small.

auricle—term used to denote an atrial *appendage* (*not* the main atrial chamber).

axis deviation—a condition in which the mean electrical axis is not within the normal range of +40° to +100°:

right axis deviation: deviation of the mean electrical axis rightward to greater than +100°, an indication of right ventricular hypertrophy or complete right bundle branch block.

left axis deviation: deviation of the mean electrical axis leftward to less than +40°, an indication of left ventricular hypertrophy.

Bailey's hexaxial lead system—system of electrocardiographic diagnosis that combines the bipolar limb leads (I, II, III) with the augmented unipolar limb leads (aVR, aVL, aVF), and is used for determining the mean electrical axis in the frontal plane.

baseline—a straight steady line produced when no electrical current is flowing. An upward deflection from the baseline is a positive deflection; a downward deflection, a negative one.

bigeminy—a condition in which every other beat is a premature beat. It may be atrial, junctional, or ventricular bigeminy, depending on which type of premature beat is present.

biphasic wave—a wave that has both positive and negative components.

bipolar limb leads—these are leads I, II, and III, which produce Einthoven's triangle and form part of Bailey's hexaxial lead system.

bradyarrhythmia—used synonymously with bradycardia.

bradycardia—a heart rate of less than 70 beats per minute. Under anesthesia, bradycardia may be considered present whenever the heart rate falls below the original baseline level.

348 / **GLOSSARY OF TERMS**

bundle branch block — disruption of impulse conduction through a branch of the bundle of His. Blockage of a major branch is called complete bundle branch block, while incomplete blockage refers to blockage of a smaller ramification.

>*right bundle branch block:* blockage of impulse conduction through the right branch of the bundle of His, resulting in a delay in right ventricular depolarization and widening of the terminal forces (S wave) on the electrocardiogram.

>*left bundle branch block:* blockage of impulse conduction through the left branch of the bundle of His, resulting in increased width of the QRS complex beyond 0.07 second.

bundle of His beat — a ventricular ectopic beat arising in or near the bundle of His, so that conduction through the ventricles is fairly normal and the QRS complex remains near-normal in configuration to those of the sinus beats. The QRS complex, however, is not associated with a P wave.

cannon "a" wave — a jugular pulse produced by a severe arrhythmia when the atria contract against closed atrioventricular valves, so that the pulse pressure of the atrial contraction moves retrograde into the jugular vein. Arrhythmias that produce a jugular pulse include ventricular premature beats, ventricular tachycardia, and complete heart block.

cardiac arrest — failure of the entire heart to produce a contraction. There are two types:

>*cardiac (ventricular) standstill (asystole):* the entire heart stops; there is no electrical activity, and the electrocardiogram records a smooth, steady baseline.

>*ventricular fibrillation:* the ventricles fibrillate but produce no contraction (see ventricular fibrillation).

cardiac standstill — (see cardiac arrest).

cardiac vector — term used synonymously with *mean electrical axis,* and signifying the direction and magnitude of the main summative electrical force produced during ventricular depolarization.

cardioversion — conversion of arrhythmias to sinus rhythm. Antiarrhythmic drugs or electrical countershock (D.C. cardioversion) may be used.

carotid sinus pressure — a technique used to increase vagal tone and slow the heart or abolish supraventricular arrhythmias by firmly massaging the area of the carotid bifurcation.

carotid sinus syndrome — as syndrome, seen in dogs with masses or irritation in the area of the carotid sinus or pharynx, or in brachycephalic dogs with stertorous respirations, in which vagal hypertonia resulting from these anatomic conditions causes bradycardia that can, in turn, result in ataxia, syncope, or seizures.

chaotic heart action — a condition in which there is ventricular tachycardia of multifocal origin with alternating bidirectional bizarre QRS complexes (see prefibrillatory rhythm).

coarse ventricular fibrillation — (see ventricular fibrillation).

compensatory pause — the pause that follows most premature beats.

complexes, electrical—those portions of the electrocardiogram that are produced by electrical activity in specific areas of the heart.

P wave: the initial deflection on the electrocardiogram, produced by depolarization of the atria.

P-R interval: portion of an electrocardiogram measured from the beginning of the P wave to the beginning of the QRS complex.

QRS complex: portion of an electrocardiogram indicating depolarization of the ventricles, and occurring in three main wave fronts: ventricular septal (Q wave), ventricular free walls (R wave), and ventricular and septal apicobasilar areas (S wave).

S-T segment: portion of a tracing between the end of the S wave and the beginning of the T wave, and represents the initial, rather slow portion of ventricular repolarization.

T wave: electrocardiographic representation of the rapid portion of ventricular repolarization.

Q-T interval: interval measured from the beginning of the QRS complex to the end of the T wave.

conduction disturbance—any interruption in the normal pathway of depolarization.

conduction velocity—the speed of impulse conduction. Normal values are: atrial tissue, 500 to 1000 mm./sec.; A-V node, 100 to 200 mm./sec.; Purkinje fibers, 2000 to 4000 mm./sec.; and ventricular muscle fibers, 200 to 400 mm./sec.

countershock (D.C. cardioversion)—the use of direct electrical current to convert various arrhythmias to sinus rhythm. The equipment is synchronized to the R wave of the electrocardiogram.

coupling—a normal beat that is followed by a premature beat at a regular repeated interval. The premature beat is "coupled" to the previous normal beat.

D.C. cardioversion—(see countershock).

defibrillator—an instrument that delivers an electric shock to the heart to convert ventricular fibrillation to sinus rhythm.

delta wave—the slow-rising, slurred, initial portion of the QRS complex seen with the Wolff-Parkinson-White syndrome.

diastolic depolarization—spontaneous discharge of pacemaker centers, without outside stimulation. During phase 4 of the membrane action potential, sodium gradually leaks into the cell until the threshold potential is reached, and then the fiber discharges.

double sensitivity recording—measurement recorded at 2 cm. = 1 mv. All height measurements must be halved to obtain their true millivoltage.

dropped beat—a phenomenon, seen in second degree heart block, in which an atrial impulse is not conducted to the ventricles, and so a P wave occurs without a QRS complex.

dysrhythmia—term used synonymously with, and probably preferential to, arrhythmia; it includes disturbances in pacemaker activity with or without an irregular heart beat.

ectopic beat—a beat that arises at a site other than the sinoatrial node; i.e., the atria, the junctional tissues, or the ventricles.

ectopic rhythm—a sustained series of ectopic beats.

electrical alternation of the heart—a regular alternation in the electrical activity of the heart in the presence of a regular rhythm. It is closely correlated with pericardial effusion, thoracic effusion, and myocardial disease. On the electrocardiogram, there is mainly variation in the height of the QRS complexes, although all portions of the electrocardiogram may be affected.

electrically vertical heart—heart that produces an electrocardiogram on which all leads are isoelectric, so that mean electrical axis cannot be determined; this is usually seen in large, thin dogs.

electrodes—the cables attached to the skin to sense the electrical impulses produced by the heart.

escape beat—a beat that arises from an inferior pacemaker site when a higher pacemaker is delayed or inactive. Escape beats may be junctional or ventricular in origin.

escape rhythm—a sustained series of escape beats.

esophageal lead—a specialized lead designed to determine the presence of P waves when their presence is in doubt. It is a long flexible electrode that is passed into the esophagus with the tip positioned over the heart. It is connected to the left arm electrode, and lead I is recorded. It produces bizarre complexes that should be simultaneously compared to a normal lead II; multichannel equipment is required for this.

excitability—the relative ease with which a myocardial fiber can be stimulated to depolarize.

extrasystole—premature beat; ideally, this term should be restricted to interpolated premature beats.

f waves—fine baseline fasciculations replacing the P waves, as seen with atrial fibrillation; f waves represent chaotic electrical activity of the atria; no atrial contraction is present (see atrial fibrillation).

F waves—baseline fasciculations, larger than "f waves," and representing the rapidly beating atria in cases of atrial flutter.

fibrilloflutter—a condition in which the atria vacillate between fibrillation and flutter.

fine ventricular fibrillation—(see ventricular fibrillation).

first degree heart block—(see atrioventricular heart block).

full sensitivity—normal sensitivity (1 cm. = 1 mv.).

half sensitivity recording—measurement recorded at $\frac{1}{2}$ cm. = 1 mv; all height measurements must be doubled to obtain the true millivoltage.

heart block—(see atrioventricular heart block).

hypertrophy—increase in length, width, and weight of the cardiac muscle fibers. Electrical activity produced is proportional to the length and diameter of the fiber, so hypertrophied fibers produce greater millivoltage, which is recorded on the electrocardiogram.

idioventricular beat—a passive ventricular beat that arises spontaneously when stimulation from a higher pacemaker center does not occur; also called ventricular escape beat.

idioventricular rhythm—a series of idoventricular beats, usually at a rate of 60 beats per minute or less, and usually a preterminal rhythm.

interpolation—a premature beat that occurs between two normal beats without disrupting the rhythm. There is no compensatory pause. This is more characteristic of ventricular premature beats.

isoelectric complex—a complex in which the sum of the positive and negative deflections is equal to 0.

isorhythmic dissociation—(see atrioventricular dissociation).

J point—the exact point at which depolarization ends and repolarization begins. The J point is seen as a small jog or notch in the terminal portion of the downstroke of the R wave.

junction—specialized fibers in the region of the atrioventricular node that possess pacemaker ability. The adjective *junctional* has replaced *nodal* when referring to beats arising in this area.

junctional escape beat—a beat that arises in the junctional area when the sinoatrial impulse is delayed or blocked (see escape beat); seen on the electrocardiogram as a PQRST complex that occurs after a pause in the rhythm, the P wave being negative.

junctional escape rhythm—a series of junctional escape beats. The heart rate is 40 to 60 beats per minute and the P waves are negative.

junctional premature beat—a type of supraventricular premature beat that occurs early, has a negative P wave (with the QRS complex remaining normal) and is followed by a pause.

junctional tachycardia—a junctional rhythm in which the heart rate is greater than 60 beats per minute. (See junctional escape rhythm.)

left axis deviation—(see axis deviation).

left bundle branch block—(see bundle branch block).

mean electrical axis—the direction of the main electrical force that is produced during ventricular depolarization. The normal axis in the dog is +40° to +100° (see axis deviation).

membrane action potential—a measurement of the changes in electrical potential that occur across the cell membrane at one exact point on the membrane during excitation of the cell.

Mobitz type I heart block—a type of second degree heart block (see atrioventricular heart block).

Mobitz type II heart block—a type of second degree heart block (see atrioventricular heart block).

multifocal premature beats—premature beats arising from more than one focus, so that the complexes indicating the beats vary in configuration.

nodal—(see junctional).

normal sinus rhythm—a sinus rhythm in which the heart rate is normal and the R-R interval is perfectly regular.

oculocardiac reflex—a vagally-mediated reflex in which compression of the eyeballs exaggerates vagal tone and slows the heart rate; it may be used like carotid sinus pressure to break episodes of supraventricular tachycardia.

orthogonal lead system—a system of leads that uses three planes to measure the cardiac impulse. When two of the planes are compared simultaneously, vector loops can be drawn.

overdrive suppression—pause occurring after a pacemaker that has been driving the heart more rapidly than the sinoatrial node quits abruptly; this pause is of about 1 second duration and occurs before the natural rhythm resumes.

P mitrale—a P wave that is wider than 0.04 second, usually is notched, and indicates left atrial hypertrophy.

P pulmonale—a P wave that is taller than 0.4 mv., usually is sharply peaked, and indicates right atrial hypertrophy.

P wave—(see complexes, electrical).

P-P interval—the distance from one P wave to the next.

P-R interval—(see complexes, electrical).

pacemaker tissue—specialized cardiac fibers that can discharge themselves automatically. These include the sinoatrial node, junction, Purkinje fibers, and, under extreme conditions, even the atrial and ventricular fibers.

pair—two premature beats in succession.

parasystole—a condition in which an ectopic focus and the normal sinus impulses occur simultaneously without interrupting each other. The ectopic focus is regular and usually much slower than the sinus impulses. Atrial or ventricular ectopic beats may be present.

paroxysmal tachycardia—bursts of tachycardia that begin and end quite abruptly, including paroxysmal atrial tachycardia, paroxysmal junctional tachycardia, paroxysmal ventricular tachycardia, paroxysmal sinus tachycardia, and paroxysmal atrial fibrillation.

paroxysmal tachycardia with block—bursts of sinus or atrial tachycardia with varying degrees of incomplete heart block.

polarity—the positivity or negativity of a lead.

prefibrillatory rhythm—an arrhythmia that precedes ventricular fibrillation, e.g., ventricular flutter or alternating bidirectional multifocal ventricular tachycardia.

preterminal rhythm—a severe bradyarrhythmia seen just prior to death, and usually an idioventricular rhythm.

pulse deficit—a condition that is seen with certain arrhythmias, in which there are more heart beats than femoral pulses.

Purkinje fibers—the part of the conduction system that is continuous with the bundle branches and terminates subendocardially in the myocardium of both ventricles.

QRS complex—(see complexes, electrical).

Q-T interval—(see complexes, electrical).

R-R interval—the distance from one R wave to the next.

refractory period—that period, following the activation of the myocardium, during which the heart's excitability is depressed or absent. Several periods comprise the refractory state:

absolute refractory period (ARP): the period following excitation when the myocardial fibers will not respond to even the highest intensity electrical impulse.

effective refractory period (ERP): the period during which impulses may appear but are too weak to be conducted.

relative refractory period (RRP): period between the end of the ERP and the end of the refractory period. The fibers respond only to impulses that are greater than the normal threshold potential, and the evoked impulses are conducted more slowly than normal.

total refractory period (TRP): the sum of the ARP and RRP.

repolarization—the flow of electrical currents as the ions return to their original positions along the surfaces of the cell membranes; seen on the electrocardiogram as the S-T segment and T wave.

resting membrane potential—the electrical potential inside a resting cardiac muscle cell. It is about −90 mv. with respect to the outside surface.

retrograde beat—conduction of the impulse backward through the atria from the junctional area toward the sinoatrial node, with the P wave negative on the lead II electrocardiogram.

right axis deviation—(see axis deviation).

right bundle branch block—(see bundle branch block).

run—three premature beats in succession.

60 cycle—an electrical artifact that causes a regular saw-toothed distortion of the baseline of a tracing.

S-T coving—(see S-T slurring).

S-T depression—occurrence of the S-T segment below the baseline on an electrocardiographic tracing. S-T depression may be caused by hypoxia, myocarditis, left ventricular hypertrophy, or hypocalcemia.

S-T elevation—occurrence of the S-T segment above the baseline on an electrocardiographic tracing. S-T elevation may be caused by hypoxia, myocarditis, or hypercalcemia.

S-T segment—(see complexes, electrical).

S-T slurring—also called S-T coving: The R wave moves directly into the T wave, and the S-T segment never straightens out along the baseline; seen with left ventricular hypertrophy.

second degree heart block—(see atrioventricular heart block).

sick sinus syndrome—a disease of the sinoatrial node and atria characterized by sinus bradycardia, sinus arrest, escape beats or rhythms, and supraventricular tachycardia.

single—one isolated premature beat.

sinoatrial block—a condition in which the sinoatrial node discharges normally, but the impulse is not conducted to the atria. The pause produced in the rhythm is usually an exact multiple of the R-R interval. Sinoatrial block is ordinarily indistinguishable from sinus arrest on the electrocardiogram.

sinoatrial node—located in the right atrium, it is the most rapid pacemaker tissue in the heart and is the normal pacemaker for the heart.

sinoatrial syncope—fainting episodes that occur as a result of excessively long pauses in the cardiac rhythm; it is seen with the sick sinus syndrome.

sinus arrest—an irregular sinus rhythm in which the pauses in the rhythm are twice or more than twice the normal R-R interval. Sinus arrest is indistinguishable from sinoatrial block on the electrocardiogram.

sinus arrhythmia—an irregular sinus rhythm in which the pauses are less than twice the normal R-R interval; it is a normal arrhythmia, present in most dogs.

sinus bradycardia—sinus rhythm at a rate of less than 70 beats per minute.

sinus rhythm—a rhythm initiated by the sinoatrial node. There are P waves for every QRS complex, the P waves and QRS complexes have definite relationship, and the P waves are positive on lead II. Examples are normal sinus rhythm, sinus arrhythmia, sinus arrest, sinus tachycardia, and sinus bradycardia.

sinus tachycardia—a sinus rhythm that is greater than 160 beats per minute (180 beats per minute in toy breeds).

spontaneous depolarization—characteristic, spontaneous discharge of pacemaker tissues. It is brought about by a gradual leakage of sodium into the cell through a semipermeable membrane during phase 4 of the membrane action potential; as a result the resting membrane potential is gradually raised until it reaches the threshold potential, and the fiber is activated.

supraventricular ectopic arrhythmia—an ectopic arrhythmia that arises either in the junctional area or in the atria elsewhere than in the sinoatrial node.

supraventricular premature beat—a premature beat from an ectopic focus either in the junctional area or in the atria elsewhere than in the sinoatrial node. The P wave is altered, but the QRS complex remains normal. One is a single, two in a row is a pair, three in a row is a run, and four or more in a row constitutes supraventricular tachycardia.

synchrony—also called isorhythmic dissociation. (See atrioventricular dissociation.)

syncope—fainting with or without seizures. When due to a cardiac cause (a severe arrhythmia), it is called Stokes-Adams syndrome.

T wave—(see complexes, electrical).

T_a wave—a depression of the P-R segment caused by right atrial hypertrophy. Pronounced "T sub a" wave, it is presumably the result of large right atrial repolarization forces.

tachyarrhythmia—any tachycardia. Includes ectopic tachycardias that may be within the limit of the normal heart rate. For example, a junctional tachycardia is a junctional rhythm with a heart rate of greater than 60 beats per minute.

tachycardia—used here to indicate that the heart rate is greater than 160 beats per minute (180 beats per minute in toy breeds).

third degree heart block—(see atrioventricular heart block).

threshold potential—that critical level to which the resting membrane potential must be raised in order to stimulate a response from an excitable tissue.

trigeminy—a condition in which every third beat is a premature beat, or in which there are two premature beats for every normal beat.

unifocal—tending to arise from one and only one source, as some types of premature beats. All such beats have an identical conformation on the electrocardiogram.

unipolar limb leads—leads aVR, aVL, and aVF. They are also called the augmented unipolar limb leads, and they comprise three leads of Bailey's hexaxial lead system.

unipolar precordial leads—leads V_{10}, CV_6LU, CV_6LL, and CV_5RL. Also called the exploring leads, these may be used to identify miscellaneous signs of ventricular hypertrophy.

ventricular bigeminy—a condition in which every other beat is a ventricular premature beat.

ventricular capture beat—a normal beat, having a normal PQRST complex but occurring between a string of ventricular premature beats; the P wave is able to "capture" the ventricles for one or several beats before the ectopic ventricular focus again dominates the rhythm; a hallmark of ventricular tachycardia.

ventricular escape beat—an impulse originated by the ventricular fibers themselves, following a long pause in the rhythm due to a failure of the higher pacemaker tissues to initiate the impulse. It is seen on the electrocardiogram as a ventricular ectopic beat that occurs after a long pause in the rhythm. The complexes are also called idioventricular beats.

ventricular escape rhythm—a series of ventricular escape beats. Also known as an idioventricular rhythm, it is usually a preterminal rhythm.

ventricular fibrillation—activity of the ventricles characterized on the electrocardiogram by chaotic baseline undulations, without organized ventricular complexes. The disorganized electrical activity of the ventricles results in totally ineffective pump action. There are two types of ventricular fibrillation, differentiated by the electrocardiogram:

coarse fibrillation: the baseline undulations are irregular in size, but fairly large. This is more susceptible to electrical defibrillation.

fine fibrillation: the baseline undulations are irregular and very small. This is less likely to respond to electrical defibrillation.

ventricular flutter—a prefibrillatory rhythm in which the ventricles contract regularly but weakly. The electrocardiogram is characterized by regular, continuous waves of large amplitude, and no distinction can be made between the QRS complex and the T wave.

ventricular fusion beat—a beat occurring as the normal impulse and an ectopic ventricular focus try to depolarize the ventricles simultaneously. It is seen on the electrocardiogram as a P wave and normal P-R interval followed by a QRS complex that is midway in form between that of the normal capture beats and that of the ventricular ectopic beats; such a fusion beat is a hallmark of ventricular tachycardia.

ventricular parasystole—a condition in which a regular sinus rhythm and a regular ectopic ventricular rhythm occur simultaneously without interfering with one another.

ventricular premature beat—a premature beat that arises in the bundle of His or in the ventricles. It is not associated with a P wave on the electrocardiogram. If the impulse arises in the bundle of His, the QRS complex is near-normal, but when it arises further out in the ventricles, the QRS complex is bizarre in form. One ventricular premature beat is a single, two in succession is a pair, three in succession is a run, and four or more in a row is ventricular tachycardia.

ventricular standstill (asystole)—(see cardiac arrest).

ventricular tachycardia—a series of four or more ventricular premature beats in a row. Capture and fusion beats may be present.

ventricular trigeminy—a condition in which every third beat is a ventricular premature beat, or in which there are two ventricular premature beats for every normal sinus beat.

vulnerable period—an interval during the relative refractory period of the heart cycle in which ventricular fibrillation is most easily produced by a single strong stimulus. It coincides approximately with the peak of the T wave. A ventricular premature beat falling at this time could possibly cause ventricular fibrillation.

wandering pacemaker—a phenomenon in which the point of origin of the beat varies within different parts of the sinus node, the atria and even the junctional tissues. It is a normal variation in the canine, and is usually associated with fluctuations in vagal tone caused by respiration. It is often seen in conjunction with sinus arrhythmia and sinus arrest. It is seen on the electrocardiogram as a variation in the height of the P wave, and the P wave may actually become negative when the pacemaker wanders into the area of the junctional tissues.

Wenckebach phenomenon—a type of second degree atrioventricular heart block (see atrioventricular heart block) seen mostly in association with digitalis intoxication.

Wolff-Parkinson-White syndrome—a possibly congenital abnormality in which there exists one or several accessory pathways that bypass the normal atrioventricular conduction pathway. It is also called pre-excitation. Patients with this syndrome are subject to episodes of supraventricular tachycardia. It is seen on the electrocardiogram as a short P-R interval and an altered ventricular complex, with the presence of a delta wave.

ABBREVIATIONS

AF: atrial fibrillation

AT: atrial tachycardia

APB: atrial premature beat

A-V dissoc: atrioventricular dissociation

A-V node: atrioventricular node

Axis: mean electrical axis

BBB: bundle branch block

CHF: congestive heart failure

ECG (or EKG): electrocardiogram

J. escape: junctional escape

J. tach: junctional tachycardia

JPB: junctional (nodal) premature beat

Junction: junctional tissues in the area of the A-V node.

LAH: left atrial hypertrophy

LBBB: left bundle branch block

LVH: left ventricular hypertrophy

NSR: normal sinus rhythm

PAT: paroxysmal atrial tachycardia

PVT: paroxysmal ventricular tachycardia

RAH: right atrial hypertrophy

RBBB: right bundle branch block

RVH: right ventricular hypertrophy

SA block: sinoatrial block

SA node: sinoatrial node

SPB: supraventricular premature beat

SSS: sick sinus syndrome

Sinus tach: sinus tachycardia

VPB: ventricular premature beat

V. escape: ventricular escape

V. fib.: ventricular fibrillation

V. tach.: ventricular tachycardia

W-P-W: Wolff-Parkinson-White Syndrome

1° HB: first degree heart block

2° HB: second degree heart block

3° HB: third degree (complete) heart block

60 cycle: sixty cycle electrical artifact

INDEX

Page numbers in *italics* indicate illustrations; (t) following a page number indicates tabular material; and (g) following a page number indicates a definition in the Glossary.

Tachycardia(s) (*Continued*)
  junctional, 124, *125, 126, 149, 331,*
      351(g)
    and ventricular premature beats, in
        digitalis intoxication, 260
    diagnosis of, 124
    etiology of, 124
    treatment of, 124
  nodal. See *junctional.*
  paroxysmal, 352(g)
    with block, 352(g)
  paroxysmal atrial, 116–119, *118, 328*
    with block, digitalis intoxication and,
        190
  right atrial, and overdrive suppression,
      208
    hemangiosarcomas and, 209
  sinus, 104, *325,* 354(g)
    atropine and, 179, 281
    diagnosis of, 106
    paroxysmal, 306
    vs. atrial, *107,* 108(t), 117
    with block, 302, *326*
  supraventricular, 204
  ventricular. See *Ventricular tachy-
      cardia.*
  vs. premature beat, 110
Terms, common, abbreviations for, 357
Therapy, for cardiac diseases, electro-
    cardiography in evaluation of, 3
Third degree heart block, 152, *157, 339,*
    347(g)
  diagnosis of, 153, 154
  etiology of, 152
  prognosis in, 158
  treatment of, 156
Thoracic radiograph(s), electrocardiog-
    raphy and, in detection of cardiac en-
    largement, 1
Threshold potential, 20, 354(g)
Total refractory period, 352(g)
Toxic myocarditis, electrocardiography in
    diagnosis of, 4
TP, 20, 354(g)
Trachea, collapsed, and P pulmonale, 292
Tranquilizers, and bradycardia, 202
  effects on electrocardiogram, 75
Trauma, routine electrocardiography in, 6
Traumatic myocarditis, 59
  and ventricular tachycardia, 269
Treatment, of cardiac disease, electro-
    cardiography for evaluation of, 3
Trembling artifact, 182, 185, *323*
Triaxial limb leads, 33(t), 34, *34*
Trigeminy, 354(g)
  atrial, 346(g)
  ventricular, 130, 280, *332,* 356(g)
Trouble shooting, electrocardiographic, 15
TRP, 352(g)
Tumor(s), heart base, electrocardiography
    in diagnosis of, 4
Twitch artifact(s), *323*

Unifocal ventricular premature beats, 131,
    331
  treatment of, 139–142, *140*

Unifocal ventricular premature beats
    (*Continued*)
  vs. multifocal ventricular
      premature beats, 131
Unipolar limb leads, 33(t), 34, 354(g)
Unipolar precordial leads, 33(t), 36,
    354(g)

V_{10} exploring lead, *12,* 33(t)
V_{10} exploring lead, positive T wave in, 61
Vagal activity, effect on heart rhythm, 29
Vagally-induced arrhythmia(s), 29, 98–
    103, 206, 230, 233
  atropine for, 256
  physical examination and, 99
Valvular heart disease, and supraventric-
    ular premature beats, 198, 250
  complications of, 299
Vector(s), cardiac, 30, 30–32, 348(g). See
    also *Mean electrical axis.*
Ventricular arrhythmia(s), 126–145. See
    also specific arrhythmia.
  myocarditis and, 126, 127
  treatment of, 139–143
Ventricular bigeminy, *130, 131, 332,*
    355(g)
  following trauma and anesthesia, 272
  multifocal, 293
Ventricular capture beat(s), 355(g)
Ventricular depolarization, *24, 25,* 27–28
Ventricular ectopic beat(s), treatment of,
    141
Ventricular escape beat(s), 149–151, *150,
    151, 337,* 355(g)
  diagnosis of, 150
  etiology of, 149, 150
  treatment of, 151
Ventricular escape rhythm, 149–151, *151,*
    306, 355(g)
  diagnosis of, 150
  etiology of, 150
  treatment of, 151
Ventricular fibrillation, 143–145, *145, 335,*
    355(g). See also *Cardiac arrest.*
  coarse, *335,* 355(g)
    vs. fine, 308
  diagnosis of, 143
  etiology of, 143
  fine, *335,* 355(g)
    vs. coarse, 144, *145,* 308
  prefibrillatory rhythm and, *144*
  prognosis of, 143
  treatment of, 143–145
  ventricular tachycardia and, 286
Ventricular flutter, *144, 335,* 355(g)
Ventricular fusion beat(s), 355(g)
Ventricular hypertrophy. See also *Left
    ventricular hypertrophy; Right ventric-
    ular hypertrophy;* and *Biventricular
    hypertrophy.*
  diagnosis of, 54(t)
  in pointer, 289
Ventricular myocarditis, and cardiac en-
    largement, 266
  multifocal ventricular tachycardia in, 264